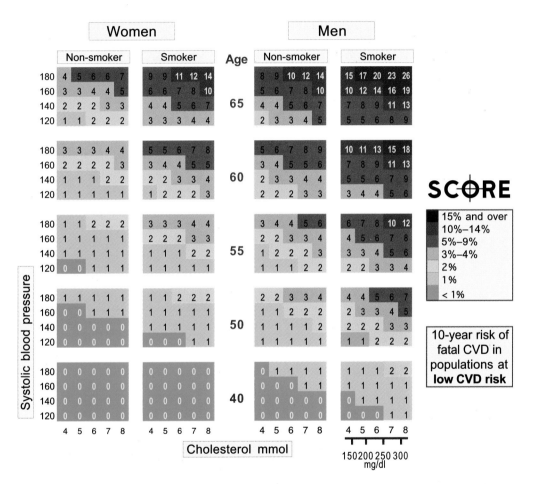

Figure 11.1 (b) The SCORE charts. 10-year risk of fatal CVD in low risk regions of Europe by gender, age, systolic blood pressure, total cholesterol and smoking status. Refer to Chapter 11 (pp. 159–72) for full discussion.

THERAPEUTIC STRATEGIES IN CARDIOVASCULAR RISK

THERAPEUTIC STRATEGIES IN CARDIOVASCULAR RISK

Edited by

Ian M. Graham
Ralph B. D'Agostino, Sr

CLINICAL PUBLISHING

OXFORD

Clinical Publishing
an imprint of Atlas Medical Publishing Ltd

Oxford Centre for Innovation
Mill Street, Oxford OX2 0JX, UK

Tel: +44 1865 811116
Fax: +44 1865 251550
Email: info@clinicalpublishing.co.uk
Web: www.clinicalpublishing.co.uk

Distributed in USA and Canada by:
Clinical Publishing
30 Amberwood Parkway
Ashland OH 44805 USA

Tel: 800-247-6553 (toll free within U.S. and Canada)
Fax: 419-281-6883
Email: order@bookmasters.com

Distributed in UK and Rest of World by:
Marston Book Services Ltd
PO Box 269
Abingdon
Oxon OX14 4YN, UK

Tel: +44 1235 465500
Fax: +44 1235 465555
Email: trade.orders@marston.co.uk

A catalogue record for this book is available from the British Library

ISBN-13 978 1 904392 64 4
ISBN-10 1 904392 64 4

The publisher makes no representation, express or implied, that the dosages in this book are correct. Readers must therefore always check the product information and clinical procedures with the most up-to-date published product information and data sheets provided by the manufacturers and the most recent codes of conduct and safety regulations. The authors and the publisher do not accept any liability for any errors in the text or for the misuse or misapplication of material in this work

Project manager: Gavin Smith, GPS Publishing Solutions, Hertfordshire, UK
Typeset by Mizpah Publishing Services Private Limited, Chennai, India
Printed and bound in Great Britain by Biddles Ltd, King's Lynn, Norfolk

Contents

Editors

RALPH B. D'AGOSTINO, SR, PhD, Professor of Mathematics/Statistics and Public Health, Director of Data Management and Statistical Analysis of Framingham Study, Mathematics and Statistics Department, Framingham Study, Boston University, Boston, Massachusetts, USA

IAN M. GRAHAM, FRCPI, FESC, Consultant Cardiologist; Professor of Cardiovascular Medicine, Trinity College, Dublin; Professor of Preventive Cardiology, Royal College of Surgeons in Ireland

Contributors

GUNILLA BURELL, PhD, Lecturer and Assistant Professor, Department of Public Health and Caring Sciences, Uppsala University, Uppsala, Sweden

RENATA CÍFKOVÁ, MD, PhD, FESC, Head, Department of Preventive Cardiology, Institute for Clinical and Experimental Medicine, Prague, Czech Republic

RONÁN M. CONROY, MusB, DSc, Senior Lecturer, Department of Epidemiology, Royal College of Surgeons in Ireland, Dublin, Ireland

MARIE THERESE COONEY, MB BCh, BAO, MRCPI, Research Fellow in Cardiology, Department of Cardiology, The Adelaide and Meath Hospital, Tallaght, Dublin, Ireland

PATRICK COUTURE, MD, FRCP(C), PhD, Associate Professor of Medicine, Lavel University, Québec City, Canada

RALPH B. D'AGOSTINO, SR, PhD, Professor of Mathematics/Statistics and Public Health, Director of Data Management and Statistical Analysis of Framingham Study, Mathematics and Statistics Department, Framingham Study, Boston University, Boston, Massachusetts, USA

GUY DE BACKER, MD, PhD, Director, Department of Public Health, Ghent University; Director, Cardiac Rehabilitation Centre, University Hospital, Ghent, Belgium

ALEXANDRA L. DUDINA, MB, Research Fellow in Cardiology, Department of Cardiology, The Adelaide and Meath Hospital, Tallaght, Dublin, Ireland

OLE FAERGEMAN, MD, DMSc, Professor, Cardiovascular Medicine, National Heart and Lung Institute, Charing Cross Campus, Imperial College, London, UK

CHIE WEI FAN, MRCP(I), DME, Lecturer in Medical Gerontology (Trinity College), Falls and Blackout Clinic, St James's Hospital, Dublin, Ireland

IAN M. GRAHAM, FRCPI, FESC, Consultant Cardiologist; Professor of Cardiovascular Medicine, Trinity College, Dublin; Professor of Preventive Cardiology, Royal College of Surgeons in Ireland

GANG HU, MD, PhD, Senior Researcher and Docent, Department of Epidemiology and Health Promotion, National Public Health Institute, Helsinki, Department of Public Health University of Helsinki, Helsinki, Finland

ERIK INGELSSON, MD, PhD, Post-Doctoral Fellow, The Framingham Study, Boston University School of Medicine, Framingham, Massachusetts, USA and Department of Public Health and Caring Sciences, Uppsala University, Uppsala, Sweden

WILLIAM B. KANNEL, MD, MPH, Professor of Medicine and Public Health, Boston University School of Medicine, Framingham Heart Study, Framingham, Massachusetts, USA

ROSE ANNE KENNY, FRCP(I), FRCP, FESC, Head, Department of Medical Gerontology, Trinity College, Dublin, Director, Falls and Blackout Clinic, St James's Hospital, Dublin, Ireland

HANNA-MAARIA LAKKA, MD, PhD, Assistant Professor, Department of Public Health and Clinical Nutrition, University of Kuopio, Department of Epidemiology and Health Promotion, National Public Health Institute, Helsinki, Finland

TIMO A. LAKKA, MD, PhD, Professor of Medical Physiology, Institute of Biomedicine, Department of Physiology, University of Kuopio, Kuopio Research Institute of Exercise Medicine, Kuopio, Finland

TORA LEONG, MB, MRCPI, Senior Reseach Fellow, Department of Cardiology, The Adelaide and Meath Hospital, Dublin, Ireland

BERNT LINDAHL, MD, PhD, Associate Professor and Senior Physician, Behavioural Medicine, Department of Public Health and Clinical Medicine, Umeå University, Umeå, Sweden

CATHERINE McGORRIAN, MRCPI, Senior Research Fellow, Department of Cardiology, The Adelaide and Meath Hospital, Dublin, Ireland

ALLAN D. SNIDERMAN, MD, FRCP(C), Edwards Professor of Cardiology, McGill University, Mike Rosenbloom Laboratory for Cardiovascular Research, Royal Victoria Hospital, Montreal, Quebec, Canada

TROELS F. THOMSEN, MD, MPH, PhD, Specialist in Publisc Health Medicine, Research Centre for Prevention and Health, Glostrup University Hospital, Glostrup, Denmark

JAAKKO TUOMILEHTO, MD, MPolSc, PhD, Professor of Public Health, Department of Public Health, University of Helsinki, Helsinki; South Ostrobothnia Central Hospital, Seinajoki, Finland

RAMACHANDRAN S. VASAN, MBBS, MD, DM, FACC, Professor of Medicine, Departments of Preventive Medicine and Cardiology, Boston University School of Medicine and Senior Investigator, The Framingham Heart Study, Framingham, Massachusetts, USA

DEIRDRE WARD, MRCPI, Consultant Cardiologist, Department of Cardiology, The Adelaide and Meath Hospital, Tallaght, Dublin, Ireland

HANS WEDEL, PhD, Professor of Epidemiology and Biostatistics, Nordic School of Public Health, Göteborg, Sweden

LARS WILHELMSEN, MD, PhD, Professor, Cardiovascular Institute, Göteborg University Göteborg, Sweden

Introduction

R. B. D'Agostino, Sr, I. M. Graham

'It is better to be healthy than ill or dead. That is the beginning and the end of the only real argument for preventive medicine. It is sufficient.' [1]

Imagine, if you will, that you will be Minister for Health for your country, starting next week. Apart from finding out how much money you have to spend, you will probably wish for certain key information –

- What is the age and sex structure of the population that you are looking after?
- What are the major causes of death and disability?
- What is known of the social and environmental determinants of health and disease in this population?
- For each cause of death and disability, how should resources be allocated between promoting changes in nutrition, exercise and tobacco consumption, screening for risk factors, early disease detection, and therapy of those with established disease?

The management of diseases with a single cause such as hypothyroidism or scurvy is straightforward. While infectious diseases such as malaria or tuberculosis appear to have one cause, the actual development of the disease in an individual may be determined by environmental, immunological and social factors.

With regard to the clinical manifestations of atherosclerotic disease (coronary heart disease, stroke, peripheral vascular disease and aneurysm) the situation is more complex again in that atherosclerosis represents the product of multiple interacting genetic and environmental influences. Epidemiological and migrant studies clearly suggest a major lifestyle contribution to aetiology, whereas within a population, genetic factors may influence both the occurrence of atherosclerosis and an individual's reaction to environmental and lifestyle factors.

It is perhaps unlikely that major new single gene determinants of atherosclerosis as important as familial hypercholesterolaemia will emerge. So far, the realization of the concept of defining a 'cocktail' of multiple polymorphisms to define an individual's total genetic risk has proved elusive. What is certain is the relentlessness with which age, male sex, rising blood pressure, rising blood cholesterol and cigarette smoking determine the mass occurrence of cardiovascular disease in multiple international studies. It will be appreciated that age is a measure of exposure time to risk factors, rather than a causal factor as such.

The term 'risk factor' was first used in the context of coronary heart disease 45 years ago by the Framingham investigators [2]. A risk factor may be defined as a characteristic of an individual that is associated with a subsequent development of disease. The criteria to decide that, beyond reasonable doubt, the relationship between a risk factor and a disease is one of cause and effect were defined by Doll and Hill [3–5] with regard to cigarette

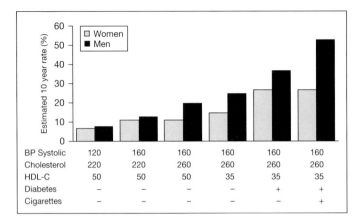

Estimated rate of coronary heart disease over 10 years according to various combinations of risk factor levels for men and women [8].

smoking. These criteria were also applied to cardiovascular disease risk factors notably by Stamler in defining the causal relationship between blood cholesterol and coronary heart disease [6, 7].

The Framingham investigators also demonstrated graphically that combinations of risk factors often exert effects that are greater than additive. This is also illustrated with data from the Systematic Coronary Risk Evaluation (SCORE) project [8] in Chapter 11. This critically important observation has led to the common factor underlying all current guidelines on the prevention of cardiovascular disease: that the management of risk in an individual requires an assessment of the combined effect of all major risk factors. This philosophy has underpinned the European recommendations on cardiovascular disease prevention from 1994 onwards [9, 10]. In the United States, while the concept of total risk is heavily stressed, its acceptance may have been impeded somewhat by the establishment of single risk factor task forces such as the National Cholesterol Education Program.

In this book, we outline the concepts of risk estimation that are summarized above, and offer simple and practical suggestions for the clinician with regard to rapid, practical total risk estimation. We then explore the lessons from major epidemiological studies of risk in more detail, and focus on the specifics of risk management, again striving to find common ground between different guidelines to, as far as possible, simplify the process of risk evaluation and management for the hard-pressed health professional.

REFERENCES

1. Rose G. The Strategy of Preventive Medicine. Oxford University Press, Oxford, 1992, p. 4.
2. Kannel WB, Dawber TR, Kagan A, Revorskie N, Sacks J. Factors of risk in the development of coronary heart disease: six year follow-up experience. The Framingham Study. *Ann Intern Med* 1961; 55:33–50.
3. Doll R, Hill AB. Smoking and carcinoma of the lung: preliminary report. *Br Med J* 1950; 2:739–748.
4. Doll R, Hill AB. The mortality of doctors in relation to their smoking habits: a preliminary report. *Br Med J* 1954; 4877:1451–1455.
5. Hill AB. The environment and disease: association or causation? *Proc R Soc Med* 1965; 58:295–300.
6. Stamler J. *Lectures on preventive cardiology*. Grune and Stratton, 1967.
7. Mitka M. Jeremiah Stamler, MD: researcher, leader in cardiovascular disease prevention. *JAMA* 2004; 292:1941–1943.

8. Conroy RM, Pyörälä K, Fitzgerald AP *et al*. Estimation of ten-year risk of fatal cardiovascular disease in Europe: the SCORE project. *Eur Heart J* 2003; 24:987–1003.
9. Pyörälä K, De Backer G, Graham I. Prevention of coronary heart disease in clinical practice: recommendations of the Task Force of the European Society of Cardiology, European Atherosclerosis Society and European Society of Hypertension. *Eur Heart J* 1994; 15:1300–1331.
10. Graham I, Atar D, Borch-Johnsen K *et al*. Fourth Joint Task Force of the European Society of Cardiology and other societies on cardiovascular disease prevention in clinical practice. European Guidelines on Cardiovascular Disease Prevention in Clinical Practice. *Eur J Cardiovasc Prev Rehabil* 2007; 14(suppl 2):S1–S113.

1

Cardiovascular epidemiology: background and principles of cardiovascular disease prevention

T. Leong, C. McGorrian, I. M. Graham

INTRODUCTION

This chapter discusses the evolution of the concepts of risk factors for atherosclerotic cardio-vascular disease (CVD) and how the criteria for causality developed. The critical roles of Ancel Keys, Jeremiah Stamler and classical epidemiological studies such as the Seven Countries Study and the Framingham Heart Study are presented. The primary importance of total risk estimation in clinical management is explained and the aspects of cardiovascular risk prediction in special groups are considered.

BACKGROUND

A *risk factor* may be defined as a characteristic of an individual that is associated with an increased risk of the development of a specific disease such as CVD. The roles of raised blood pressure, increased cholesterol level and smoking as risk factors for CVD are now firmly established. Multiple randomized controlled trials have proven that treatment of raised serum cholesterol and blood pressure reduces mortality, and observational studies indicate that those who do not smoke or stop smoking are at greatly reduced risk.

It was Ancel Keys (1904–2004) who initiated what was probably the first prospective study of CVD in 286 clinically healthy businessmen and professional men aged 40–55 in Minneapolis, St. Paul, Minnesota in 1945 [1]. This was done after the observed fall in coronary heart disease rates in Northern Europe during and after the Second World War. These Minnesota businessmen were followed up for 15 years and Keys observed high levels of myocardial infarctions amongst the higher socioeconomic groups. These findings were also found in comparative observational studies done on contrasting populations, particularly in terms of diet, in Italy, Spain, England and New Zealand. The link between diet and cholesterol was made when low cholesterol levels were found in studies of firemen in Naples and of the poor in Madrid, whereas a study of 50 professional men in Madrid revealed high cholesterol levels on a par with their American counterparts. Other important findings in Keys' early studies included the high prevalence of coronary heart disease observed in Finland and its relative rarity in Mediterranean countries such as Crete.

Tora Leong, MB, MRCPI, Senior Reseach Fellow, Department of Cardiology, The Adelaide and Meath Hospital, Dublin, Ireland

Catherine McGorrian, MRCPI, Senior Research Fellow, Department of Cardiology, The Adelaide and Meath Hospital, Dublin, Ireland

Ian M. Graham, FRCPI, FESC, Consultant Cardiologist; Professor of Cardiovascular Medicine, Trinity College, Dublin; Professor of Preventive Cardiology, Royal College of Surgeons in Ireland

Keys' early work and his interest in diet culminated in the famous Seven Countries Study [2]. This is widely accepted as the beginning of modern cardiovascular epidemiology. The Seven Countries Study was the first study to systematically examine the relationship of diet, lifestyle and risk factors with coronary heart disease and stroke in contrasting populations. The study included 16 cohorts from seven countries – the United States, Finland, the Netherlands, Italy, Yugoslavia, Greece and Japan. Perhaps more than any other study, the Seven Countries Study has documented differences in risk factor levels, in particular cholesterol and diet, between populations and their corresponding differences in CVD rates. Keys was also among the first to use mathematical regression and prediction equations in biology in the 1920s – the relationship betweeen weight and length of fishes [3]. This is the basis for modern cardiovascular risk prediction equations.

Another investigator who has devoted his career to cardiovascular epidemiology and prevention is Jeremiah Stamler [4], who examined the role of cholesterol and other risk factors such as blood pressure, smoking, obesity, physical inactivity, adverse eating patterns and diabetes [5]. Stamler's pioneering work consolidated the concept of risk factors, and established the possibility of using interventions such as better nutrition, exercise and non-smoking in order to reduce CVD. His early work in the 1940s showed that feeding cholesterol and fat to chickens produced atherosclerotic lesions [6], while raising blood pressure concomitantly resulted in intensified atherosclerosis [7]. Stamler demonstrated that multifactorial lifestyle intervention, especially diet, can reduce risk factor levels in both the Chicago Coronary Prevention Evaluation Program [8] and Multiple Risk Factor Intervention Trial (MRFIT) [9].

RISK FACTORS

It was the Framingham Heart Study that confirmed raised blood pressure, serum cholesterol and smoking as risk factors of coronary heart disease [10]. This landmark study was undertaken by the United States Public Health Service in order to investigate possible biological and environmental factors that might explain the epidemic of CVD in the United States during the 1930s [11, 12]. The town of Framingham, Massachusetts was chosen and 5209 healthy residents between the ages of 30 and 60 were recruited in 1948. The Framingham Heart Study was also the first major cardiovascular study to enrol women recruits. Later, in 1971, the Framingham Offspring Study recruited 5124 men and women between the ages of 5 and 70, consisting of the spouses and children of the Framingham Heart Study. The Third Generation Study in 2002 enrolled about 3900 grandchildren of the original cohort to provide data on three generations. The Framingham Heart Study has constantly evolved to study potential new risk factors, including genetics, in partnership with local, national and international partners.

Before the Framingham Heart Study, the role of cholesterol in CVD was neither fully understood nor widely accepted. In particular, the Framingham Heart Study established a strong association between low density lipoprotein (LDL) cholesterol and coronary heart disease, and the protective effect of high density lipoprotein (HDL) cholesterol. The Framingham Heart Study also established the role of blood pressure in the development of CVD, and dispelled the myths that blood pressure may be less harmful in women, and that the elderly may tolerate higher blood pressures. Smoking was also found to be associated with increased risk of myocardial infarction in the Framingham population, and the risk increased with the number of cigarettes smoked. The fact that filters in cigarettes gave no protection for coronary heart disease was also another finding from the Framingham Heart Study. Other important findings also associated with the Framingham Heart Study are summarized in Table 1.1.

THE RATIONALE FOR THE PREVENTION OF CARDIOVASCULAR DISEASES

CVD remains the leading cause of death worldwide, accounting for 16.7 million deaths (29.2% of total mortality) worldwide in 2003 [13]. It is now recognized that atherosclerosis is

Table 1.1 Some associations found in the Framingham Heart Study [10, 11]

Coronary heart disease
  Smoking (1970)
  Cholesterol (1971)
  Blood pressure (1971)
  ECG abnormalities (1971)
  Diabetes (1974)
  Menopause (1976)
  Triglycerides (1977)
  Psychosocial factors (1978)
  Type A behaviour (1988)
  Isolated systolic hypertension (1988)

Stroke
  Blood pressure (1970)
  Atrial fibrillation (1978)
  Smoking (1988)
  Left ventricular enlargement (1994)

Possible new risk factors for coronary heart disease
  Fibrinogen (1978)
  Homocysteine (1990)
  Lipoprotein (a) (1994)
  Apolipoprotein E (1994)

the background disease process which culminates in CVD – the clinical presentation of which includes acute coronary syndromes, ischaemic stroke and peripheral vascular disease. Once CVD manifests itself, e.g. as myocardial infarction and stroke, it is associated with high morbidity and mortality.

Significant atherosclerosis has been demonstrated in fit and healthy young men in autopsy studies such as those of the veterans who died during the Korean [14] and Vietnam Wars [15]. This process begins early in life as autopsies done on children as young as 9 months old have shown fatty streaks in their coronary arteries. The Pathological Determinants of Atherosclerosis in Youth (PDAY) study showed that significant atherosclerosis is associated with risk factors such as cholesterol and smoking [16]. The Bogalusa Heart Study further showed that the extent of atherosclerosis in the aorta and coronary arteries is related to the number of risk factors present [17]. These risk factors include body mass index, systolic blood pressure (SBP), LDL cholesterol, triglycerides and smoking. Does this matter, one may ask, as arteries have a great ability to adapt to atherosclerotic changes? Findings from the Framingham Heart Study, Chicago Heart Association Detection Project [18] and multiple other studies suggest that risk factors present early in life predict future coronary heart disease events. Primary prevention studies such as the Air Force/Texas Coronary Atherosclerosis Prevention Study (AFCAPS/TexCAPS) have shown the mortality benefit of reducing cholesterol in the primary prevention setting [19].

CRITERIA FOR CAUSALITY

In 1965 Austin Bradford Hill suggested nine viewpoints to consider before an association can be considered causal. Hill's guidelines are commonly referred to as the Bradford Hill criteria for causality [20] and are summarized in Table 1.2. Although Hill himself did not consider these criteria as indisputable for cause and effect, they nevertheless provide us with a framework to examine an association. Perhaps Hill's greatest contribution to epidemiology was the pioneering use of the randomized controlled trial design to study the

Table 1.2   Bradford Hill criteria for causality

(1) *Strength*: A large increase in risk when exposed to a factor is easier to detect and supports causation. However, it does not follow that a modest association excludes causality
(2) *Consistency*: Findings which are repeatedly observed by different persons, in different places, circumstances and times make the association less likely due to chance and strengthen the likelihood of an effect
(3) *Specificity*: Causation is more likely if only a certain population exposed to the risk factor develops the disease, assuming that that population does not have any other reason for developing the disease
(4) *Temporality*: The effect has to occur after the cause, and this is particularly important if there are several factors involved
(5) *Biological gradient*: The association is more likely to be causal if there is a dose-dependent response of the disease to dose of the risk factor exposed. Lack of this relationship may weaken but does not exclude causality
(6) *Plausibility*: A biological plausible mechanism between cause and effect is helpful but this could be limited by present knowledge
(7) *Coherence*: New findings on the association of the risk factor should not seriously conflict known facts about the disease
(8) *Experiment*: If an intervention to reduce the risk factor in question prevents the disease, then this may be the strongest argument in favour of causality
(9) *Analogy*: In some circumstances, it may be possible to judge through previous similar experiences

treatment of tuberculosis using streptomycin in the 1940s [21]. The randomized controlled trial is now considered the highest level of evidence in cardiovascular epidemiology. Austin Hill, along with his protégé Richard Doll, was also best known for being the first to show the association between cigarette smoking and lung cancer in the 1950s [22, 23].

RISK ESTIMATION SYSTEMS

A healthy individual's risk may be estimated on the basis of various risk factors present. Although many risk estimation systems exist, the risk equations based on the Framingham Heart Study [24, 25] and the SCORE (Systematic Coronary Risk Evaluation) project [26] are recommended by the American Third Adult Treatment Plan (ATP III) of the National Cholesterol Education Program (NCEP) [27] and the European Fourth Joint Task Force on Cardiovascular Disease Prevention in Clinical Practice [28], respectively. The Framingham risk equation suggested by ATP III uses age, gender, total cholesterol, HDL cholesterol, SBP, smoking and antihypertensive treatment as risk factors to estimate an individual's 10-year risk of developing coronary heart disease – the 'hard' coronary endpoints which are fatal and non-fatal myocardial infarctions. The SCORE system [26] estimates an individual's 10-year risk of death from CVD from risk factors such as age, gender, SBP, smoking, total and/or HDL cholesterol.

TOTAL OR GLOBAL RISK

The modern approach to managing cardiovascular risk is to reduce an individual's total or global risk, rather than grading risk on individual risk factors alone. This is because risk factors may interact to produce a greater than additive risk, and because risk factors tend to cluster together. The European Fourth Joint Task Force on Cardiovascular Disease Prevention in Clinical Practice [28] stresses the need for total risk estimation, and has shifted from coronary heart disease to total atherosclerotic CVD prevention, since the same risk factors may result in coronary heart disease, stroke, peripheral vascular disease or aneurysm. Situations may arise where management decisions based on single risk factors may be misleading,

Table 1.3 Impact of combinations of risk factors on 10-year risk of cardiovascular death

Sex	Age	Cholesterol	Blood pressure	Smoker	SCORE 10-year risk (%)
Female	60	8	120	No	2
Female	60	7	140	Yes	5
Male	60	6	160	No	9
Male	60	5	180	Yes	21

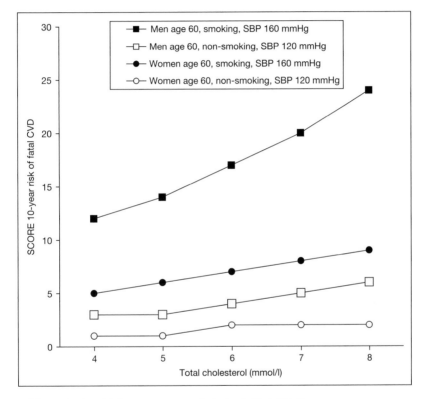

Figure 1.1 Effects of other risk factors on serum cholesterol: High Risk Europe.

with some instances described in Table 1.3 above. For instance, a male smoker with a cholesterol of 6 mmol/l, and SBP of 160 mmHg can be at four times higher risk than a female non-smoker with a cholesterol of 8 mmol/l and SBP of more than 120 mmHg (10-year absolute risk of CVD death at age 60 using the SCORE system is 9% vs. 2%) (Table 1.3). If risk had been assessed by using cholesterol alone, then a woman with a cholesterol of 8 mmol/l would have been treated with higher priority than that of a man with cholesterol of 5 mmol/l when clearly the man had the higher global risk. Figure 1.1 further illustrates how individuals with a single cholesterol level can have a range of cardiovascular risks depending on the presence of other risk factors, and how smoking and hypertension can override the risk advantage of being female.

THE DEFINITION OF HIGH RISK

A 10-year risk of developing 'hard' coronary heart disease (fatal and non-fatal events) of greater than 20% using the Framingham risk score is considered high risk. Individuals with a 10-year risk of fatal total cardiovascular death of 5% or greater, now or extrapolated to age 60, estimated using the SCORE system are considered to be at high risk. The European Fourth Joint Task Force suggests the following individuals as priorities for risk evaluation and management:

(1) Those with established CVD.
(2) Those who have a SCORE risk of 5% or greater, markedly raised levels of individual risk factors and those with Type 1 diabetes or Type 2 diabetes with microalbuminuria.
(3) Close relatives of those with premature CVD or asymptomatic individuals at particularly high risk.
(4) Those encountered routinely in clinical practice.

THE STRATEGY OF PREVENTION – THE POPULATION AND HIGH-RISK APPROACH

It is natural for clinicians to direct treatment to those at greatest need. In the case of CVD, those who have established CVD deserve the highest priority. However, while the 'high-risk' approach is efficient, preventive efforts in CVD should also be complemented with the mass or 'population' approach, because *a large number of people exposed to a small risk may generate many more cases than a small number exposed to a high risk*. This means that a measure that can bring large benefits to the population as a whole often offers little to each individual – the 'prevention paradox' described by Geoffrey Rose [29, 30]. Figure 1.2 illustrates this point.

Those with an estimated 10-year risk of cardiovascular death of 5% or greater under the SCORE system are considered high-risk, and thus, prioritized to receive intervention in the form of either lifestyle changes or drugs. This is highly successful and efficient at an individual level. However, a substantial number of deaths from CVD occur in those who have a predicted risk of less than 5% – those classified as 'low risk' – simply because they are much more numerous.

In the example in Figure 1.2, where men aged 50–59 in the SCORE cohorts are concerned, a substantial number of deaths from CVD occur in those who have a predicted risk of less than 5%. Therefore, the high-risk strategy in this situation will miss a significant proportion of cardiovascular deaths. These individuals will have cholesterols or blood pressures that are slightly above normal, and may be smokers who may not get the prevention advice that they need. Although their individual risk may be low, their cumulative contribution to the total population risk is high. Therefore, effective CVD prevention should be approached at both the high-risk [27, 28] and the population [31] levels.

The other difficulty with the population approach is that most of us are generally motivated by a benefit that is visible. In the case of CVD, the effects of reducing cholesterol and blood pressure are not immediately visible or tangible, as the conditions are asymptomatic in the vast majority of individuals.

RISK ESTIMATION AT THE EXTREMES OF AGE

Special problems in cardiovascular risk assessment arise in both extremes of age – the young and the elderly. For example, the SCORE system presents its results in the form of easy-to-use risk charts which start at age 40 and end at 65. In the case of young adults, their absolute risk of CVD is extremely low, and hence, they have relatively few cardiovascular events.

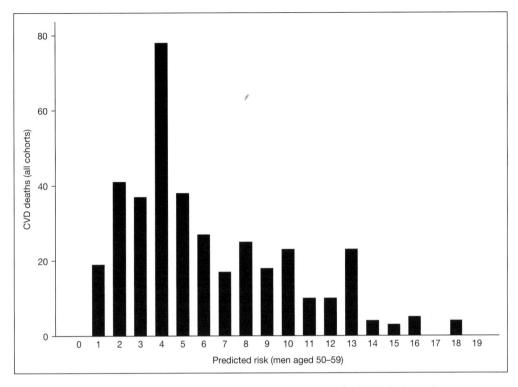

Figure 1.2 The expected number of CVD deaths in men aged 50–59 in the SCORE Project cohorts at increasing levels of predicted risk: Illustration of the fact that a significant number of deaths occur in low-risk subjects (Courtesy of Dr Anthony P Fitzgerald).

Although at low absolute risk, this group may have markedly different relative risks, which may be important for stimulating early preventive lifestyle advice.

The fourth European Task Force recommendations on the prevention of CVD [28] deal with this issue by using a relative risk chart which can be used to show a younger person that, although at low absolute risk, they may be at high relative risk if they carry a heavy burden of risk factors. If not managed, this will translate into a high relative risk as the person ages. These issues are discussed in chapter 11 and in the sections on management. A risk score for coronary heart disease risk in young adults (aged 15–34) was recently published based on data from the PDAY study [32]. This risk scoring system estimates the probability of having atherosclerotic lesions in the coronary arteries and abdominal aorta using risk factors such as age, gender, non-HDL and HDL cholesterol categories, smoking, hypertension, obesity and hyperglycaemia [32]. Another solution used by many clinical trials is the use of carotid intima–media thickness measurement as a surrogate for early atherosclerosis. It is known that cardiovascular risk factors in childhood influence arterial changes leading to the development of atherosclerosis [33, 34].

In high-risk countries, virtually all men aged 65 years or older are at 'high risk' as defined by the SCORE system and, of course, on the day of one's death, absolute risk becomes 100%. Conventional and other risk factors may operate differently in the elderly; e.g. a raised plasma homocysteine may also predict dementia or osteoporosis. Randomized controlled trials have confirmed the benefit of cholesterol lowering to 82 years of age [35, 36]. However, the age at which risk factor modification becomes useless is still unknown. Both new cohort and intervention studies in the elderly are still needed.

GENDER AND CARDIOVASCULAR RISK

In general, women are less likely than men to receive adequate risk evaluation [37] and treatment [38, 39]. While the SCORE risk charts suggest that women are at lower risk than men, this is misleading. Risk in women is delayed by 10 years compared to men but eventually, more women than men die of coronary heart disease [40, 41]. In contrast, women with single risk factors are at low absolute risk and may be subjected to unnecessary drug treatment but insufficient help with regard to nutrition, exercise and avoidance of tobacco.

ETHNICITY AND CARDIOVASCULAR RISK

Middle-aged Caucasian men have been the most studied group in cardiovascular studies. There can be ethnic differences both in the relative effect of risk factors, and in response to therapeutics. For example, the role of the renin–angiotensin system in hypertension is probably less important in Afro-Caribbeans than Caucasians, and hence the use of β-blockers and angiotensin-converting enzyme (ACE) inhibitors is less efficacious in this group. Even cut-points for the relationship of body mass index to cardiovascular risk may be different in different ethnic groups. This has led the International Diabetes Federation to suggest a lower waist circumference cut-point when detecting the metabolic syndrome in South Asian or Indian, Chinese, and Japanese populations [42].

We also know that the Framingham risk score which is derived from a predominantly Caucasian population has tended to over-predict risk in some southern European populations and a Chinese population [43]. There are also important population differences in CVD incidence to consider, as the Seven Countries Study and the World Health Organization (WHO) MONitoring trends and determinants in CArdiovascular disease (MONICA) study have shown. One of the main reasons for this is the differences in risk factor levels between populations. There is evidence that the Framingham functions can be recalibrated by adjusting for incidence levels resulting in valid risk functions [24, 43].

The predominant types of CVD are also different in different parts of the world. Some Southern European countries have a higher proportion of stroke than coronary heart disease, as with most Asian countries. Stroke is a more common form of CVD than coronary heart disease in China. In Asian countries, the proportion of haemorrhagic stroke is also greater than ischaemic stroke. Haemorrhagic stroke carries a higher mortality than ischaemic stroke. These differences are important because it means that preventive strategies that work in one region may not be equally as effective in another. The Omni Study, which started recruitment of Framingham's minority community in 1995, will allow investigators to examine whether the risk factors for CVD are the same in this group compared to the other Framingham cohorts. Other worldwide studies which may help answer these questions may include studies done in Asian populations such as the Asia Pacific Cohort Studies Collaboration. Nevertheless, the INTERHEART case–control study shows that the major classical risk factors are strongly associated with CVD in diverse populations in 52 countries [44].

THE ISSUE OF BLOOD SUGAR AND DIABETES

The current WHO definition of diabetes is a fasting plasma glucose of 7.1 mmol/l or more, or a 2-h post-prandial blood glucose of 11.1 mmol/l or more. Having a cut-point is useful for clinicians to direct treatment but, in fact, the relationship of glucose with cardiovascular risk is continuous, and a 2-h post-prandial blood sugar is an even better predictor of risk than fasting glucose. The definition of diabetes has changed over time and the heterogeneity of definitions of diabetes makes it hard to quantify its contribution to risk. Nevertheless, there is general agreement that diabetes doubles the risk in men and increases it three- to five-fold in women.

Table 1.4 Criteria for widespread use of a risk marker

(1) *Standardized and reproducible*: At the moment, most diagnostic assays for novel risk markers are not standardized, and hence, values obtained from one laboratory cannot be compared with those obtained elsewhere, with the exception of C-reactive protein and homocysteine

(2) *Added predictive value*: Measurement of the risk marker should add information on top of conventional risk factors in terms of risk assessment. At this time, this is only true for risk markers such as C-reactive protein, homocysteine and fibrinogen

(3) *Prospectively assessed*: The risk markers should have been assessed in prospective cohort studies. This is true of C-reactive protein and homocysteine

(4) *Intervention produces benefit*: Therapy should be available for the risk factor in question, and it should be demonstrated that treating these risk markers will reduce the hard endpoints of CVD such as myocardial infarction, stroke and mortality. Ideally, this benefit of treatment should offer advantages over current methods used to treat conventional risk factors such as blood pressure, cholesterol and diabetes. At this point in time, none of the novel risk markers have definitive evidence in this respect

(5) *Applicability*: Diagnostic and treatment criteria must be applied to the correct population from which the evidence is based. For example, secondary prevention data may not be applicable to healthy asymptomatic individuals. The issue of applying data to different ethnic populations has been previously discussed

NEWER RISK FACTORS

A significant proportion of people develop atherosclerosis and CVD in the absence of the established conventional risk factors. Historically, it was thought that half of people who present with acute myocardial infarctions have no discernible risk factors. Larger studies such as the MRFIT and the more recent INTERHEART study [44] suggest that as much as 90% of coronary heart disease and acute myocardial infarctions, respectively, may be attributable to conventional risk factors, the definition of which may vary from study to study. Since INTERHEART was a case–control study it cannot generate definite population attributable risk estimates and as such must be interpreted with some caution. The choice of cut-points used for risk factors such as cholesterol, blood pressure and blood sugar may also affect estimates of attributable risk. If, as in many epidemiological studies, a risk factor such as blood pressure is only measured on one occasion, it may be spuriously high or low, thus reducing the real relationship with risk, a phenomenon known as regression dilution bias [45].

On the basis of more recent epidemiological studies and new knowledge of vascular biology, new risk markers have been sought to refine cardiovascular risk prediction. Some risk markers such as high-sensitive C-reactive protein, homocysteine, fibrinogen and lipoprotein (a) have been extensively studied. Newer risk markers may be relevant not only because they may explain some of the 10% or more of unexplained CVD, but they may also modify the effects of conventional risk factors, e.g. homocysteine and cigarette smoking [46, 47], C-reactive protein and total cholesterol:HDL ratio [48]. Table 1.4 illustrates some other points which need consideration before a test is used widely for public screening. This is particularly relevant to the evaluation of newer risk markers.

UTILITY – RISK PREDICTION SYSTEMS AND GUIDELINES

Effective CVD prevention can only occur if there is a good partnership between the doctor and the patient. Even the best risk prediction system will be useless if there is no one using it. It should be easily accessible, easy to use and utilize risk factors that are simple and measured universally. Clear, up-to-date guidelines should be available for the clinician to manage modifiable risk factors as appropriate based on evidence from best practice. Electronic risk calculators based on the Framingham risk score are available from various sources. The

HeartScore® program [49] is an example of an electronic web-based risk prediction and management system recommended for use by the European Fourth Joint Task Force. Risk factor levels are entered by the user and the 10-year absolute risk of fatal CVD for that country is calculated based on data derived from the SCORE Project, calibrated where possible from national mortality statistics and risk factor levels based on approved local or regional surveys. HeartScore® is also a risk management system which gives advice on both lifestyle and pharmaceutical intervention based on the European Fourth Joint Task Force guidelines.

Ultimately, the prevention of cardiovascular disease depends upon social and economic factors coupled with individual knowledge and motivation. Most individuals are not 'patients' in the traditional setting. They do not exhibit symptoms and signs of their high cholesterol and blood pressure, and hence, the motivation for lifestyle change is difficult for most. Last but not least, key decision makers for the health service must take an interest in making CVD prevention a priority.

Let Geoffrey Rose have the last word:

'The primary determinants of disease are mainly economic and social, and therefore its remedies must also be economic and social. Medicine and politics cannot and should not be kept apart.'

REFERENCES

1. Keys AB, Taylor HL, Blackburn H, Brozek J, Anderson JT, Simonson E. Coronary heart disease among Minnesota business and professional men followed fifteen years. *Circulation* 1963; 28:381–395.
2. Keys AB. *Seven Countries: A Multivariate Analysis of Death and Coronary Heart Disease*. Harvard University Press, London, 1980.
3. Keys AB. The weight-length relation in fishes. *Proc Natl Acad USA* 1928; 14:922–925.
4. Mitka M. Jeremiah Stamler, MD: researcher, leader in cardiovascular disease prevention. *JAMA* 2004; 292:1941–1943.
5. Stamler J, Stamler R, Neaton JD *et al*. Low risk-factor profile and long-term cardiovascular and noncardiovascular mortality and life expectancy: findings for 5 large cohorts of young adult and middle-aged men and women. *JAMA* 1999; 282:2012–2018.
6. Stamler J, Katz LN. Production of experimental cholesterol-induced atherosclerosis in chicks with minimal hypercholesterolemia and organ lipidosis. *Circulation* 1950; 2:705–713.
7. Stamler J, Katz LN. The effect of salt hypertension on atherosclerosis in chicks fed mash without a cholesterol supplement. *Circulation* 1951; 3:859–863.
8. Stamler J, Berkson DM, Levinson MJ *et al*. A long-term coronary prevention evaluation program. *Ann N Y Acad Sci* 1968;149:1022–1037.
9. Stamler J, Caggiula A, Grandits GA, Kjelsberg M, Cutler JA. Relationship to blood pressure of combinations of dietary macronutrients. Findings of the Multiple Risk Factor Intervention Trial (MRFIT). *Circulation* 1996; 94:2417–2423.
10. Kannel WB, Dawber TR, Kagan A, Revotskie N, Stokes J 3rd. Factors of risk in the development of coronary heart disease – six year follow-up experience. The Framingham Study. *Ann Intern Med* 1961; 55:33–50.
11. http://www.framingham.com/heart
12. http://www.nhlbi.nih.gov/about/framingham/
13. World Health Organization Statistics. http://www.who.int/
14. Enos WF, Holmes RH, Beyer J. Coronary disease among United States soldiers killed in action in Korea; preliminary report. *J Am Med Assoc* 1953; 152:1090–1093.
15. Strong JP. Landmark perspective: coronary atherosclerosis in soldiers. A clue to the natural history of atherosclerosis in the young. *JAMA* 1986; 256:2863–2866.
16. Wissler RW, Strong JP. Risk factors and progression of atherosclerosis in youth. PDAY Research Group. Pathological Determinants of Atherosclerosis in Youth. *Am J Pathol* 1998; 153:1023–1033.
17. Berenson GS, Srinivasan SR, Bao W, Newman WP 3rd, Tracy RE, Wattigney WA. Association between multiple cardiovascular risk factors and atherosclerosis in children and young adults. The Bogalusa Heart Study. *N Engl J Med* 1998; 338:1650–1656.

18. Navas-Nacher EL, Colangelo L, Beam C, Greeland P. Risk factors for coronary heart disease in men 18 to 39 years of age. *Ann Intern Med* 2001; 134:433–439.

19. Downs JR *et al*. Primary prevention of acute coronary events with lovastatin in men and women with average cholesterol levels: results of AFCAPS/TexCAPS. Air Force/Texas Coronary Atherosclerosis Prevention Study. *JAMA* 1998; 279:1615–1622.

20. Hill AB. The environment and disease: association or causation? *Proc R Soc Med* 1965; 58:295–300.

21. Hill AB. Suspended judgment. Memories of the British Streptomycin Trial in Tuberculosis. The first randomized clinical trial. *Control Clin Trials* 1990; 11:77–79.

22. Doll R, Hill AB. Smoking and carcinoma of the lung; preliminary report. *Br Med J* 1950; 2:739–748.

23. Doll R, Hill AB. The mortality of doctors in relation to their smoking habits; a preliminary report. *Br Med J* 1954; 4877:1451–1455.

24. D'Agostino RB, Sr, Grundy S, Sullivan LM, Wilson P; CHD prediction group. Validation of the Framingham coronary heart disease prediction scores: results of a multiple ethnic group investigation. *JAMA* 2001; 286:180–187.

25. Wilson PW, D'Agostino RB, Levy D, Belanger AM, Silbershatz H, Kannel WB. Prediction of coronary heart disease using risk factor categories. *Circulation* 1998; 97:1837–1847.

26. Conroy RM, Pyörälä K, Fitzgerald AP *et al*. Estimation of ten-year risk of fatal cardiovascular disease in Europe: the SCORE project. *Eur Heart J* 2003; 24:987–1003.

27. Executive Summary of the Third Report of The National Cholesterol Education Program (NCEP) Expert Panel on Detection, Evaluation, and Treatment of High Blood Cholesterol In Adults (Adult Treatment Panel III). *JAMA* 2001; 285:2486–2497.

28. Graham I, Atar D, Borch-Johnsen K *et al*. Fourth Joint Task Force of the European Society of Cardiology and other societies on cardiovascular disease prevention in clinical practice. European Guidelines on Cardiovascular Disease Prevention in Clinical Practice. *Eur J Cardiovasc Prev Rehabil* 2007; 14(suppl 2):S1–S113.

29. Rose G. *The Strategy of Preventive Medicine*. Oxford University Press, Oxford, 1992.

30. Rose G. Strategy of prevention: lessons from cardiovascular disease. *Br Med J (Clin Res Ed)* 1981; 282:1847–1851.

31. Carleton RA, Dwyer J, Finberg I *et al*. Report of the Expert Panel on Population Strategies for Blood Cholesterol Reduction. A statement from the National Cholesterol Education Program, National Heart, Lung, and Blood Institute, National Institutes of Health. *Circulation* 1991; 83:2154–2232.

32. McMahan CA, Gidding SS, Fayad ZA *et al*. Risk scores predict atherosclerotic lesions in young people. *Arch Intern Med* 2005; 165:883–890.

33. Li S, Chen W, Srinivasan SR *et al*. Childhood cardiovascular risk factors and carotid vascular changes in adulthood: the Bogalusa Heart Study. *JAMA* 2003; 290:2271–2276.

34. Raitakari OT, Juonala M, Kahonen M *et al*. Cardiovascular risk factors in childhood and carotid artery intima-media thickness in adulthood: the Cardiovascular Risk in Young Finns Study. *JAMA* 2003; 290:2277–2283.

35. Shepherd J, Blauw GJ, Murphy MB *et al*. Pravastatin in elderly individuals at risk of vascular disease (PROSPER): a randomised controlled trial. *Lancet* 2002; 360:1623–1630.

36. Collins R, Armitaqe J, Parish S *et al*. MRC/BHF Heart Protection Study of cholesterol-lowering with simvastatin in 5,963 people with diabetes: a randomised placebo-controlled trial. *Lancet* 2003; 361:2005–2016.

37. Bartys S, Baker D, Lewis P, Middleton E. Inequity in recording of risk in a local population-based screening programme for cardiovascular disease. *Eur J Cardiovasc Prev Rehabil* 2005; 12:63–67.

38. Daly C, Clemens F, Copez Sendon JL *et al*. Gender differences in the management and clinical outcome of stable angina. *Circulation* 2006; 113:490–498.

39. Anand SS, Xie CC, Mehta S *et al*. Differences in the management and prognosis of women and men who suffer from acute coronary syndromes. *J Am Coll Cardiol* 2005; 46:1845–1851.

40. Stramba-Badiale M, Fox KM, Priori SG *et al*. Cardiovascular diseases in women: a statement from the policy conference of the European Society of Cardiology. *Eur Heart J* 2006; 27:994–1005.

41. Bello N, Mosca L. Epidemiology of coronary heart disease in women. *Prog Cardiovasc Dis* 2004; 46:287–295.

42. Alberti KG, Zimmet P, Shaw J. The metabolic syndrome – a new worldwide definition. *Lancet* 2005; 366:1059–1062.

43. Liu J, Hung Y, D'Agostino RB *et al*. Predictive value for the Chinese population of the Framingham CHD risk assessment tool compared with the Chinese multi-provincial cohort study. *JAMA* 2004; 291:2591–2599.

44. Yusuf S, Hawken S, Ounpuu S *et al.* Effect of potentially modifiable risk factors associated with myocardial infarction in 52 countries (the INTERHEART study): case-control study. *Lancet* 2004; 364:937–952.

45. Emberson JR, Whincup PH, Morrs RW, Walker M. Re-assessing the contribution of serum total cholesterol, blood pressure and cigarette smoking to the aetiology of coronary heart disease: impact of regression dilution bias. *Eur Heart J* 2003; 24:1719–1726.

46. O'Callaghan PA, Fitzgerald A, Fogarty J *et al.* New and old cardiovascular risk factors: C-reactive protein, homocysteine, cysteine and von Willebrand factor increase risk, especially in smokers. *Eur J Cardiovasc Prev Rehabil* 2005; 12:542–547.

47. O'Callaghan P, Meleady R, Fitzgerald T, Graham I, European COMAC Group. Smoking and plasma homocysteine. *Eur Heart J* 2002; 23:1580–1586.

48. Ridker PM, Glynn RJ, Hennekens CH, C-reactive protein adds to the predictive value of total and HDL cholesterol in determining risk of first myocardial infarction. *Circulation* 1998; 97:2007–2011.

49. http://www.heartscore.org/

2

From epidemiological risk to clinical practice by way of statistics – a personal view

R. M. Conroy

'The power and elegance of the logistic function make it an attractive and elegant statistical instrument, but in the end we cannot push a button and hope that everything will come out all right. Because frequently it will not'. Tavia Gordon [1]

'The new and personalized era of medicine is one in which risk assessment can be individualized early in life with precision. Validation will require large populations with integrated collection of phenotypic and genomic data, and long follow-up for key endpoints. The current risk scores for coronary disease are a helpful foundation to be enriched and refined in the years ahead. In the meantime, when an individual asks 'should I take low-dose aspirin?' we have rudimentary tools with intrinsic limitations but which are nonetheless useful'. Eric Topol [2]

INTRODUCTION

In the 30 years between Tavia Gordon's remarks and those of Eric Topol, the considerable promise that multivariate statistical methods seemed to offer proved slow to translate into clinical practice. As Tavia Gordon makes clear, there is a considerable gap between calculating a risk estimation function and implementing risk estimation as part of routine clinical practice. Statisticians and epidemiologists have tended to be dismayed that their work has not been enthusiastically embraced by clinicians, but in the three decades that separate Gordon's remarks and the publication of the first widely-adopted clinical methods of coronary (later cardiovascular) risk estimation, we have learned a lot about the process of building models that will work in clinical practice. Topol's editorial, occasioned by the publication of the SCORE (Systematic Coronary Risk Evaluation) cardiovascular risk estimation system [3], was entitled *'The rudimentary phase of personalised medicine: coronary risk scores'*. The implication is clear: it has taken three decades for the clinical use of risk estimation methods, foreseen by Tavia Gordon, to become a reality. Why did it take so long? This chapter, based on the experience of the SCORE project, examines some of the reasons, in the hope that the lessons learned may speed the process in other applications of statistical risk estimation to clinical practice.

It is also a personal journey. The SCORE risk chart would not have been possible without the work and ideas of many people. I have tried to sketch the history of risk estimation, to show where these ideas and tools came from. This is not intended to be a history of risk estimation systems, but of the underlying ideas and problems. I have tried to give credit where

Ronán M. Conroy, MusB, DSc, Senior Lecturer, Department of Epidemiology, Royal College of Surgeons in Ireland, Dublin, Ireland

it is due, but I am conscious that there are many researchers and many assessment systems that I have omitted.

A NOTE ON TERMS

I use the expression 'risk estimation' throughout, as we have used it in the original publication of the SCORE algorithm. The expression 'risk prediction' implies a precision which is misleading, and gives the impression that the risk function 'knows' something about the person or the future. A risk function estimates risk in the person based on risk in the population. It is important for users to be aware of Neils Bohr's dictum: *prediction is very difficult, especially about the future.* (http://www.quotationspage.com/quote/26159.html)

THE PIONEERS

From the outset, the investigators of large epidemiological studies were aware that their data had the potential to allow the identification of people at elevated risk of heart disease and stroke, and the potential – the necessity, even – of computers in carrying out the requisite analyses. As far back as 1963, Thomas Dawber [4] was arguing that epidemiological data could not be exploited properly without a computer. Tellingly, he published the paper in the journal 'Progress in Cardiovascular Diseases', feeling that, of all practitioners, it was cardiologists who needed to be briefed on the potential benefits that would come from turning the power of computers on large epidemiological databases.

The history of cardiovascular risk estimation owes a particular debt to the investigators of the Framingham study [5]. In 1961, Kannel and Dawber [6] presented 6-year mortality data from the Framingham study in which they related mortality to levels of individual risk factors. However, the goal of integrating this information into a predictive model awaited developments in both statistics and computing. A landmark paper from Cornfield [7] used a discriminant function to model the relationship of heart disease risk to cholesterol and blood pressure simultaneously. However, it was clear that the calculations involved in multivariate models would only become feasible if computers could be brought to bear on the problem.

The increasing availability of mainframe computers towards the end of the 1960s encouraged statisticians to attempt to program multivariate models of risk. The first such models were based on discriminant analysis. Early attempts to program logistic regression models were hampered by the amount of computer time they required to run and the consequent expense of running them. Discriminant function analysis, pioneered by Cornfield, was frequently used in lieu of logistic regression because of the cost of computer time [8]. Ancel Keys [9] and his collaborators from the Seven Countries Study, describing their analytic methods, state 'Solving the multiple logistic equation by the Walker and Duncan method (what we would now term logistic regression) is costly and requires sequestration of a block of uninterrupted time on an extremely powerful computer, such as the CDC 6600. Accordingly, in the present study, after some parallel runs with both methods, we have concentrated on the methods of Truett et al., using a CDC 3300 computer.' The Truett method referred to is nowadays called discriminant function analysis, and has largely disappeared, since it makes restrictive assumptions about the distributions of the predictors: that they are multivariate normal and have equal variances and covariances. The CDC 6600 mentioned in the quotation has likewise disappeared into history, but was the world's first supercomputer, and, until 1971, the world's fastest computer. It was about as fast as an IBM 486. (By the time we came to calculate the SCORE risk functions, Stata, running on my Macintosh G4, was spending less than 35 seconds solving Weibull models with a quarter of a million observations.)

Rapid advances in programming were soon to reduce the computer overheads in calculating risk functions. Pioneering programs were written in the 60s at National Heart Lung

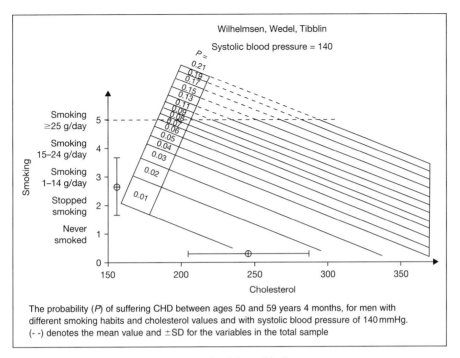

The probability (*P*) of suffering CHD between ages 50 and 59 years 4 months, for men with different smoking habits and cholesterol values and with systolic blood pressure of 140 mmHg. (- -) denotes the mean value and ±SD for the variables in the total sample

Figure 2.1   An early attempt to show cardiovascular risk graphically.

and Blood Institute (NHLBI) by Joel Verter. He wrote both a discriminant function program and then, soon after the Walker and Duncan paper appeared, in 1967 he wrote one for the maximum likelihood approach. The program was sent to anyone, anywhere, who had a FORTRAN compiler and wanted it. A significant advance came when Hans Wedel, the Swedish statistician and long-term collaborator of Lars Wilhelmsen *et al.* [10] developed a FORTRAN routine which was capable of solving a logistic regression model in less than 10 min (Wilhelmsen and Wedel, personal communications). Wilhelmsen, Wedel and Tibblin published their multivariate analysis of almost 1000 Swedish men in 1973. Another fruit of the Wilhelmsen, Wedel and Tibblin collaboration was an ingenious chart giving the 10-year risk of CHD at various levels of cholesterol and smoking, in a man with a systolic blood pressure of 140. Despite its obvious limitation to a single discrete blood pressure value, the chart is a pioneering and ingenious attempt to translate epidemiological models into clinical risk estimation. It is shown in Figure 2.1.

In the years that followed, many more models, based on epidemiological cohort studies were published. These risk estimation models were also indebted to the work of the Seven Countries Study investigators, who, as early as 1972, had pointed out the over- and under-estimation of risk when functions from one cohort were used to estimate risk in another [9]. Alessandro Menotti took this finding further, developing the first risk functions intended for use with low-risk populations. In 1975, he developed a model for use in Italy [11] which recommended risk estimation based on age, systolic blood pressure, serum cholesterol, consumption of cigarettes and physical activity.

The early pioneers, however, were not primarily interested in risk estimation in individuals. First, epidemiologists had to demonstrate that risk factors were associated with coronary heart disease (CHD) in a consistent way across different populations. They were concerned with establishing causal links between risk factors and disease and showing that no matter where you were, the impact of a unit of cholesterol on your risk was the same. Initially, too much of the research concerned CHD. The realization that a family of risk factors drive rates of not just CHD, but also stroke and dementias has been slow in arriving and, as we shall see, has had important implications for the limitations of risk estimation models in clinical practice.

FROM EPIDEMIOLOGY TO OUTPATIENTS

Although the first multivariate models relating coronary disease to risk factors were primarily concerned with establishing the role of the risk factors, a number of the more far-sighted (and practical) epidemiologists had been alive to the possibility that the resulting mathematical models might provide a basis for identifying those at highest risk of disease. As early as 1976, Kannel, McGee and Gordon made the point that: *'One general function for identifying persons at high risk of cardiovascular disease is also effective in identifying persons at risk for each of the specific diseases, CHD, atherothrombotic brain infarction, hypertensive heart disease and intermittent claudication, even though the variables used have a different impact on each particular disease. The 10 percent of persons identified with use of this function as at highest risk accounted for about one-fifth of the 8 year incidence of CHD and about one-third of the 8 year incidence of atherothrombotic brain infarction, hypertensive heart disease and intermittent claudication. Hence the function provides an economic and efficient method of identifying persons at high cardiovascular risk who need preventive treatment and persons at low risk who need not be alarmed about one moderately elevated risk characteristic'* [12]. Gordon and Kannel later put the matter even more bluntly: *'the fifth of the population with the highest risk function score had six times the risk of those who scored in the lowest fifth. It would not seem wise to leave such high-risk persons undetected and unprotected by preventive measures'* [13].

RISK ESTIMATION SYSTEMS: THE EARLY DAYS

The earliest risk estimation systems were, in effect, multiple regression equations. Each risk factor was entered into a complex equation and the resulting risk calculated. Keys *et al.* [9] were impressed with the ability of a small number of risk factor measurements to estimate risk. *'A high degree of discrimination of future risk is possible from only age, a casual systolic blood pressure measurement, a single serum cholesterol value and an answer to a query about current cigarette smoking.'* Furthermore, he goes on to say, a physician, given this information *'can enter these numbers into the multiple logistic equation, together with the constant and the coefficients [in Table 2], and calculate his probability of developing CHD in 5 years . . . Actually, the calculation is exceedingly simple with modern programming calculators no bigger than a typewriter.'* However, Keys' enthusiasm for modern programming calculators no bigger than a typewriter was not shared by his clinical colleagues, leading many people to consider other ways of simplifying the process of risk estimation to make it more likely to be used in the management of the individual patient.

One alternative to having the clinician do all the calculation was to supply ready-reckoner tables, and the first comprehensive attempt to do so was made by the Framingham investigators. Their Section 27 Report [14] contained 14 pages of tables giving the 8-year risk of developing CHD at six levels of cholesterol and of blood pressure, at 5-year ages between 35 and 70, for smoking and non-smoking men and women with and without left ventricular hypertrophy and glucose intolerance – a total of over 4500 individual risk factor combinations. Furthermore, anyone glancing at this large tabulation will be struck by the similarity in format to the SCORE risk chart. The information is presented coherently and in small regular blocks, a principle adopted for the European Task Force risk charts and, indeed, by many others in the intervening years. Figure 2.2 shows a sample page of the chart. The use

PROBABILITY* OF DEVELOPING CORONARY HEART DISEASE IN EIGHT YEARS BY SEX, AGE, SYSTOLIC BLOOD PRESSURE, CHOLESTEROL, LEFT VENTRICULAR HYPERTROPHY BY ECG, CIGARETTE SMOKING AND GLUCOSE INTOLERANCE: THE FRAMINGHAM STUDY, 16-YEAR FOLLOW-UP

35 YEAR OLD MAN**

DOES NOT SMOKE CIGARETTES   SMOKES CIGARETTES

--LVH-ECG NEGATIVE--

GLUCOSE INTOLERANCE ABSENT

CHOL	SBP 105	120	135	150	165	180		SBP 105	120	135	150	165	180
185	4	5	6	7	9	11		7	8	10	12	15	18
210	6	7	8	10	13	15		9	11	14	17	20	24
235	8	10	12	14	17	21		13	16	19	23	28	34
260	11	13	16	20	24	29		18	22	26	32	38	46
285	15	19	23	27	33	40		25	30	36	44	53	63
310	21	26	31	38	45	55		34	41	50	60	72	86

GLUCOSE INTOLERANCE PRESENT

CHOL	SBP 105	120	135	150	165	180		SBP 105	120	135	150	165	180
185	5	6	8	9	11	14		8	10	12	15	18	22
210	7	9	11	13	15	19		12	14	17	21	25	31
235	10	12	15	18	22	26		16	20	24	29	35	42
260	14	17	20	25	30	36		22	27	33	40	48	58
285	19	23	28	34	41	50		31	37	45	54	65	78
310	27	32	39	47	56	68		42	51	62	74	89	106

--LVH-ECG POSITIVE--

GLUCOSE INTOLERANCE ABSENT

CHOL	SBP 105	120	135	150	165	180		SBP 105	120	135	150	165	180
185	9	11	13	16	19	23		14	17	21	25	30	37
210	12	15	18	22	26	32		20	24	29	35	42	50
235	17	20	25	30	36	43		27	33	39	47	57	69
260	23	28	34	41	49	59		37	45	54	65	78	93
285	32	39	47	56	67	81		51	61	74	88	105	125
310	44	53	64	76	91	109		69	83	99	118	140	166

GLUCOSE INTOLERANCE PRESENT

CHOL	SBP 105	120	135	150	165	180		SBP 105	120	135	150	165	180
185	11	13	16	20	24	29		18	21	26	31	38	46
210	15	18	22	27	33	39		24	30	36	43	52	63
235	21	25	31	37	45	54		34	41	49	59	71	85
260	29	35	42	51	61	74		46	56	67	80	96	114
285	40	48	58	70	83	100		63	76	91	108	129	152
310	55	66	79	94	112	133		86	102	122	145	170	200

*PROBABILITY IS SHOWN IN THOUSANDTHS.
**FRAMINGHAM MEN AGED 35 YRS HAVE AN AVERAGE SBP OF 128 MM HG AND AN AVERAGE SERUM CHOL OF 221 MG%. 70 PERCENT SMOKE CIGARETTES, 0.0 PERCENT HAVE DEFINITE LVH BY ECG AND 2.1 PERCENT HAVE GLUCOSE INTOLERANCE. AT THESE AVERAGE VALUES THE PROBABILITY OF DEVELOPING CORONARY HEART DISEASE IN EIGHT YEARS IS 13/1000.

Figure 2.2 A page from the original Framingham risk tables. The layout of the SCORE risk chart owes a clear debt to these tables.

of a computer line-printer is another reminder of the growing importance of computers in epidemiology.

TWO APPROACHES: AUTOMATION AND SIMPLIFICATION

AUTOMATION

The vastness of the Framingham investigators' risk estimation table, and the apparent unwillingness of clinicians to do anything that resembled calculation or involved turning over pages, led to two approaches to the simplification of risk estimation. The first of these attempted to use technology to build a user-friendly calculator (and ideally one that would be smaller than a typewriter). The second entailed simplifying the process by reducing or eliminating calculation. A number of slide-rule-like calculators were developed, but with the steady decline in the cost of pocket calculators during the 1970s attention turned to the development of dedicated calculators. Several pharmaceutical companies manufactured calculators in which the risk was calculated by entering values for each risk factor and then pressing a specific key to identify which risk factor had been entered. The calculator finally displayed the 10-year risk. The first of these was based on a risk function developed by Professor Dan McGee, based on a model in Section 28 of the Framingham monographs,

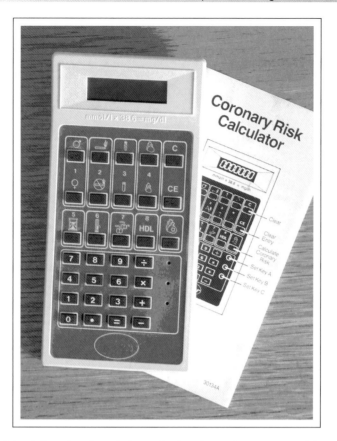

Figure 2.3   One of the dedicated pocket calculators developed to estimate coronary risk.

with a modification which allowed for the addition of high-density lipoprotein (HDL) cholesterol. Despite significant numbers of these calculators being given away free, there is no evidence that they were used in clinical practice on a significant scale, and the author has a small collection of them, donated by clinical colleagues with the comment 'It probably only needs a new battery.' One of these is shown in Figure 2.3.

I never encountered a clinician who had replaced the battery. The increasing availability of computers also led to the development of a number of stand-alone applications, or add-ins for spreadsheet packages, which calculated risk. While many of these were relatively easy to use, and produced a risk estimate in a matter of minutes, none has had a lasting impact on clinical practice. I will discuss possible reasons for this later in the chapter.

Another ingenious piece of automation was the coronary risk disk. The original risk disk was developed by Henry Blackburn, one of the principal investigators of the Seven Countries Study. The risk disk resembled a slide rule, but was circular, with concentric disks, one for each risk factor, which were turned to register the risk factor levels. The total risk could then be read off a printed scale. The idea was pioneered almost single-handedly, however, by Hugh Tunstall-Pedoe, who developed the Dundee Coronary Risk Disk, for the UK Coronary Prevention Group [15, 16]. The Dundee Risk Disk displays relative rather than absolute risk, in line with its brief as a means of health promotion and doctor–patient communication, and calculates risk based on the modifiable risk factors. It has an important place in the evaluation of risk estimation in clinical practice in that it was the first system to be developed around the needs of a physician who is trying both to estimate risk and to motivate the patient. That is, it was the first system to incorporate both clinical management and health promotion functions.

Finally, no history would be complete without the advent of the PDA. The development of handheld computers has placed a significant amount of computer power in the average doctor's pocket. In the US, the Adult Treatment Panel III (ATP III) of the National Cholesterol Education Program issued a PDA application which combined risk assessment, based on a new Framingham function [17] – the sixth risk function produced by the group since 1973 – with treatment guidelines. Bear in mind that the very small screen size of a PDA means that the resolution is necessarily quite low. Nevertheless, the ability of PDAs to start working instantly when powered on, combined with their extreme lightness, makes them considerably more useful to doctors than laptop or desktop computers. Small wonder then that the European Society of Cardiology (ESC) also adapted their task force guidelines for use on a PDA.

PRECARD and Heartscore

It is not my purpose to describe these developments in detail. This will be covered elsewhere. However, logically they also belong here. The Danish PRECARD program [18, 19] was the first national system of cardiovascular risk management to be computer-based, have an integral risk estimation system (which was based on Danish data) and a database system for individual patient tracking. It combined the strengths of risk estimation with the value of the Dundee system by using both absolute and relative risk and, innovatively, it also showed attributable risk in the form of a pie chart. The contribution of each risk factor to the patient's risk was shown on the chart.

PRECARD was designed with the clinician in mind. Risk factor data, for example, had to be capable of being entered within a minute, so data entry screens were streamlined and risk factors were narrowed down to the most informative. PRECARD's success in Denmark was in a very large measure due to the firm grasp that its principal investigator, Troels Thomsen, showed of the realities of clinical practice and the information needs (and IT skills!) of clinicians. Its success led to its adoption in other countries and, here too, Troels' foresight was shown. The program had been designed from the outset to be customized using different languages and different risk estimation functions.

Subsequently, the PRECARD package became the template for the European Heartscore package, which makes online risk estimation and risk factor management available to health professionals all over Europe. While the Heartscore system is a product of the input of many individuals, it still carries the hallmarks of Troels' design specification for PRECARD, which marked a giant step in bridging the gap between epidemiological modelling and clinical practice.

SIMPLIFICATION

The second strand involved simplifying the calculation process by replacing complex formulae with simple systems in which points were allocated for risk factor levels, then added up. The risk was read from a table that converted point scores into risk levels. While there were numerous attempts to develop such scoring systems, few made it to large-scale evaluation. One which did was the British Regional Heart Study score [20], but despite extensive work calibrating the score for the British population [21], this seems to have fallen into neglect. The approach continues to have its advocates, and as recently as 1998, the Framingham investigators published a risk estimation method based on point scores [22] and such a system was incorporated into an American Heart Association/American College of Cardiology (AHA/ACC) statement on assessment of risk, which published a table allocating points for risk factors and a small chart in which these were converted to absolute risk [23]. Stuart

Pocock and his colleagues have extended this risk assessment method in several useful ways. They published a risk score system for people with raised blood pressure [24] and, more recently, one for people with stable angina [25]. These have been based on analysis of patients enrolled in therapeutic trials, a data source which has been generally neglected in developing risk estimation methods.

Special mention must be made of GREAT (General Rule to Enable Atheroma Treatment) which is a simple treatment decision system which seems to work as well in practice as other more complex systems [26, 27]. I asked the developer, Tony Wierzbicki, how the algorithm had been developed, and he replied by email, that: *'It was thought up in a bar and written down based on clinical experience of what Tim Reynolds, Martin Crook and I do in clinical practice as we never use computers in outpatients.'* I find it heartening to note that, despite the countless hours of computer time that have been turned upon the problem, a couple of clinicians can work out on a beer mat a useful risk assessment system that performs just as well.

Despite the simplicity of these approaches, clinicians have proved reluctant to take out a pen and paper and calculate a risk score, however simple (perhaps because they, like everyone else, distrust their arithmetic skills). Their main drawback, however, is that only one calculation at a time can be done. To see the effects of risk factor change or of advancing age another calculation has to be done. While each calculation is short, the total time taken can increase greatly.

THE FIRST EUROPEAN TASK FORCE RISK CHART

PRECARD was still in the future when I was given the brief to design a simple risk estimation system for use with the First Joint Task Force guidelines on CHD prevention in clinical practice. (Troels and I met at an early planning meeting for the SCORE project and discussed how PRECARD and SCORE could develop harmoniously, and Troels was an active and influential member of the SCORE scientific committee.)

The system was to be based on a model which had just been published by Andy Avins of the Framingham group [28] which was powerful, accurate and flexible (it could be used for calculating risk at varying lengths of follow-up) but which was mathematically complex and well beyond the calculational skills (and patience) of a busy clinician.

Discussing the brief with members of the Task Force, it became clear that the system would have to be simple. I drew up a list of what I considered the criteria for a workable system:

- the patient's risk could be read instantly;
- no calculations whatsoever were involved;
- the effect of change in risk factors, including the effect of increasing age, could be seen without any recalculation;
- it did not require a computer;
- there was no instruction manual necessary;
- it could be reproduced by photocopying.

The original version of the chart met all of these criteria and displayed risk, in five categories, for 320 combinations of the 'classical' risk factors. It was indebted to the pioneering work done by Rodent Jackson and the New Zealand group [29], who had published a brilliantly simple chart, based on one of the many Framinghan risk functions, to be used in the management of hypertension. The chart was inspired by the principles of graphic design advocated by Edward Tufte [30, 31]. It was also shamelessly based on the layout of the original 14-page Framingham risk tabulation in Section 27 [14]. Although the chart was often reproduced at A4 size or larger, it was successfully reduced in size to fit on a snowscraper

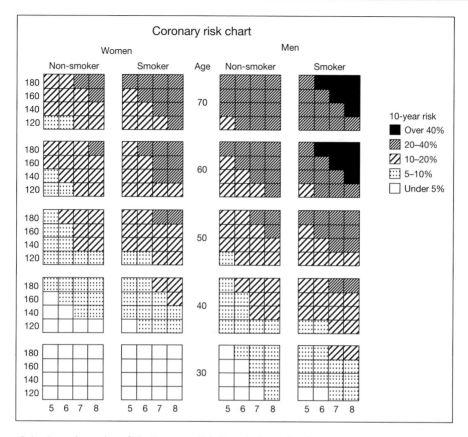

Figure 2.4 An early version of the European Risk Chart (redrawn for clarity).

by one enterprising pharmaceutical company. The original chart was monochrome, with shading indicating the level of risk. It could be photocopied badly and repeatedly and yet remain legible (I tested this by repeatedly faxing it to myself and then re-faxing the copies). It was, in short, designed to be user-friendly, robust low-technology. The chart was incorporated into the Task Force guidelines [32] and used as the basis for risk estimation and management. My original version is shown in Figure 2.4.

The chart was what Tufte calls a 'small multiple' [31] – a chart made up by repeating a smaller chart several times. The fact that age ascended and women were on the left while smokers were on the right meant that the whole chart showed a pattern of increasing risk from bottom left (young, non-smoking women) to top right (old smoking men) while each component cell echoed this pattern, with low cholesterol and low blood pressure at bottom left and high cholesterol and high blood pressure at top right. The chart showed, on a flat surface, data in seven dimensions: level of risk, gender, smoking, age, cholesterol and blood pressure. Adding colour to depict risk, with a 'traffic light' system running from deep green (low risk) through amber to dark red (high risk) reinforced the risk gradient dramatically, and made the chart take on a unified appearance.

The chart was used as the basis for coronary prevention guidelines in a number of countries in Europe. In the UK, however, the joint British guidelines were based on a rather elegant variant, which used curving lines to show the shape of the risk associations, rather than the rectangular boxes of the European chart [33]. The Sheffield group also developed a table which gave detailed risk estimation at 2-year age intervals in men and women [34] which they subsequently modified to bring it into line with recommended thresholds for clinical intervention [35]. However, the Sheffield chart scored poorly in user tests, with nurses using it less well than family doctors, and users preferring the simpler format of the New Zealand and Joint British charts [36, 37].

The second version of the European Risk Chart [38] which accompanied the Second Joint Task Force guidelines differed in the addition of an extra cholesterol category, bringing to 400 the number of risk factor combinations it displayed. Colour was now used as standard. However, the design company engaged by the Task Force added detailed instructions for use, extra text, duplicate axis labels, gridlines and tick marks, quadruplicated the conversion grid for cholesterol, transposed the risks for men and women and added pictorial symbols beside the words 'men' and 'women', festooning the chart with what Tufte refers to as chartjunk. These were removed in the SCORE risk chart, which, while continuing to use colour to depict risk, reverted to the more simple appearance of the original design. As a piece of trivia, I designed and produced the risk charts using AppleWorks. They are nothing but spreadsheets, with colour added.

THE SCORE PROJECT

Having designed a risk chart which was now being printed by the thousand, and that underpinned guidelines on CHD prevention which had been adopted by all European countries, I grew concerned that if the chart were wrong or misleading, errors in treatment were being committed all over Europe. The members of the Third Joint Task Force had similar concerns. The chart was, after all, based on data from the Framingham project. All the evidence suggested that it would overestimate risk in European countries where levels of risk in the population were lower than in Framingham, i.e., over a significant proportion of European countries. Furthermore, the Framingham group at the time of the publication of the original Task Force chart were continuing to use an idiosyncratic definition of acute coronary heart disease, which included unstable angina and new-onset stable angina. Few other cohort studies could reproduce this endpoint, so it was difficult to evaluate the fit of the Framingham function to European cohorts. And, finally, it was clear that a European risk function would have to be capable of being recalibrated for use in different European countries based on national data. This would include mortality statistics, but would not generally include significant data from cohort studies, especially in low-risk regions of Europe.

These issues were clearly articulated by a Spanish epidemiologist, Dr Susana Sans, who brought a proposal to the Board of the European Society of Cardiology that a European risk prediction system be developed. Under the leadership of Professor Ian Graham, the SCORE project was born. It was based on a pool of cohort studies from around Europe. It is not my intention to describe the project in detail, but to concentrate on the key decisions that were made in developing the SCORE risk assessment system.

KEY QUESTIONS IN DEVELOPING A RISK ASSESSMENT SYSTEM

The issues which arose in the course of the SCORE project can be discussed under four headings:

(1) Asking the right question.
(2) Finding the right data.
(3) Using the right statistical methods.
(4) Developing the system in the context of therapeutic guidelines.

ASKING THE RIGHT QUESTION

Statisticians talk about type 1 (false-positive) and type 2 (false-negative) errors. However, the most important error in science is the type 3 error – asking the wrong question.

By the time of the SCORE project, there was no shortage of risk estimation methods published. However, these still betrayed their epidemiological origins by being disease-specific. The clinical reality, however, is that the same factors which lead to the development of CHD also produce stroke. From the perspective of the clinician managing risk, as well as from the perspective of the patient, calculating risk of CHD in isolation misrepresents the total burden of risk. This is especially important in regions in which the rates of cardiovascular risk are low. In these regions, the proportion of all cardiovascular events accounted for by stroke is considerably higher than in regions at high cardiovascular risk, making the underestimation of total risk even more clinically significant [39–42].

The SCORE group, responding to the enthusiastic advocacy of Dr Susanna Sans, adopted total cardiovascular risk as the endpoint for estimation. This entailed some negotiation with the Third European Task Force, who were at the same time preparing their guidelines. However, the arguments for total risk were persuasive enough to win out [43–45]. We soon realized that health economic calculations would need total risk to be broken down into CHD risk and risk of other vascular events. As a solution, we made the original SCORE risk model a two-part formula, calculating each component of the risk separately before combining them.

Even so, the full impact of the cardiovascular risk factors is not adequately captured by limiting our attention to heart attack and stroke. They are also at the basis of the development of vascular dementias, which are one of the leading causes of disability in older age. Unfortunately, while this sort of endpoint is of great significance for those who provide healthcare – not just the medical profession but in society as a whole – it is hard to find sources of data which can be factored into risk estimation models.

THE RIGHT DATA

Availability of data

Any risk function applied to patient management should be capable of being tailored to fit the population to which the patient belongs. The variation in cardiovascular risk between countries is so significant that there is no value in a one-size-fits-all risk estimation system. While relative risks are stable across populations, absolute risks are not. Comparing the high-risk and low-risk regions of Europe, the difference between a Finn and an Italian with the same risk factor levels is equivalent to 4 mmol of cholesterol. It was clear from the outset that the SCORE system would have to be a European solution which was capable of responding to the diversity of the continent.

This requirement, however, was hard to fulfil in practice, and had a profound impact on the final risk estimation system. Though there are many cohort studies based on population samples from countries in which incidence of coronary disease is high, there are many fewer data from low-incidence regions. Initially, the SCORE project aimed to use only population studies, but we realised we would have to include occupational cohorts from low-risk regions to help to make good the shortfall of data. This lack of data from low-risk countries also acted as a warning signal. If SCORE was going to be capable of being adapted for use in any European country, it could not afford to rely exclusively on cohort study data. We had no data from many European countries simply because there were no cohort studies in these countries. Any risk estimation method that relied on using national cohort data would be useless in these countries. Any practical risk estimation system would have to be capable of being recalibrated using nationally-available data, which meant, in practice, mortality data.

The decision to base risk estimation on mortality data was a difficult one to sell to the European Task Force. They had grown used to the idea of managing risk based on risk of fatal and non-fatal events. However, the need to adapt risk estimation to national levels of risk was a deciding factor and, in the end, the Task Force agreed to switch to management recommendations based on risk of fatal events.

Clinically appropriate measurements: diabetes and acute CHD

Epidemiological datasets may be collected using protocols that are not the same as those used to collect clinical data. The use of different protocols for blood pressure measurement, for instance, may cause levels measured in epidemiological studies to differ from those read in a clinical setting [46]. More telling, however, is the case of diabetes. The original Task Force risk charts, based on the Framingham function, included a chart for persons with diabetes. The Framingham investigators wisely included a measure of impaired glucose tolerance in their data. However, for many cohort studies, including most of those available to the SCORE project, diabetes was measured by asking people if they had even been told by a doctor that they had any of a list of medical conditions. People simply ticked the ones they thought they had. Some of the studies which made up the SCORE database had followed up anyone who claimed to have diabetes and checked with their family doctor, which verified the cases, but, of course, did nothing about the many people who would have had diabetes unknown to themselves.

This left us with a problem: diabetes, as measured by a self-report question, is clearly not the same as clinically diagnosed diabetes. Many people with type 2 (late-onset) diabetes are unaware that they have it. Having a diagnosis of diabetes, as opposed to just having diabetes, may reflect the frequency with which the person visits the doctor, which, in turn, may reflect their general state of health. Women, who visit the doctor more often than men, will, or ought to have, higher detection rates. Taken together, this suggests that self-reported diabetes should carry a different prognosis to clinically-diagnosed diabetes, and that this effect might well be different in the two sexes. So when epidemiological studies model risk using self-reported diabetes, they are using the word in a very different sense to the clinician, and the fit between the two entities may be far from perfect.

There is a further problem with diabetes, which compounds the issue. Diabetes is actually two separately-defined syndromes: the American (ADA) definition, based on fasting blood sugar, and the World Health Organization (WHO) definition, based on a glucose tolerance test. Of the two, the WHO definition is associated with a worse prognosis [47], but the ADA definition is far more suited to screening in clinical practice. It can be made on the basis of a single fasting measurement. The WHO diagnosis requires the patient to wait for 2 hours following a glucose load, making it very impractical for widespread use. The two types of diabetes have similar prevalences, but there is a considerable non-overlap: some people meeting the ADA definition meet the WHO definition also, but a significant number do not [48, 49]. So even at the clinical level, there are two different definitions of diabetes, which are neither equivalent in terms of risk nor in terms of the people they identify. Adopting one definition or another has profound implications for clinical prevention. The ADA system is easy to integrate into opportunistic screening, while the WHO system is more informative about prognosis at the cost of being a cumbersome procedure. And, importantly, neither definition corresponds to the self-reported diabetes in many epidemiological studies.

Deciding on how to define diabetes and how to incorporate it into risk estimation is, clearly, an issue which goes well beyond statistics into the realms of health service planning. It underlines the importance of developing statistical risk estimation models hand-in-hand with the planning of clinical management of risk.

Another important mismatch between epidemiological and clinical practice concerned the definition of non-fatal events which was used by the Framingham investigators in their earlier functions. These functions included the ones which underlay the original European Task Force risk chart, as well as many other risk estimation systems. The original Framingham definition of non-fatal CHD [50] included non-fatal myocardial infarction, new-onset angina and 'coronary insufficiency'. This rather wide definition was useful in the early years of the study as it increased the number of endpoints in the data analysis. However, it is at variance with many epidemiological studies, which would not classify the onset of angina as an acute event, and, more importantly, with current clinical practice. The diagnosis of myocardial infarction has, of course, changed over the years with the avail-ability of more sensitive markers of myocardial necrosis, such as troponin T, making it no longer compatible with the definitions used in older epidemiological studies. But the addi-tion of new-onset angina had important consequences for the Framingham endpoint. Angina accounted for 41% of all events in men and 56% in women [51], making the Framingham definition of acute CHD not only different to the understanding that clini-cians would have of the term, but also different between men and women. It worried me that I had published a risk chart which estimated risk of fatal and non-fatal CHD when the diagnosis that it used was so much at variance with clinical practice. I would bet that most clinicians using it were unaware of this problem. A letter in the *BMJ* from a number of prominent British cardiovascular epidemiologists, pointing out the problem, seems to have fallen on deaf ears [52].

Of course, the Framingham investigators were aware of this problem also, and have sub-sequently published risk estimation methods based on a more conventional definition of acute CHD [17].

More and more risk factors – better and better risk estimation?

People used to come up to me gesticulating in exasperation, demanding to know why the SCORE risk chart did not include whatever their pet risk factor was. Lipidologists seem especially prone to becoming convinced that a proper assessment of risk cannot be carried out without measuring LLLs (lots of little lipoproteins). But their numbers are swelled by those who want risk assessment to include other risk factors too. These people can all point to epidemiological analyses that show that their pet risk factor is a 'significant independent risk predictor'. So why do we ignore all these vitally important factors?

The first reason is terribly simple: the risk chart shows five risk factors: age, sex, blood pressure, cholesterol and smoking. This results in a six-dimensional graph which still fits conveniently onto a smallish flat surface. There seems to be no way to include another risk factor while keeping the simplicity of the chart. I have experimented with all sorts of 'clever' design features (and I even threw the problem open to Edward Tufte's internet forum). The result has inevitably been a chart that was cumbersome and hard to read.

The second reason is just as important: statistically significant does not mean clinically important. Just because a factor is statistically associated with cardiovascular disease (CVD) does not mean that it will give a clinically significant improvement in the clinical perform-ance of a risk assessment system. And despite a lot of research into 'new' risk factors (which seems to cover anything from 1980 onwards) there is little evidence to demonstrate the clinical utility of including them in risk assessment.

Also, for each additional risk factor you include in the assessment process, the cost and complexity of screening goes up. Specialized laboratory facilities are needed. And, of course, you have to evaluate how well the risk assessment method works when all the risk factor information is not available, something that gets more and more likely the more risk factors that have to be measured.

The literature on patient compliance with medical treatment is clear on this point: com-pliance drops for every additional piece of complexity. Patients are more likely to take one 10 mg tablet than two 5 mg ones. For this reason, I have defended the simplest possible risk estimation. There is no point in having complex systems if we have great difficulty in getting even the simplest systems accepted in practice.

At this point, I feel, I have to say why there is a risk chart based on the HDL:cholesterol ratio, a thing that Sarah Lewington of the Oxford Prospective Studies Collaboration once described to me as 'not a risk factor but a nightmare'. The answer is because I was told that clinicians demanded it. I am not sure anyone ever uses it, and there are serious reasons for not doing so. The most important of these is that the evidence base for cardiovascular risk reduction is based on cholesterol, not HDL ratio. The therapeutic literature on cholesterol is largely based on trials which have recruited and treated patients on the basis of their total cholesterol. To me, it makes sense to assess risk using the risk factors that will be used to set therapeutic targets. But to a body of clinicians, nothing would do but that we make a parallel risk assessment system based on HDL ratio. We did so. It performs no better and no worse than the cholesterol-based one. That is to say, if you are going to have one measure of lipid level (and this is all you can have, given the physical limitations of the risk chart) then the HDL ratio does no better than total cholesterol. This is an important point, as it is not the same as saying that the HDL cholesterol does not add significant prognostic information to the information in total cholesterol.

The HDL ratio chart, after all the fuss, was greeted with utter silence. No-one has ever enquired about it, asked for the formula, asked to reproduce it. No-one seems to be using it. Sometimes you have to do exactly what the client wants in order to prove that it did not need doing.

If there is a shortcoming of the SCORE system that I regret, it is that it is an all-in-one method. It requires using all the risk factor information at once. I would like to see the development of a sequential method of risk assessment that begins with the things that people know about themselves: their age, sex, height, weight and smoking. This could be used to identify people in whom it would be beneficial to measure blood pressure, and this information could be used in turn to identify people in whom it would be beneficial to measure cholesterol and glucose. This sort of system could be used in health promotion campaigns aimed at the general public, and would act as a set of filters, triaging the population and allocating screening resources optimally.

No, there is no such system. But we do need one.

Single measurements versus clinical practice: regression dilution bias

Another major difference between epidemiological data and clinical data lies in the use of single measurements in epidemiology. The risk factor levels which are used to estimate subsequent risk in epidemiological models are collected at a single screening, while the practitioner typically has access to repeated measurements when she or he is contemplating risk factor intervention. No practitioner would classify a patient as mildly hypertensive on the basis of a single reading, and treatment of all but the highest levels of blood pressure requires repeatedly elevated readings over a period of weeks. Epidemiological studies can generally provide no analogous models based on multiple measurements.

This problem has given rise to an underestimation of the true strength of the relationship between risk factors and diseases, because of the effect of regression dilution bias [53–57]. Regression dilution bias occurs when a single measurement is a poor proxy for continual measurements. There are two factors which contribute to the problem: first, the presence of measurement error in the predictor variable will cause the strength of the relationship to be underestimated [58]. This problem has been long recognized in statistical modelling [59]. While modelling was concerned with testing hypotheses about relationships more than quantifying these relationships accurately, the problem was of incidental interest. However, as Tavia Gordon pointed out in a 1974 editorial [1], when linear models are used to estimate the risk of developing a disease, measurement error will have the effect of reducing the gradient of predicted risk.

More importantly, however, some risk factors vary over time in a way that is not easily predictable from a single measurement. A single reading of cholesterol is a good indicator of the previous and subsequent levels of cholesterol, but a single reading of blood pressure is a much poorer indication of the person's previous and subsequent blood pressure. For this reason, regression dilution bias affects the relationship of blood pressure to CVD more than the relationship of cholesterol.

Regression dilution bias therefore distorts the risk factor relationships which would be found using clinical data The epidemiological model is literally true: these are the risk factor relationships that you would find using a single set of risk factor measurements, but they misrepresent the strengths of the relationship and, in particular, under-represent the effect of potentially modifiable risk factors on risk. In the case of risk estimation, they cause us to overestimate the risk in those with below-average risk factor levels and to underestimate it in those above the mean.

One part of the analytic work of the SCORE project was directed towards investigating the effect of this 'flattening out' of the risk factor gradient on the risk estimation system which we were developing. To our relief, correcting for regression dilution bias, though theoretically important, turned out to have little practical significance for the construction of a risk evaluation system. The effect of correcting for the bias was to make risks that were already very low lower still, and risks that were very high became correspondingly higher. However, in the mid-range of risk, where the interest of the clinician would be focused, there was no visible difference to the risk chart when a regression dilution bias correction was introduced. (This makes sense when we remember that the effect of regression dilution bias will be to underestimate the effects of risk factors, thus shrinking the real range of risk associated with the risk factor.) In the end, we did not use a correction for regression dilution bias in the finally published risk estimation system, feeling that the extra complexity introduced would not affect individuals at or near intervention thresholds. In addition, there is some concern about the validity of applying regression dilution bias corrections to multivariate models, and at least one review [58] has come out against the practice.

I should, of course, point out that epidemiological studies were originally set up to document levels of disease and to identify risk factors, which they have done successfully. I am not criticizing the methods they adopted so much as pointing out that these methods lead to problems when epidemiological data are being used to generate clinical estimation models.

STATISTICAL METHODS

Risk estimation, almost since its inception, has been dominated by two models: logistic regression and Cox regression. Despite the development of many more complex models for dealing with data representing the occurrence of a disease over a follow-up period, logistic regression provides an excellent fit to a wide variety of medical datasets and, in comparative analyses, emerges as only slightly less powerful than complex (and computer-intensive) methods [60]. It has the additional advantage of transparency: the risk factor coefficients can be (and are best) expressed as odds ratios. Unlike methods such as piecewise regression, spline functions and neural networks, the risk model generated by logistic regression is an easily-explainable linear function. Though the logistic function is most commonly used in medicine, there are other models, such as the complementary log–log regression, which differ from logistic regression in the shape of the function which links the risk factors to the occurrence of the disease. Though none has shown a clear potential to replace logistic regression in cardiovascular risk modelling, it is also fair to say that epidemiologists have rarely tried to evaluate their usefulness.

The one drawback of the logistic model is that odds ratios are less easy to explain than relative risks. For this reason, generalized linear models for the binomial family are a useful alternative, since they are capable of estimating relative risks. There is, unfortunately, a drawback: they do not always produce a solution. While logistic regression cannot produce a risk estimate that falls outside the range of 0–1, the same is not true of binomial models. Where the outcome being modelled is relatively common, odds ratios can give a misleading impression to the casual reader, and binomial models are worth trying. In the case of CVD, the difference between odds ratios and relative risks is not usually large enough to worry about.

Cox regression, however, is the standard procedure used to construct risk estimation models, as it can be used when participants have been followed for a variable amount of time. The model is constructed in two parts: in the first, the survival function is calculated empirically (in other words, making no assumptions about its shape); in the second, the effect of change in risk factor levels on the survival function is calculated. There is a strong advantage in making no assumption about the shape of the survival function. Rather than having to be modelled explicitly, the survival function becomes, in effect, a complicated piece of calculation which will have to be got out of the way before the main business of model estimation.

This has made the Cox model popular in epidemiology. Epidemiologists are more concerned, typically, with measuring the effects of risk factors than with measuring the actual risk function. The reverse, however, is true in clinical practice. Therefore, it is clear that the effect of the risk factors is to vary the person's risk above or below the population risk, but variation in risk between populations is highly significant and has to be taken into account in any risk estimation system. As I pointed out earlier, comparing the high-risk and low-risk charts shows how small the effect of individual risk factors can be in comparison with the effects of the absolute risk in the population.

The Cox model, then, is a two-step process. First, it calculates the risk over the whole sample. Then it uses the individual risk factor information to calculate how much each risk factor modifies an individual's risk above or below the average. Research has tended to confirm that the second part of the model is 'portable' i.e., the effects of risk factors such as smoking and cholesterol on a person's risk are pretty constant from one setting to another. However, the first part of the model – the absolute risk – is not. There have been many papers looking at the performance of models derived in one population when applied to another population. The general conclusion is that models get the relative risk right, but can be very wrong about the absolute risk. In a seminal paper in 2001, D'Agostino showed how models could be 'tuned' to fit different populations using a process of recalibration [17].

With a Cox model, the first decision to be made concerns the time variable used in calculating the hazard function. Although epidemiologists have traditionally used time since initial risk factor measurement as the hazard variable, Ed Korn [61] proposed that using age has a number of significant advantages. For the development of risk estimation models, the most important of these is the ability to construct a hazard function over the entire range of observed ages, rather than being restricted to the length of available follow-up. This is the approach we adopted in the SCORE system, allowing us to use datasets in which follow-up was less than 10 years to build 10-year risk estimates. This greatly increased the amount of data available, and reduced the complexity of the model by having only a single term for age, rather than dividing it into time-on-study (incorporated into the hazard function) and time-before-study, modelled as a risk factor.

The second decision to be made when building a Cox model is which categorical risk factors to use as covariates and which are better represented as stratum variables. If the shape of the hazard function differs between groups, the variables are better treated as stratum variables. For these reasons, Cox regression is far from a turnkey estimation system. Our experience on the SCORE project was that differences in the shape of the hazard function between men and women resulted in significant estimation errors in women in their fifties, and we ended up estimating separate models for men and women, improving model fit appreciably. We were fortunate in having so many data; small studies rarely have enough endpoints among women, especially at younger ages, to estimate separate models for the two sexes.

Beyond Cox

Although the Cox model is overwhelmingly the most popular method for generating risk estimation models from data with varying lengths of follow-up, it is not the only possibility. The most frequent alternative to Cox models is the family of parametric survival models in which there is an explicit time variable – accelerated failure time models. Although many such models exist with differing shapes for the time function, the one which appears to fit cardiovascular data best is the Weibull model, a modified form of which was the basis for the original European Risk Chart. The advantage to the Weibull model is that estimates can be generated for any length of follow-up. This was put to good use by Keaven Anderson, who developed flexible models, based on Framingham data, which could be used to generate predictions for any length of time [62]. (Anderson's model was also the basis of the very first European Risk Chart.) This approach allowed the SCORE project to assess the goodness of fit of the Framingham function in databases with varying lengths of follow-up. The SCORE risk assessment system was based on a Weibull model, since this allows the hazard function to be calculated for any desired length of time. However, the subsequent adaptation of the SCORE system for use in individual countries has used the Cox model. We ran numerous Cox and Weibull models side by side and could find no material advantage of one over the other. The choice was based on expediency. Use of a Cox model allows national mortality data to be used to calculate an empirical hazard function, without the need to estimate a Weibull parameter, which would make the calculation slightly more complex and potentially more open to inaccuracy.

Data mining, neural networks and other complex models

In recent years, more complex mathematical approaches to estimation have become widespread in commercial application. The fundamental difference between these 'data mining' exercises and epidemiological data analysis is that epidemiology has traditionally been concerned with identifying the factors which cause diseases and with quantifying their effects. In business, on the other hand, the primary goal is correct estimation, rather than demonstration of a scientific theory. Data mining is well suited to the situation where there are many candidate predictors, most of which are uninformative or collinear, and no good previous research or theory that will help to winnow out a useful subset. Indeed, theories are often built *post hoc* on the basis of identification of predictive characteristics, rather than determining the characteristics which are used as predictors. These approaches may be divided into three main types, depending on the final model produced.

Neural network approaches use computer-intensive algorithms to develop a classification function which is frequently of considerable complexity. Predictor variables may recur frequently in the calculation, making it difficult to assess or express the significance of the variable in the final risk score. Typically, neural network algorithms require careful development if they are not to produce a function which perfectly reproduces the pattern of endpoints in the training dataset, but which cannot be generalized to new data. Unlike linear models, there is no formula which allows the model shrinkage to be calculated (shrinkage is the loss of predictive accuracy when the model is applied to a new dataset).

Clustering methods attempt to identify groups of patients who share a similar risk profile and a similar prognosis. This approach, generating groupings rather than placing patients on a continuum of risk, has an immediate clinical advantage. Conventional risk functions derived from logistic or Cox regression do not attempt to make clinically coherent groups. Patients whose risk falls over the 20% level on the European Risk Chart have diverse combinations of risk factors and ages. Using clustering methods, on the other hand, high-risk groups with distinctive clinical profiles can be identified, making it potentially easier to link the results of the risk assessment to recommendations about risk factor management. Clustering methods are surprisingly neglected in medicine in view of the excellent results reported from recent applications in the business sector.

Finally, *tree-structured methods* attempt to split the population repeatedly into subgroups on the basis of risk factors so as to yield prognostically homogenous subgroups. The difference between tree-structured methods and clustering methods is that clustering methods make use of all the information at once, while tree-structured methods can be developed to suggest the optimum order for measuring risk factors. For instance, some persons may be classifiable as low- or high-risk on the basis of a very small number of risk factors, allowing clinical management to be initiated rapidly with a minimum of extra testing, while others may require further measurements (such as fasting lipids or lipid fractions) in order to make an informed clinical decision on management. Tree-structured methods can be programmed to parallel the process of diagnosis and management, with additional tests being ordered only for those patients in whom the result would throw valuable light on their management. Since epidemiological models tend to use all available factors, their use in clinical practice may result in unnecessary testing and delay.

All of these methods, however, have shown their greatest potential in areas in which the amount of potential predictor variables is very large and traditional methods for selecting the most useful candidate predictors (such as stepwise methods) are fraught with statistical problems.

These computer-intensive methods suffer from the problem of model shrinkage. When the model is applied to a new population, the predictive ability declines sharply. For stepwise methods, this shrinkage is proportional not to the number of variables in the model, but to the number of candidate variables that were examined. For other approaches, numerous algorithms for model validation which are aimed at reducing model shrinkage have been developed. It is fair to say, however, that these models have not resulted in any useful applications when applied to epidemiological datasets. Typically, epidemiological datasets are made up of small numbers of measurements, and so the main advantage of these methods – their ability to wade through many uninformative predictors – is lost. While there have been some interesting developments in risk assessment based on neural network models, these models often require the availability of specialized lipid assessments, making them impractical for many clinicians. More important, their ability to transfer to different settings remains unproven. And, to make matters worse, there does not seem to be a simple, clinically realistic way of implementing them in practice.

The SCORE project evaluated a number of statistical approaches. We were reassured, in the process, that all yielded very similar results. Cardiovascular risk is well-behaved enough to be capable of being modelled well using a variety of models, and none of the more arcane approaches we tried resulted in a significant improvement in model fit, or, indeed, significantly different model estimates. The choice of model, we concluded, was more a pragmatic one than a statistical one.

Sparse data

One further statistical problem arises when models from epidemiological data are applied to patient management. Examination of the SCORE Risk Chart shows risks tabulated for risk factor combinations which are so rare in (or entirely absent from) both the cohort studies and the population that they represent extrapolation of the risk function beyond the data space in which it was calculated. This has unfortunate repercussions for calculation of risk in people with unusual risk factor combinations, but also in the extension of risk functions to estimate risk in younger persons. The original European Risk Chart contained risk estimates for persons aged 30. The shapes of the statistical functions used in calculating these risk scores inevitably result in the overestimation of risk at the extreme low end of the observed distribution of the data, a phenomenon which was commented upon regularly by the pioneers in the field [1] but which has been mentioned less frequently, if at all, in more recent publications. When a function is extended beyond the range of the data, as happened when the Framingham function was used to calculate risk for 30-year-olds, the estimates will be considerably higher than they ought to be.

Following publication of the original risk chart, quite a number of people pointed out to us in private correspondence that the CHD rate for persons aged 30 is so small that the risks portrayed in the original European Risk Chart must surely have been wrong. Hugh Tunstall-Pedoe, in a personal communication, compared the UK national death rates for persons aged 30–40 with the estimates of CHD risk in the chart and came to the same conclusion. He expanded these observations in a subsequent paper [63]. Based on the SCORE databases, we found that these fears were justified. The risk of fatal CHD in women aged under 35 is never higher than 1 event per 10 000 person-years and the risk in men never higher than 5 events per 10 000 person-years. Although the associations between cholesterol, blood pressure and smoking are clear in young people, use of extrapolation to estimate absolute risk results in nonsensical estimates.

It was Dirk de Bacquer, a member of the SCORE steering group, who pointed out that the original risk chart wasted space on risk estimates for young people, in whom risk was universally low and, as I have just admitted, estimated very badly wrong, and on older people, in whom risk was almost universally high. We should be concentrating, he said, on the intermediate age range: 40 to 65, with a closer age spacing. In this age range, risk is changing rapidly with age, and it is here that the chart can be of most value. Once said, this was obvious, and we acted on it. This removed the embarrassment of the nonsense risk estimates for the 30-somethings, and provided more clinically useful information for the ages at which cardiovascular disease prevention becomes clinically important.

Assessment of goodness of fit
Epidemiological risk models have traditionally been concerned with establishing rates of disease, identifying risk factors and exploring differences between groups of people. Their application to the estimation of risk in the individual, however, is by no means automatic. One drawback of models which estimate risk of events based on characteristics is that there is no simple, direct test of goodness of fit. A person either will or will not have a coronary event, so the model estimation is either right or wrong at the level of the individual. One solution has been to divide the sample into deciles on the basis of predicted probability of experiencing an event and to examine the relationship between the number of events predicted and observed, a procedure known as a Hosmer-Lemeshow Chi-squared test. This can be used to identify badly fitting models, but of itself does not indicate a useful model. A good model also has to show a sharp gradient of increasing risk with increasing predicted risk. The ability of the risk score to discriminate high-risk from low-risk groups is often assessed by comparing the rates in the first and fifth quintiles of risk.

In parallel with the realization among epidemiologists that estimation models, to be useful, will have to concentrate on correct allocation of patients to treatments has come a swing from the use of significance testing as the basis for model construction to the use of classification statistics. The most frequently used of these is the area under the receiver operator characteristic (ROC) curve. This shows the relationship between the sensitivity of the risk estimation system and its specificity. The area under the ROC curve has a simple and intuitive interpretation, which is the probability that a person who later develops CHD will have a higher score than a person who does not. More recently, Avins [28] has proposed a modification to the conventional presentation of the ROC curve to show the relationship between positive and negative predictive value, which is more appropriate when the feature to be optimized is the correct estimation of the risk assessment system when a threshold score is used as the basis for a decision to intervene or not. An equivalent statistic, C, which could be used with survival models was proposed by Harrell, and developed by D'Agostino [64].

However, there is no single mathematical criterion for diagnostic utility; test performance may be assessed using sensitivity, specificity, positive and negative predictive values, and positive and negative likelihood ratios. Each index reflects a different aspect of the performance of the test. Since the use of risk assessment will entail allocating interventions, we may expect these systems to be assessed increasingly on the basis of the proportion of the population who will receive intervention, the type of intervention they will receive, the costs of the intervention and the likely health benefits if the interventions are delivered. Clearly, these evaluation exercises are complex and will require epidemiologists and statisticians to work closely with clinicians and economists. Equally clearly, they are real-life measures of model performance rather than simple mathematical indices.

The central obstacle to defining goodness of fit of an estimation model is the variety of uses to which the model can be put. Assessing goodness of fit, in the statistical sense, is less important than assessing fitness for purpose in the real-life sense. Without knowing the purpose of the model, its fitness for this purpose cannot be calculated. In the case of the risk function used in the current European Task Force Risk Chart, treatment is based on a threshold of 5% predicted risk of fatal CVD. The chart must therefore be assessed primarily as a diagnostic tool, and its errors quantified in terms of false negatives and false positives: persons who experience subsequent CVD but fall below the treatment threshold and persons above the threshold who do not subsequently experience CVD. Since the purpose of diagnosis is the correct allocation of treatments to patients, the utility of a diagnostic tool is primarily in its ability either to identify those who will benefit from treatment or to identify those in whom treatment is unnecessary. Misestimation of risk is of less consequence than misapplication of treatment. It matters little if a person whose risk is estimated at 25% has actually got a 35% risk – they will receive treatment in any event; and likewise a person whose risk is estimated at 1% while it is actually 10% will not receive treatment. The whole crux of model performance is its performance in the region around the cutpoint for clinical intervention.

Clearly, defining the cutoff point which ought to be used for clinical intervention is not simply a statistical issue. This will be a product of the healthcare resources available, the competing health needs in the population and opportunity costs of interventions, and the proportion of the population who will require treatment as a result of the adoption of a specific cutpoint. This latter criterion once again exposes the weakness of the use of a cutpoint derived from a multivariate model as a threshold for intervention; depending on the risk factor profile of the section of the population above the intervention threshold, the implications for healthcare may vary widely. Evaluating the utility of a cutpoint purely by means of positive and negative predictive value ignores the interventionary purpose of risk evaluation. Persons whose high risk derives from unmodifiable risk factors such as previous CHD, diabetes and age may give a risk function a high positive predictive value without giving it a high clinical utility. For this reason, it is important to evaluate risk functions primarily on those whose risk is most dependent on modifiable risk factors: younger persons without previous CHD or diabetes.

This sort of health economic and health service planning evaluation is not a trivial task, but as CVD prevention accounts for a significant and rising component of healthcare costs, it is an exercise that will become more and more important.

RELATIONSHIP WITH THERAPEUTIC GUIDELINES

It should be clear by now that the SCORE risk assessment system was developed hand-in-hand with the development of the guidelines of the Third Joint Task Force, in the same way that in the US the ATP III guidelines were linked to a newly-developed Framingham risk function which, for the first time, used coronary disease endpoints comparable with those used in treatment trials [17]. The use of SCORE as the risk estimation system is continued in the Fourth European Joint Task Force guidelines [65]. This linkage is important for several reasons. First, it ensures a risk assessment system which fits with the guidelines, but second it made sure that the guidelines were based on good epidemiology as well as good clinical practice. The decision of the SCORE group not to produce a separate chart for diabetics, for example, was one that was taken only after a lot of debate, some of which I have already described. One additional clinical consideration in this decision was the fact that once diabetes is diagnosed, the clinical management and prognosis will depend on factors which are not available in epidemiological data, such as measures of diabetic control. It seemed to be confusing at best, and unethical at worst, to try to develop a system which ignored this vital and routinely available clinical data, which had already been integrated into specific risk assessment systems such as the UKPDS system [66].

The central lesson which emerged from the SCORE project was that statistical modelling of risk is capable of producing an almost unlimited number of useless models. Useless not because they are wrong, but because they are not what is needed. The task of understanding the needs of the clinician is the first step in model building, and provides the ultimate test of model utility. Without this, we risk doing better and better something that we are simply doing wrong.

ACKNOWLEDGMENTS

I have spent many entertaining hours in the company of colleagues, whose ideas, reminiscences and whimsies have made their way into this chapter. I would like to record my indebtedness to my friend and mentor, Prof. Kalevi Pyörälä, whose compelling vision of a unified, concerted and evidence-based European approach to cardiovascular risk management underpinned the development of the SCORE project.

This chapter has benefited from the reminiscences of Prof. Dan McGee of the Medical University of South Carolina, and from the encyclopaedic knowledge of Prof. Ralph D'Agostino, to both of whom I owe a debt of gratitude.

The SCORE project was supported by a EU Concerted Action grant under the Biomed programme, contract number BMH4-CT98-3186. More recent developments are being supported by a grant from the Irish Heart Foundation.

The SCORE project is guided by a scientific committee, and is the product of their dedication, enthusiasm and interactive input. Its members are:

SCORE Project Leader: Prof. Ian M. Graham
Chairman of the Scientific Committee: Prof. Kalevi Pyörälä
Principal Investigator: Dr Ronán Conroy
Scientific Committee: Prof. Kalevi Pyörälä, Prof. Ian M. Graham, Prof. Ulrich Keil, Prof. Alessandro Menotti, Prof. Lars Wilhelmsen, Prof. David Wood, Dr Troels Thomsen, Dr Ronán Conroy and Ms Jane Ingham.

The project would not have been possible without the generosity of the partners who contributed both their data and their considerable intellectual input. The partners are: Prof. Guy de Backer, Dr Dirk De Bacquer, Dr Troels Thomsen, Dr Michael Davidsen, Dr Knut Borch Johnsen, Prof. Kalevi Pyörälä, Prof. Jaakko Tuomilehto, Prof. Erkki Vartiainen, Prof. Pekka Jousilahti, Dr Pierre Duciemetière, Prof. Ulrich Keil, Dr Paul Cullen, Dr Helmut Schulte, Prof. Ian M. Graham, Dr Ronán Conroy, Dr Tony Fitzgerald, Prof. Leslie Daly, Prof. Alessandro Menotti, Prof. Daan Kromhout, Dr Inger Njolstad, Dr Aage Tverdal, Dr Randi Selmer, Prof. David Nebieridze, Dr Susana Sans, Prof. Hans Wedel, Prof. Lars Wilhelmsen, Prof. David Wood, Prof. Michael Marmot, Prof. Shah Ebrahim, Prof. Hugh Tunstall-Pedoe, Prof. Philip Poole-Wilson, Ms Jane Ingham, Prof. Peter Whincup, Dr Goya Wannamethee and Dr Mary Walker.

REFERENCES

1. Gordon T. Hazards in the use of the logistic function with special reference to data from prospective cardiovascular studies. *J Chronic Dis* 1974; 27:97–102.
2. Topol EJ, Lauer MS. The rudimentary phase of personalized medicine: coronary risk scores. *Lancet* 2003; 362:1776–1777.
3. Conroy RM, Pyörälä K, Fitzgerald AP *et al.* Estimation of ten-year risk of fatal cardiovascular disease in Europe: the SCORE project. *Eur Heart J* 2003; 24:987–1003.
4. Dawber TR, Kannel WB, Friedman GD. The use of computers in cardiovascular epidemiology. *Prog Cardiovasc Dis* 1963; 5:406–417.
5. Dawber TR, Meadors GF, Moore FE. Epidemiological approaches to heart disease: the Framingham Study. *Am J Public Health* 1951; 41:279–286.
6. Kannel WB, Dawber T, Kagan A, Revotskie N, Stokes J. Factors of risk in the development of coronary heart disease – six-year follow-up experience. *Ann Intern Med* 1961; 55:33–50.
7. Cornfield J. Joint dependence of risk of coronary heart disease on serum cholesterol and systolic blood pressure: a discriminant function analysis. *Fed Proc* 1962; 21:58–61.
8. Truett J, Cornfield J, Kannel WB. A multivariate analysis of the risk of coronary heart disease in Framingham. *J Chronic Dis* 1967; 20:511–524.
9. Keys A, Aravanis C, Blackburn H *et al.* Probability of middle-aged men developing coronary heart disease in five years. *Circulation* 1972; 45:815–828.
10. Wilhelmsen L, Wedel H, Tibblin G. Multivariate analysis of risk factors for coronary heart disease. *Circulation* 1973; 48:950–958.
11. Menotti A, Corradini P, Capocaccia R, Farchi G, Mariotti S, Puddu V. The prediction of coronary heart disease. A mathematical model applied to Italian field studies (authors transl). [Italian]. *G Ital Cardiol* 1975; 5:843–849.
12. Kannel W, McGee D, Gordon T. A general cardiovascular risk profile: The Framingham Study. *Am J Cardiol* 1976; 38:46–51.
13. Gordon T, Kannel WB. Multiple risk functions for predicting coronary heart disease: the concept, accuracy and application. *Am Heart J* 1982; 103:1031–1039.
14. Kannel WB, Gordon T. The Framingham Study: an epidemiological investigation of cardiovascular disease. In: Gordon T, Sorlie P, Kannel WB (eds). *Section 27. Coronary Heart Disease, Atherosclerotic Brain Infarction, Intermittent Claudication – A Multivariate Analysis of Some Factors Related to their Incidence: Framingham Study, 16-year followup.* US Government Printing Office, Washington DC, 1971.
15. Tunstall-Pedoe H. The Dundee coronary risk-disk for management of change in risk factors. *BMJ* 1991; 303:744–747.
16. Tunstall-Pedoe H. Value of the Dundee coronary risk-disk: a defence. *BMJ* 1992; 395:231–232.
17. D'Agostino RB, Grundy S, Sullivan LM, Wilson P. CHD Risk Prediction Group. Validation of the Framingham coronary heart disease prediction scores: results of a multiple ethnic groups investigation. *JAMA* 2001; 286:180–187.
18. Thomsen TF, Davidsen M, Jorgensen HIT, Jensen G, Borch-Johnsen K. A new method for CHD prediction and prevention based on regional risk scores and randomized clinical trials; PRECARD and the Copenhagen Risk Score. *J Cardiovasc Risk* 2001; 8:291–297.
19. Bonnevie L, Thomsen T, Jørgensen T. The use of computerized decision support systems in preventive cardiology – principal results from the national PRECARD survey in Denmark. *Eur J Cardiovasc Prev Rehabil* 2005; 12:52–55.
20. Shaper AG, Pocock SJ, Phillips AN, Walker M. A scoring system to identify men at high risk of a heart attack. *Health Trends* 1987; 19:37–39.
21. Thompson SG, Pyke SD, Wood DA. Using a coronary risk score for screening and intervention in general practice. British Family Heart Study. *J Cardiovasc Risk* 1996; 3:301–306.
22. Wilson PF, D'Agostino RB, Levy D, Belanger AM, Silbershatz H, Kannel WB. Prediction of coronary heart disease using risk factor categories. *Circulation* 1998; 97:1837–1847.
23. Grundy SM, Pasternak R, Greenland P, Smith SJ, Fuster V. Assessment of cardiovascular risk by use of multiple-risk-factor assessment equations: a statement for healthcare professionals from the American Heart Association and the American College of Cardiology [Review] [115 refs]. *Circulation* 1999; 100:1481–1492.
24. Pocock SJ, McCormack V, Gueyffier F, Boutitie F, Fagard RH, Boissel JP. A score for predicting risk of death from cardiovascular disease in adults with raised blood pressure, based on individual patient data from randomised controlled trials. *BMJ* 2001; 323:75–81.

25. Clayton TC, Lubsen J, Pocock SJ et al. Risk score for predicting death, myocardial infarction, and stroke in patients with stable angina, based on a large randomized trial cohort of patients. BMJ 2005; 331:869–872.

26. Wierzbicki AS, Reynolds TM, Gill K, Alg S, Crook MA. A comparison of algorithms for initiation of lipid lowering therapy in primary prevention of coronary heart disease. J Cardiovasc Risk 2000; 7:63–71.

27. Reynolds TM, Twomey PJ, Wierzbicki AS. Concordance evaluation of coronary risk scores: implications for cardiovascular risk screening. Curr Med Res Opin 2004; 20:811–818.

28. Avins AL, Browner WS. Improving the prediction of coronary heart disease to aid in the management of high cholesterol levels: what a difference a decade makes. JAMA 1998; 279:445–449.

29. Jackson R, Barham P, Bills J et al. Management of raised blood pressure in New Zealand: a discussion document. BMJ 1993; 307:107–110.

30. Tufte ER. The Visual Display of Quantitative Information. Graphics Press, Cheshire, Connecticut, 1983.

31. Tufte ER. Envisioning Information. Graphics Press, Cheshire, Connecticut, 1990.

32. Pyörälä K, de Backer G, Graham I, Poole-Wilson P, Wood D. Prevention of coronary heart disease in clinical practice. Recommendations of the Task Force of the European Society of Cardiology, European Atherosclerosis Society and European Society of Hypertension. Eur Heart J 1994; 15:1300–1331.

33. Anonymous. Joint British recommendations on prevention of coronary heart disease in clinical practice: summary. British Cardiac Society, British Hyperlipidaemia Association, British Hypertension Society, British Diabetic Association. BMJ 2000; 320:705–708.

34. Haq IU, Jackson PR, Yeo WW, Ramsay LE. Sheffield risk and treatment table for cholesterol lowering for primary prevention of coronary heart disease. Lancet 1995; 346:1467–1471.

35. Wallis EJ, Ramsay LE, Ul Haq I et al. Coronary and cardiovascular risk estimation for primary prevention: validation of a new Sheffield table in the 1995 Scottish health survey population [published erratum appears in BMJ 2000; 320:1034]. BMJ 2000; 320:671–676.

36. Isles CG, Ritchie LD, Murchie P, Norrie J. Risk assessment in primary prevention of coronary heart disease: randomized comparison of three scoring methods. BMJ 2000; 320:690–691.

37. Jones AF, Walker J, Jewkes C et al. Comparative accuracy of cardiovascular risk prediction methods in primary care patients. Heart 2001; 85:37–43.

38. Wood D, de Backer G, Faergeman O, Graham I, Mancia G, Pyörälä K. Prevention of coronary heart disease in clinical practice: recommendations of the Second Joint Task Force of European and other Societies on Coronary Prevention. Atherosclerosis 1998; 140:199–270.

39. Ramos R, Solanas P, Cordón F et al. Comparison of population coronary heart disease risk estimated by the Framingham original and REGICOR calibrated functions. Med Clin (Barc) 2003; 121:521–526.

40. Marrugat J, D'Agostino R, Sullivan L et al. An adaptation of the Framingham coronary heart disease risk function to European Mediterranean areas. J Epidemiol Community Health 2003; 57:634–638.

41. Menotti A, Puddu PE, Lanti M. Comparison of the Framingham risk function-based coronary chart with risk function from an Italian population study. Eur Heart J 2000; 21:365–370.

42. Kent DM, Griffith J. The Framingham scores overestimated the risk for coronary heart disease in Japanese, Hispanic, and Native American cohorts. ACP J Club 2002; 136:36.

43. De Backer G, Ambrosioni E, Borch-Johnsen K et al. European guidelines on cardiovascular disease prevention in clinical practice. Third Joint Task Force of European and other Societies on Cardiovascular Disease Prevention in Clinical Practice (constituted by representatives of eight societies and by invited experts). Atherosclerosis 2004; 173:381–391.

44. De Backer G, Ambrosioni E, Borch-Johnsen K et al. European guidelines on cardiovascular disease prevention in clinical practice: third joint task force of European and other societies on cardiovascular disease prevention in clinical practice (constituted by representatives of eight societies and by invited experts). Eur J Cardiovasc Prev Rehabil 2003; 10:S1–S10.

45. De Backer G, Ambrosioni E, Borch-Johnsen K et al. European guidelines on cardiovascular disease prevention in clinical practice. Third Joint Task Force of European and Other Societies on Cardiovascular Disease Prevention in Clinical Practice. Eur Heart J 2003; 24:1601–1610.

46. Conroy RM, O'Brien E, O'Malley K, Atkins N. Measurement error in the Hawksley random zero sphygmomanometer: what damage has been done and what can we learn? BMJ 1993; 306:1319–1322.

47. Qiao Q, Pyörälä K, Pyörälä M et al. Two-hour glucose is a better risk predictor for incident coronary heart disease and cardiovascular mortality than fasting glucose. Eur Heart J 2002; 23:1267–1275.

48. Qiao Q, Nakagami T, Tuomilehto J et al. Comparison of the fasting and the 2-h glucose criteria for diabetes in different Asian cohorts. Diabetologia 2000; 43:1470–1475.

49. Anonymous (The DECODE Study Group). Is fasting glucose sufficient to define diabetes? Epidemiological data from 20 European studies. European Diabetes Epidemiology Group. Diabetes epidemiology: collaborative analysis of Diagnostic Criteria in Europe. Diabetologia 1999; 42:647–654.

50. Dawber TR, Kannel W, Revotskie N, Kagan A. The epidemiology of coronary heart disease – the Framingham Enquiry. *Proc R Soc Med* 1962; 55:265–271.

51. D'Agostino RB, Russell MW, Huse DM *et al*. Primary and subsequent coronary risk appraisal: new results from the Framingham study. *Am Heart J* 2000; 139:272–281.

52. Lampe FC, Walker M, Shaper AG, Brindle PM, Whincup PH, Ebrahim S. End points for predicting coronary risk must be clarified. *BMJ* 2001; 323:396–397.

53. Lewington S, Thomsen T, Davidsen M, Sherliker P, Clarke R. Regression dilution bias in blood total and high-density lipoprotein cholesterol and blood pressure in the Glostrup and Framingham prospective studies. *J Cardiovasc Risk* 2003; 10:143–148.

54. Jousilahti P, Vartiainen E, Korhonen HJ, Puska P, Tuomilehto J. Is the effect of smoking on the risk for coronary heart disease even stronger than was previously thought? *J Cardiovasc Risk* 1999; 6:293–298.

55. Clarke R, Shipley M, Lewington S *et al*. Underestimation of risk associations due to regression dilution in long-term follow-up of prospective studies. *Am J Epidemiol* 1999; 150:341–353.

56. Verschuren WM, Jacobs DR, Bloemberg BP *et al*. Serum total cholesterol and long-term coronary heart disease mortality in different cultures. Twenty-five-year follow-up of the seven countries study. *JAMA* 1995; 274:131–136.

57. MacMahon S, Peto R, Cutler J *et al*. Blood pressure, stroke, and coronary heart disease. Part 1, Prolonged differences in blood pressure: prospective observational studies corrected for the regression dilution bias. *Lancet* 1990; 335:765–774.

58. Knuiman MW, Divitini ML, Buzas JS, Fitzgerald PE. Adjustment for regression dilution in epidemiological regression analyses. *Ann Epidemiol* 1998; 8:56–63.

59. McNemar Q. *Psychological Statistics*. Wiley, New York, 1949.

60. Lim T-S, Loh W-Y. A comparison of prediction accuracy, complexity and training time of thirty-three old and new classification algorithms. *Mach Learn* 2000; 40:203–229.

61. Korn EL, Graubard BI, Midthune D. Time-to-event analysis of longitudinal follow-up of a survey: choice of the time-scale. *Am J Epidemiol* 1997; 145:72–80.

62. Anderson KM, Odell PM, Wilson PW, Kannel WB. Cardiovascular disease risk profiles. *Am Heart J* 1991; 121:293–298.

63. Tunstall-Pedoe H. How cardiovascular risk varies with age, sex and coronary risk factors: do standard risk scores give an accurate prospective? *Eur Heart J Suppl* 1999; 1(suppl D):D25–D31.

64. Pencina MJ, D'Agostino RB. Overall C as a measure of discrimination in survival analysis: model specific population value and confidence interval estimation. *Stat Med* 2004; 23:2109–2123.

65. Graham I, Atar D, Borch-Johnsen K *et al*., Fourth Joint Task Force of the European Society of Cardiology and other Societies on Cardiovascular Disease Prevention in Clinical Practice. European Guidelines on Cardiovascular Disease Prevention in Clinical Practice. *Eur J Cardiovasc Prev Rehabil* 2007; 14(suppl 2):S1–S113.

66. Stevens RJ, Kothari V, Adler AI, Stratton IM. The UKPDS risk engine: a model for the risk of coronary heart disease in Type II diabetes (UKPDS 56). *Clin Sci (Lond)* 2001; 101:671–679.

3

Endpoints, mortality and morbidity

C. McGorrian, T. Leong, I. M. Graham

INTRODUCTION

The term 'endpoint' is used to describe the event of a disease manifestation in epidemiological studies and trials. An endpoint may be unequivocal, or 'hard', such as death; or subjective or 'soft', such as ill-defined chest pain. An intermediate endpoint would be myocardial infarction (MI) defined on the basis of pre-defined criteria.

The definition of endpoints is of paramount importance to both cardiovascular risk estimation, where we need to know what exactly is being predicted and why, and in the evaluation of therapies. For example, in the recent trials in lipid-lowering therapy, a number have shown impressive reductions in composite endpoints, but with no discernible impact on mortality rates. Other theraputic trials (of heart failure and dysrhythmias) showed improvements in soft endpoints but a substantial increase in the much more important endpoint of mortality.

The need to clearly define endpoints has been a learning process that has exercised the intellect of those responsible for the inception and design of cohort studies such as the Seven Countries Study [1], the Framingham Study [2] and the MONitoring trends and determinants in CArdiovascular disease (MONICA) study [3], as well as intervention studies such as the Multiple Risk Factor Intervention Trial (MRFIT) [4] and multiple subsequent drug trials. Some, such as the Seven Countries Study and MONICA, had to deal with cultural, language and ethnic differences. The Systematic Coronary Risk Estimation (SCORE) project [5] has had to try to find common ground in terms of endpoint definition between its 12 constituent cohorts. As treatments in cardiology become ever more efficacious, therapeutic trialists have been faced with diminishing returns as major new therapeutic benefits become less likely. The result is a demand for ever larger multicentre studies to demonstrate ever smaller therapeutic improvements, and a temptation to describe a reduction in softer endpoints as proof of benefit. These studies often span continents, and recruit and randomize many thousands of subjects. In investments of time, money and effort of this magnitude, it is imperative that the research question is answered clearly and appropriately – but this is not always so.

Little wonder that health professionals become confused and overwhelmed by the myriad studies and trials. The practising clinician needs answers to the following questions:

▥ If I wish to advise a person as to their risk of cardiovascular disease, can I reliably predict the mix of total mortality, cardiovascular mortality, or a non-fatal event for that individual?

Catherine McGorrian, MRCPI, Senior Research Fellow, Department of Cardiology, The Adelaide and Meath Hospital, Dublin, Ireland

Tora Leong, MB, MRCPI, Senior Reseach Fellow, Department of Cardiology, The Adelaide and Meath Hospital, Dublin, Ireland

Ian M. Graham, FRCPI, FESC, Consultant Cardiologist; Professor of Cardiovascular Medicine, Trinity College, Dublin; Professor of Preventive Cardiology, Royal College of Surgeons in Ireland

▓ Are the results of therapeutic trials valid (i.e. true) and applicable (i.e. related to the kinds of people I see in my own day-to-day practice)?
▓ Can I clearly explain the risks and benefits accruing to my patient from the treatment I want to prescribe?

None of these questions can be adequately assessed unless the studies concerned define clearly the endpoint(s) under consideration.

This chapter will examine the problems and usefulness of hard and soft endpoints such as mortality and morbidity in cardiovascular studies, and comment on the appropriateness of composite endpoints.

DEATH AS AN ENDPOINT

Hard endpoints give a study 'real world' validity and reproducibility. All-cause mortality is a hard endpoint that is clearly easy to define, and ascertainment of mortality rates is straightforward in most countries. It is when we come to subdivide all-cause mortality into different causes of death that we experience some problems. Cause of death is usually taken from data from the death certificate, and these death certificates are often filled out by doctors who have received little or no tuition in how to complete them, and who may not have had much knowledge of the patient's final illness. One study revealed that in a review of 50 death certificates, 34% had a serious error reporting the wrong cause or manner of death [6]. Another study found that general practitioners and pathologists were most accurate at filling out death certificates [7]. In everyday hospital practice, the more junior doctors, who have a weaker understanding of disease processes, may have less knowledge of the patient, and may not attribute much importance to the death certification, are the ones who fill out these forms.

Declining autopsy rates mean that modern clinicians have little chance to correlate their diagnosis of cause of death with actual pathological findings, so that some death certification must be at best an educated guess. Attems and colleagues correlated autopsy results and clinical diagnosis in 1594 geriatric patients, and found very poor levels of accuracy in the clinical diagnoses, including only 56% accuracy in those who had autopsy-proven cardiovascular death [8]. Death certification is an area of medical practice where feedback is not yet routine.

Use of the International Classification of Diseases (ICD) coding system has helped to ensure that hospital records and death certifications have a single, worldwide coding system for events. The ICD was most recently updated in 1989, and this ICD-10 classification came into use in the World Health Organization (WHO) member states in 1994. ICD-10 has significantly more codes than ICD-9 (12 420 codes, in place of 6969 in ICD-9), allowing for better specificity in coding. The format of the codes has also been changed, to provide a more flexible structure for further revisions. Indeed, yearly revisions are produced, so the ICD system can be seen as a coding method that is able to change to deal with changes in diseases and changes in data collection systems.

Changing from ICD-9 to ICD-10 has, however, added a complication to cohort studies that are collecting follow-up data spanning both systems. The codes for ICD-9 cannot be directly converted to ICD-10: there have been changes, particularly in the classification for cardiac death and so-called 'sudden cardiac death'. Changes in endpoints like these may adversely affect the validity of outcome data. Furthermore, ICD coding in developing nations such as those of Sub-Saharan Africa is not uniform. It is in these countries that accurate morbidity and mortality figures would be most useful. An appropriate goal for the WHO would be to support rollout of ICD coding in these developing nations, to foster morbidity and mortality reporting where mortality from cardiovascular causes is changing rapidly.

However, although the use of death certificates and hospital ICD coding has its flaws, it nevertheless provides an accessible and theoretically reproducible source of follow-up data, particularly for those studies which are not industry funded, and in countries or studies where resources are tight. To these, one can quote Major Greenwood: *'The scientific purist, who will wait for medical statistics until they are nosologically exact, is no wiser than Horace's rustic waiting for the river to flow away'* [9].

Thus, endpoint data from cohort studies using death certification notices are open to more biases than data that are collected and validated prospectively. This is particularly so in the field of cardiology: when death occurs with no obvious single cause, and no autopsy is performed, a diagnosis of coronary heart death may be used as a 'default' by physicians looking for what they deem to be the likeliest cause of death. Some authors have deemed 'all-cause mortality' to be the only real 'hard' endpoint, because of potential biases in other classifications of mortality. All-cause mortality is easily ascertained, does not require adjudication and is objective [10]. Subclassifying cause of death into 'cardiovascular mortality' or 'arrhythmic death' endpoints is subjective, and relies on a degree of accuracy in the death certification which may not be present [11]. These issues have been particularly relevant to the SCORE risk evaluation project, which collated data from 216 000 subjects from 12 European cohorts. The utility and accuracy of both fatal and non-fatal events in these data has been the source of considerable debate.

NON-FATAL ENDPOINTS

It is in the definition of the non-fatal endpoints that we really run into problems. Two in particular, which we apply to both cohort studies and case–control studies, are MI and stroke. Defining stroke in the older studies is fraught with difficulty, as the diagnosis was mostly clinical until the advent of widespread computed tomography scanning in the 1990s. MI has long been defined using the WHO 'two out of three' definition – namely, that two of the following features are present: typical chest pain for greater than 20 min, raised cardiac enzyme levels and typical electrocardiograph (ECG) changes [12]. This definition has formed the cornerstone of the definitions used in the MONICA and Framingham studies. In particular, MONICA classified proposed fatal and non-fatal coronary ischaemic events into five groups: definite acute MI, possible acute MI or coronary death, ischaemic cardiac arrest with successful resuscitation not fulfilling criteria for definite or possible MI, no acute MI, and fatal cases with insufficient data [13].

However, the advent of troponin T and I testing, both of which are highly specific and sensitive for myocardial ischaemia, has allowed us to detect very small infarcts, which previously would not have been classified as such. This presents a significant problem for epidemiological studies, in which the incidence of MI will be seen to increase substantially: the use of troponin testing doubled the incidence of new MIs in one study [14], while case fatality rates inevitably fall. In an attempt to clarify the classification of MI, the European Society of Cardiology (ESC) and the American College of Cardiology (ACC) released a consensus document with a new definition of MI [15]:

Either one of the following criteria satisfies the diagnosis for an acute, evolving or recent MI:

(1) Typical rise and gradual fall (troponin) or more rapid rise and fall (CK-MB) of biochemical markers of myocardial necrosis with at least one of the following: (a) ischaemic symptoms; (b) development of pathologic Q waves on the ECG; (c) ECG changes indicative of ischaemia (ST segment elevation or depression); or (d) coronary artery intervention (e.g. coronary angioplasty).

(2) Pathologic findings of an acute MI. Criteria for established MI. Any one of the following criteria satisfies the diagnosis for established MI: (a) development of new pathologic Q

waves on serial ECGs. The patient may or may not remember previous symptoms. Biochemical markers of myocardial necrosis may have normalized, depending on the length of time that has passed since the infarct developed; (b) pathologic findings of a healed or healing MI.

Unsurprisingly, this definition, which is indeed quite different from the earlier WHO definition, has caused much controversy [16, 17]. Critics will say that troponin testing is still not widespread enough to justify this change (and in the case of developing nations, troponin assays may not yet be feasible at all). The crux of this definition of MI is a blood test, in contrast to the WHO definition, in which blood assays were not necessary to diagnose a MI. Because of the high sensitivity of troponins for even tiny myocardial events, many more people will be diagnosed with myocardial injury or infarction than before, with implications for their working life and their ability to get insurance – even though their prognosis may in fact be excellent, if the event was only a minor one.

Even if the ESC/ACC definition of MI is taken at face value to be used as an endpoint in clinical trials, there are some questions left unanswered. The guidelines do not recommend which troponin assay to use, and indeed one author reports that only one out of the seven assays available adequately meets the performance criteria suggested (acceptable imprecision of the troponin measurement at the 99th centile should be <10% coefficient of variation) [18]. It is unclear how re-infarction should be defined, as this is a commonly surveyed outcome in post-MI therapeutic trials, and given that troponin T in particular can remain elevated for up to 2 weeks after a single event, diagnosing a second MI inside of that time using these criteria could be challenging. Also, elevated troponins are indicators not only of MI, but also of myocardial necrosis from any cause, including such causes as pulmonary embolism, drug toxicity and sepsis. Therefore, more clinical information than a simple dichotomous answer for troponin should be considered.

In order to try and resolve some of these issues, a second working group met in 2002 and published their case definitions for acute coronary heart disease in epidemiology and clinical research studies in 2003 [19]. In this paper, ischaemic coronary heart disease was defined as definite, probable, possible or not diagnosed, depending on biomarker status, symptoms and signs, and ECG findings. This diagnostic schema provides a lot more information on ECG coding, and allows a diagnostic option for subjects where biomarkers of ischaemia were not assayed. It also provides a classification of cause of out of hospital death, something which was not included in the ECS/ACC guidelines. When this 2003 definition for acute coronary syndromes (ACS) was examined in a large Finnish MI register with troponin information and compared with the WHO MONICA MI definition, 83% more subjects were diagnosed with definite MI. These subjects were older, more often had diabetes mellitus, and had a higher risk of cardiovascular death at 1 year, than those subjects who were diagnosed with definite MI by both definitions [20].

Recently, these issues have been comprehensively re-visited by the Joint ESC/ACCF/AHA/WHF Task Force for the redefinition of myocardial infarction with a new 'universal definition of myocardial infarction' [21], and the reader is referred to this for a comprehensive review of these issues. They can also be viewed on the ESC (escardio.org) and American Heart Association (my.americanheart.org) websites.

The completeness of the 2003 and 2007 definitions is laudable, and the classifications will be an invaluable tool in future studies. However, with this level of completeness comes the downside that instead of one 'yes/no' definition for MI/ACS, we now have a number of grades of likelihood of disease, and therefore the system is immediately less user-friendly for day-to-day clinical use. Nevertheless, it is acknowledged that myocardial necrosis represents a continuum of damage, and there is no troponin threshold at which MI can be declared 'definite'.

With these new MI definitions, the implications for the major epidemiological studies already published on cardiovascular outcomes are unclear – it is quite obvious that a MI, as described in the MONICA or Framingham studies, is quite different to a small troponin-positive MI, which occurs in the setting of an otherwise uncomplicated coronary angioplasty procedure. New cohort studies will need to be undertaken, with prospective gathering of non-fatal event information. These issues have been highly relevant to the SCORE risk stratification system and its development [5]. SCORE uses traditional atherosclerotic risk factors to estimate individual 10-year risk of cardiovascular death, and cardiovascular death was defined using appropriate ICD-9 coding from death certification. In response to calls for a European system to estimate risk of non-fatal cardiovascular events, a project is underway to use the same risk factors to estimate 10-year risk of both fatal and non-fatal cardiovascular disease. The Finnish cohort, which used the MONICA definition for MI, forms the basis of this project. However, like other epidemiological studies, the changing face of MI remains a challenge when evaluating this project, and changes in the natural history of the disease due to changing risk factor distribution and newer therapies are hard to represent when using older cohort data.

In summary, in modern clinical practice, troponin testing has become a fundamental tool in the evaluation of patients with suspected ACS [22]. Using troponins as diagnostic criteria may cause an apparent increase in the incidence of acute MI, but these were cases that we were missing with the old WHO definition – and there is evidence that 6-month re-admission and mortality rates are at least as bad in this new MI group as in those already defined by the WHO criteria [23]. The preferred definition of MI for the 21st century is not yet clear, but there is no doubt that diagnosing MI by troponin level is here to stay – we must work with its strengths and accept the challenge to epidemiological and clinical trials.

COMPOSITE ENDPOINTS AND SHIFTING ENDPOINTS IN TRIALS

The primary endpoint in clinical trials is usually the method by which a trial therapy is deemed to be efficacious or not. Therefore, choosing an appropriate endpoint for which a significant result can be proven is a vital step in planning a clinical trial. One of the most controversial topics in considering endpoints in clinical trials is that of the composite endpoint. This is a phenomenon that is on the increase in randomized controlled trials (RCTs). Although death is an excellent primary endpoint, it is not a frequent enough outcome in many conditions to make it feasible to use on its own. For this reason, and given the ever smaller gains made by new treatments or combinations of treatments in clinical trials, composite endpoints can be required. These will result in a higher event rate than death alone, allowing a smaller sample size to be followed for a shorter period of time. Although larger trials are more statistically 'pure', there are some benefits to these smaller sample sizes: more information can be gathered on the smaller groups, and the methodologies can be more strictly adhered to. A commonly used composite endpoint is cardiovascular mortality, non-fatal MI and stroke. In this context, presentation of total mortality is important in case a reduction in cardiovascular mortality is offset by an increase in non-vascular causes of death.

In many of the medical device trials, such as those looking at the outcomes for different types of coronary stents, there is pressure both from industry and clinicians to obtain results quickly on new technologies. For this reason, and because of the low morbidity now associated with percutaneous coronary stenting procedures, endpoints such as 'death, non-fatal MI and 30-day need for revascularization' are being used. The problem with such an endpoint is that all three events have such different implications for the patient: even if the individual endpoint results lack significance, they should be individually reported. A discussion on the results of the Controlled Abciximab and Device Investigation to Lower Late Angioplasty Complications (CADILLAC) study [24], where patients underwent either optimal percutaneous transluminal balloon angioplasty (PTCA) or PTCA and routine stenting, commented on the 1-year composite endpoint of death, re-infarction, disabling stroke and target vessel revascularization (TVR) [25]. This endpoint was greater in the PTCA only group, but was driven by the TVR endpoint, whereas the risks of death, re-infarction and disabling stroke showed a non-significant trend to be higher in the stenting group. The CADILLAC investigators acknowledged the inequity of these endpoints, and their differing contributions to the total composite.

Another study, a review of the evidence for glycoprotein IIb/IIIa inhibitors in acute coronary syndromes [26] pooled the all-cause mortality data from four major RCTs. Despite these four trials individually reporting a favourable outcome for a composite endpoint, including death, when the review authors examined the risk of all-cause mortality they found an odds ratio (OR) of 1.00; 95% confidence interval (CI) 0.82–1.22. Often, the result for the composite endpoint only is reported, and no information is provided on the individual endpoints. This can lead to adverse events or trends, which may later turn out to be significant, being overlooked.

Furthermore, the use of this composite endpoint infers that the effect of the risk factor or treatment is equivalent on all the outcomes in the composite. This is clearly not the case, when one considers the factors that may be at play between the outcomes of death and re-admission at 30 days! A positive effect of a therapy on one outcome may be masked in a composite primary endpoint, if one part of that composite is a frequent event but is not affected by that therapy. Therefore, valuable information may be hidden in a seemingly negative trial result. There is also the bias involved with competing risks when multiple endpoints, including both fatal and non-fatal outcomes, are used.

Composite endpoints often provide very nice 'soundbites' – a one-liner describing the trial's outcome. However, few trials are that simple, and these soundbites can mask the complexities of the results and any weaknesses in the methodologies. The endpoints used in clinical trials should be made explicit in both the abstract and the text. We should take our cue from the Consolidated Standards of Reporting Trials (CONSORT) guidelines for reporting of RCTs, which suggests reporting of:

'Clearly defined primary and secondary outcome measures and, when applicable, any methods used to enhance the quality of measurements...For each primary and secondary outcome, a summary of results for each group, and the estimated effect size and its precision (e.g. 95% CI).... Interpretation of the results, taking into account...the dangers associated with multiplicity of analyses and outcome.' [27]

FUTURE CHALLENGES

The world of the cardiovascular RCT is becoming ever more complex. Populations are changing: the developed world countries are seeing an explosion in obesity and type 2 diabetes mellitus. Meanwhile, patterns of disease in the 'developing' nations are also changing, with a shift from communicable diseases as the primary cause of morbidity and mortality, to non-communicable and cardiovascular diseases. The implications for cohort studies that commenced 40 and 50 years ago are unclear, but we have to acknowledge that the changes in diet and activity levels must make some impact.

Similarly, the 'greying' of our population presents us with a number of difficulties. The vast majority of RCTs selected only younger patients for their studies. As we age, so must the pharmacokinetics and dynamics of drug treatments change, and the evidence base for many treatments is simply not available for the very elderly. With the improvements in therapies for cardiovascular diseases, the case fatality rate has dropped, but the prevalence is on the increase, as we live through these diseases, gradually accruing more and more comorbidities. Again, in many RCTs these patients with multiple comorbidities were not included, and so we do not have direct evidence for many treatments in this subgroup.

Early cardiovascular RCTs used a simple double-blind approach, with patients randomized to either treatment or placebo. However, with the multitude of proven treatments now available for acute coronary syndromes and heart failure, for example, it is not ethical to deprive a patient of treatment in order to give him a placebo for a clinical trial. RCTs now are examining combinations of therapies, with ever more complicated designs and smaller therapeutic yields. In this context, it behoves the reader to examine the endpoints chosen to see if they are clinically relevant.

REFERENCES

1. Anonymous. Coronary heart disease in seven countries. *Circulation* 1970; 41(suppl):I186–I195.
2. Dawber TR, Kannel WB. The Framingham Study. An epidemiological approach to coronary heart disease. *Circulation* 1966; 34:553–555.
3. Tunstall-Pedoe H, Kuulasmaa K, Mahonen M, Tolonen H, Ruokokoski E, Amouyel P. Contribution of trends in survival and coronary-event rates to changes in coronary heart disease mortality: 10-year results from 37 WHO MONICA project populations. Monitoring trends and determinants in cardiovascular diseases. *Lancet* 1999; 353:1547–1557.
4. Anonymous. The Multiple Risk Factor Intervention Trial (MRFIT). A national study of primary prevention of coronary heart disease. *JAMA* 1976; 235:825–827.
5. Conroy RM, Pyörälä K, Fitzgerald AP *et al*. Estimation of ten-year risk of fatal cardiovascular disease in Europe: the SCORE project. *Eur Heart J* 2003; 24:987–1003.
6. Pritt BS, Hardin NJ, Richmond JA, Shapiro SL. Death certification errors at an academic institution. *Arch Pathol Lab Med* 2005; 129:1476–1479.
7. James DS, Bull AD. Death certification: is correct formulation of cause of death related to seniority or experience? *J R Coll Physicians Lond* 1995; 29:424–428.
8. Attems J, Arbes S, Bohm G, Bohmer F, Lintner F. The clinical diagnostic accuracy rate regarding the immediate cause of death in a hospitalized geriatric population; an autopsy study of 1594 patients. *Wien Med Wochenschr* 2004; 154:159–162.
9. Greenwood M. *Medical Statistics from Graunt to Farr*. Cambridge University Press, Cambridge, 1948.
10. Topol EJ, Califf RM, Van de Werf F *et al*., The Virtual Coordinating Center for Global Collaborative Cardiovascular Research (VIGOUR) Group. Perspectives on large-scale cardiovascular clinical trials for the new millennium. *Circulation* 1997; 95:1072–1082.
11. Lauer MS, Blackstone EH, Young JB, Topol EJ. Cause of death in clinical research: time for a reassessment? *J Am Coll Cardiol* 1999; 34:618–619.
12. Nomenclature and criteria for diagnosis of ischaemic heart disease: Report of the Joint International Society and Federation of Cardiology/World Health Organization Task Force on Standardization of Clinical Nomenclature. *Circulation* 1979; 59:607–609.
13. From CD-ROMs Part 2. In: Tunstall-Pedoe T (ed.). *MONICA Monograph and Multimedia Sourcebook*. World Health Organization, Geneva, 2003.
14. Ferguson JL, Beckett GJ, Stoddart M, Walker SW, Fox KAA. Myocardial infarction redefined: the new ACC/ESC definition, based on cardiac troponin, increases the apparent incidence of infarction. *Heart* 2002; 88:343–347.
15. Alpert JS, Thygesen K, Antman E, Bassand JP. Myocardial infarction redefined – a consensus document of The Joint European Society of Cardiology/American College of Cardiology Committee for the redefinition of myocardial infarction. *J Am Coll Cardiol* 2000; 36:959–969.
16. Tunstall-Pedoe H. Redefinition of myocardial infarction by a consensus dissenter. *J Am Coll Cardiol* 2001; 37:1472–1474.
17. Norris RM. Dissent from the consensus on the redefinition of myocardial infarction. *Eur Heart J* 2001; 22:1626–1627.
18. Apple FS, Murakami MM. Serum 99th percentile reference cutoffs for seven cardiac troponin assays. *Clin Chem* 2004; 50:1477–1479.
19. Luepker RV, Apple FS, Christenson RH *et al*. Case definitions for acute coronary heart disease in epidemiology and clinical research studies: a statement from the AHA council on Epidemiology and

Prevention; the AHA Statistics Committee; World Heart Federation Council on Epidemiology and Prevention; the European Society of Cardiology Working Group on Epidemiology and Prevention; Centers for Disease Control and Prevention; and the National Heart, Lung and Blood Institute. *Circulation* 2003; 108:2543–2549.

20. Salomaa V, Koukkunene H, Ketonen M *et al.* A new definition for myocardial infarction: what difference does it make? *Eur Heart J* 2005; 26:1719–1725.

21. Thygesen K, Alpert JS, White HD, on behalf of the Joint ESC/ACCF/Task Force for the redefinition of myocardial infarction. Universal definition of myocardial infarction. *Eur Heart J* 2007; 28: 2525–2538.

22. White HD. Things ain't what they used to be: impact of a new definition of myocardial infarction. *Am Heart J* 2002; 144:933–937.

23. Meier MA, Al-Badr WH, Cooper JV *et al.* The new definition of myocardial infarction: diagnostic and prognostic implications in patients with acute coronary syndromes. *Arch Intern Med* 2002; 162:1585–1589.

24. Cox DA, Stone GW, Grines CL *et al.* Outcomes of optimal or 'stent-like' balloon angioplasty in acute myocardial infarction: the CADILLAC trial. *J Am Coll Cardiol* 2003; 42:971–977.

25. Massel D. Composite confusion. *J Am Coll Cardiol* 2004; 43:1926–1927.

26. Freemantle N, Calvert M, Wood J, Eastaugh J, Griffen C. Composite outcomes in randomized trials: greater precision but with greater uncertainty? *JAMA* 2003; 289:2554–2560.

27. Moher D, Schulz KF, Altman D, The CONSORT group. The CONSORT statement: revised recommendations for improving the quality of reports of parallel-group randomized trials. *JAMA* 2001; 285:1987–1991.

4

Genetics, family history and risk estimation in the young

O. Faergeman

INTRODUCTION

In the early 1950s, the unexpected finding of frank atherosclerosis in the coronary arteries of young Americans, killed in action in the Korean War, helped us realize that we had an epidemic of atherosclerotic disease on our hands [1]. Later, pathological studies in Louisiana (Pathological Determinants of Atherosclerosis in Youth) showed not only how the disease evolves from adolescence throughout young adulthood; they also revealed some of the behavioural, pathophysiological and genetic determinants of the disease [2], and it is now possible to pick out some of the children and young adults who, before their time, but mostly years down the road, will succumb to atherosclerotic and thrombotic disease. They identify themselves by eating unwisely, by smoking or by being fat and sedentary. Their risk is greater if close family members have had an early stroke or heart attack, and greater still if a physician finds blood pressure, plasma cholesterol or plasma glucose to be high.

In this chapter, we shall first recapitulate the simplest way to quantify cardiovascular risk in the young, and we will then discuss some options for refining risk assessment. They include arterial imaging, new biochemical markers of risk, and molecular genetic analysis. Emphasis will be on discussions of the latter.

CLASSICAL RISK ASSESSMENT

The simplest approach, already sketched above is to identify high-risk patterns of behaviour, perform the appropriate clinical assessments, and advise the young person about the consequences of maintaining a high-risk pattern of behaviour and pathophysiology over many years. A formal version of this approach is the one adopted in the Joint European Recommendations for cardiovascular prevention. An individual's risk of dying of cardiovascular disease over the next ten years can be read from the chart given as Figure 11.1(b). To assess risk over the longer time span relevant for young people, identify the cell to which the person now belongs (up to age 40) and follow the table upwards, e.g. to age 60, to see how risk increases with age if the pattern of risk factors is maintained. In general, risk will actually increase more than indicated by this exercise, because risk factor levels also tend to increase with age.

Ole Faergeman, MD, DMSc, Professor, Cardiovascular Medicine, National Heart and Lung Institute, Charing Cross Campus, Imperial College, London, UK

REFINING RISK ASSESSMENT

In older as well as younger persons, this classical approach to risk assessment does fairly well at the extremes of risk: persons at very low and at very high risk are identified with acceptable accuracy. In the intermediate range of risk, however, risk assessment based on classical risk factor patterns may be less accurate [3]. Since most people are at intermediate risk, there is a real need for better risk assessment tools. Other approaches to risk assessment may include relative risk (easily estimated from the chart), years of life lost, lifetime risk [4] and rate advancement periods [5].

ARTERIAL IMAGING

One approach is arterial imaging of some sort. A recent study suggested that measurements of coronary calcium by computer tomography differentiated quite well between persons destined and not destined to have atherosclerotic cardiovascular disease (CVD) events, even in the intermediate range of risk as defined by the Framingham risk function [3]. The European and US guidelines for prevention of CVD [6, 7] have already recognized that techniques such as measurements of coronary calcium or ultrasonic measurement of the thickness of the carotid intima-media can be employed in sophisticated risk assessment of individual patients, but the guidelines have not incorporated imaging formally into their algorithms [6, 7]. Scott Grundy has suggested a way to do that [8], and there are good arguments for arterial imaging in older persons as part of, or even as the basis for, risk assessment [3]. Whether future guidelines committees will recommend imaging for routine risk assessment should depend, therefore, primarily on answers to questions about safety, availability and costs. In adolescents and young adults, however, atherosclerotic lesions, demonstrable at autopsy, are below the detection limits of available appropriate techniques, and arterial imaging is currently not an option for risk assessment in the young.

BETTER BIOCHEMICAL MARKERS OF RISK

Another option is better biochemical markers of risk. They include thrombogenic factors, markers of inflammation, homocysteine and better indices of dyslipidaemia. Discussions of the latter, which probably are the most relevant for assessments of long-term risk, have for quite some time been focused on ways to combine different measurements of lipoprotein components in a simple number conveying maximal information about cardiovascular risk. One idea is to replace measurements of the cholesterol content of low-density lipoproteins (LDL) and high-density lipoproteins (HDL) by measurements of the major protein components of these lipoproteins, apolipoprotein B (apoB) and apolipoprotein A1 (apoA1), respectively, and to combine the measurements in the ratio of apoB to apoA1.

The ratio makes good sense, at least intuitively, since it combines an apparently harmful with an apparently protective lipoprotein variable. Concentrations of apoB are a true measure of concentrations of atherogenic lipoproteins such as LDL and the smaller varieties of very low-density lipoprotein (VLDL), and apoA1 is the major apolipoprotein of HDL, low concentrations of which are associated with high risk of disease. Thus, the higher the ratio, the higher is the risk.

The idea is not new. In its original form, it was the ratio of total cholesterol (or LDL cholesterol) to HDL cholesterol, and that version of the ratio is well supported by observational epidemiology [9–11]. It has therefore been widely used to assess risk and, indeed, it is included in the current European guidelines [6]. Nevertheless, the arguments for the version of the ratio based on protein measurements are supported by results of recent epidemiological studies [12, 13], better understanding of lipoprotein metabolism, and improvements in laboratory technology and standardization.

There are problems, of course. If one wants to define a particular value of the ratio as a target of drug therapy to affect plasma lipoproteins, does it make a difference whether apoB/apoA1 is lowered by decreasing the numerator or by increasing the denominator? The evidence to support the lowering of the numerator, apoB, is very strong, *inter alia* because lowering the apoB lipoproteins is what statins do [14]. In large clinical trials of statins to lower LDL, the association of high concentrations of apo B with cardiovascular events in both the placebo and treatment groups is stronger than that of LDL [15]. In some of these trials, the apoB/apoA1 ratio does even better [16]. Nevertheless, it's a tricky business translating these observations into lowering ratios, be they apoB/apoA1 or total choles-terol/HDL cholesterol, as new targets of therapy. These ratios could be lowered with unchanged concentrations of LDL if only concentrations of HDL are increased, but the proposition that patients will benefit from drug therapy to increase HDL, or apoA1, is sup-ported mainly by *in vitro* and animal experimentation [17], and the evidence from clinical trials to test the hypothesis explicitly is very limited [18].

We also do not know whether we should increase HDL or whether, irrespective of HDL concentrations, we should try to increase flux of cholesterol through the various routes of 'reverse cholesterol transport' from arteries, arterial macrophages in particular, and other organs to the liver. The two are not necessarily proportional, just as the amount of water (concentration of HDL) in a bath tub is not a measure of how much water is flowing into and out of the tub (flux of cholesterol). One of the methods of increasing concentrations of HDL (and apoA1) is to inhibit the transfer of cholesterol from HDL to VLDL by cholesteryl ester transfer protein (CETP), and CETP inhibition therefore almost certainly decreases reverse cholesterol transport. The merits of this kind of drug therapy are currently being tested in clinical trials [19], and at this time we still do not have a fully satisfactory answer to the question of whether to use the ratio of apoB to apoA1 (or total cholesterol to HDL cholesterol) as a target of therapy as well as a measure of risk.

FAMILY HISTORY AND MOLECULAR GENETIC ANALYSIS

A third option, molecular genetic analysis, can extend the information obtained by taking a family history. It is particularly relevant for young people, since genetic variations herald-ing early-onset cardiovascular disease are present from birth.

The potential of family history has been most clearly demonstrated in twin studies. In a classical Swedish study of several thousand monozygotic and dizygotic twin pairs, born between 1886 and 1925, Marenberg *et al.* showed that a person's risk of death from coronary artery disease was much higher if he or she had lost a twin to the disease before the age of 55 (for men) or 65 years (for women). Risk of a coronary death was especially high if the twin pair was monozygotic rather than dizygotic (hazard ratios 8.1 vs. 3.8 for men and 15.0 vs. 2.6 for women), indicating that genetic factors strongly affect risk of dying of coronary artery disease in both men and women. The importance of genetics was attenuated by ageing, however, since the surviving twin's risk decreased with increasing age at the cor-onary death of his or her twin [20, 21].

The clinical utility of a family history depends on what the patient knows and how well the physician elicits that knowledge. We seem to know less and less about our families in urbanized than in traditional societies. Many Danes, for example, know almost nothing about their extended families. Fortunately, and consistent with the twin studies, the import-ance of a history of CVD is greater when the family relationship is closer. Disease in a parent is more important than disease in a grandparent or uncle. The importance of the informa-tion is also greater the younger the family member was at disease inception. Since a myocar-dial infarction or a coronary death is not necessarily the first manifestation of coronary artery disease, the physician must be sure to ascertain age at first symptoms, e.g. angina pectoris. Finally, importance of family history of disease increases with the percentage of family members afflicted [4], and that percentage is more accurately determined as more is known about the extended family.

Uncommon variations in DNA structure (prevalence <1%) are arbitrarily termed mutations, whereas more common variations (prevalence >1%) are called polymorphisms. The results of molecular genetic analyses are used in two ways. First, the variation, be it rare or common, can be considered an important part of interacting agents of disease if the relationship to disease is sufficiently strong and consistent. It is common in such cases to speak of molecular genetic diagnosis, even though this concept is based on a misunderstanding to be discussed below. Second, some genetic variations are less directly related to disease, and it is necessary to make no assumptions about causality. Instead, the relationship is associational. A genetic variation could be used as a risk factor in risk assessment if the association of the variation to disease is sufficiently common (a polymorphism) and consistent.

The spectrum from causality to association is continuous, and any distinction between them is arbitrary. In a very broad sense, moreover, the environment modulates how early and how strongly any particular genetic variation can contribute to a young person's risk of clinically apparent disease in the long term. For the gene's point of view, of course, environment is everything from gene–gene interaction to the agricultural policies of government.

MOLECULAR GENETIC ANALYSIS, SCREENING AND COUNSELLING

Molecular genetic analysis and genetic counselling are relevant for a small minority of young people, and this section is devoted to a discussion of the current possibilities, limitations and requirements of this approach.

Genotypic or phenotypic disease definitions?

If a physician wants to base clinical decisions on finding or excluding a variation in the DNA of a particular gene, he must understand how that variation is related to disease and the possibilities of treatment. He must, in other words, understand what is known about the relationship of the phenotype (the disease) to the genotype (the mutation).

At present, molecular genetics makes sense mainly in advising patients with monogenetic disorders of clotting of blood, of myocardial function and of metabolism, dyslipidaemias in particular. An example is the relationship between familial hypercholesterolaemia (FH) and deficiency or absence of the LDL receptor, the discovery of which began the era of molecular medicine [22].

In FH, concentrations of LDL cholesterol can vary from 4 to 10 mmol/l (~150–390 mg/dl) when only one of the two alleles of the gene for the LDL receptor is dysfunctional. This is the heterozygous state. When both alleles of the gene are affected, LDL cholesterol can be much higher, ranging from 6 to 20 mmol/l (~230–780 mg/dl). This is the homozygous state. In most western societies, heterozygous FH occurs in about 1 in every 500 persons, and homozygous FH therefore occurs only once in a million births ($1/500 \times 1/500 \times 1/4$). Untreated, heterozygous FH can cause myocardial infarction in early adulthood, whereas patients with the homozygous form can die of atherosclerosis in childhood. Cholesterol deposition occurs not only in the arteries as atherosclerosis, but also in the eyelids as xanthelasmata, in the cornea as corneal arcus, and in tendons as tendinous xanthomata.

For historical reasons, the term 'FH' has become synonymous with mutations in the LDL receptor, and that is the way the disease is presented in most textbooks. That identity has become less and less tenable, however, as we have learned more about the genetics of the clinical picture of familial hypercholesterolaemia (cf. Online Mendelian Inheritance in Man, www.ncbi.nih.gov/omim).

First, the clinical picture of FH can be due to mutations in genes coding for proteins other than the LDL receptor. Apolipoprotein B is the structural protein in LDL, and it serves as a ligand for the LDL receptor. A mutation in the gene for apoB, just like mutations in the gene for the receptor, disrupts binding of LDL to the receptor. The condition has been called 'familial defective apolipoprotein B'. The resulting hypercholesterolaemia is, on average, only slightly less severe than that associated with LDL receptor defects, but there is so much overlap that the distinction is irrelevant for the many physicians who do not have access to a molecular genetics laboratory. Even for those who do, it makes no difference when making therapeutic decisions. It is the degree and duration of hypercholesterolaemia that matter, not the molecular diagnosis. Rare variations in genes coding for still more proteins are also related to the clinical picture of familial hypercholesterolaemia. Thus, the phenotypic clinical picture does not allow us to predict the results of molecular genetic analysis. Different genotypes can underlie the same phenotype.

Second, the reverse holds true. The same genetic variation can be associated with quite different clinical pictures. It depends on the environment. Pimstone *et al.* [23] identified mutations in the LDL receptor gene in 16 patients of Chinese origin with heterozygous FH living in Canada, and they compared the clinical picture with that of 18 individuals with the same or similar mutations living in China. Average concentrations of LDL cholesterol were 4.35 in the patients in China and 7.46 mmol/l in the patients in Canada. Although average age and sex were the same (about 39 years, about half women), none of the patients in China had coronary artery disease or tendon xanthomata, which afflicted a quarter and almost half, respectively, of the patients living in Canada. The authors suggested that these substantial differences in clinical phenotype could be ascribed to differences in intake of dietary fat (about 20% and 34% of calories in China and Canada, respectively). It should be obvious from this example that treatment decisions based on knowledge only of the genotype could be quite mistaken.

The nature of genotype/phenotype relationships can also be more fully appreciated by a careful look at the patients referred for FH to a lipid clinic. By analysis of the genes for apolipoprotein B gene and the LDL receptor, including sequencing of the 18 exons, the flanking intronic regions and the promotor region of the LDL receptor gene, we were able to detect mutations in less than 65% of families with a clinical diagnosis of definite FH according to the criteria of the Simon Broome register in London or of the Dutch Lipid Clinic Network. Conversely, we had to analyse the genes of many families with a less typical clinical picture (probable or possible FH) to find most of the mutations in the LDL receptor gene that, in fact, were present in patients and families referred to us. We concluded, therefore, that the relationship between genotype and phenotype, even in the fairly homogeneous atherogenic environment of Denmark, is much more tenuous than generally appreciated [24].

These considerations, based on studies of familial hypercholesterolaemia, can be extended to the genetics of other conditions affecting risk of coronary artery disease or other heart disease. Indeed, there are few, if any, invariant relationships between genotype and phenotype in clinical medicine, as there are in embryology. Results of molecular genetic analysis should therefore not be considered diagnosis, and they should not, on their own, become the basis for clinical decisions. Rather, they should be collated with individual and family history, clinical and paraclinical examination, therapeutic options, etc., and careful integration of as much information about the patient and his family as possible should underlie diagnosis, counselling and therapy.

The most responsible way to use molecular genetic analysis in clinical work is to base diagnosis, and thereby clinical decisions, on conferences between clinician and molecular biologist, much like conferences between clinicians and pathologists should underlie therapeutic decisions on behalf of patients with cancer. Some gene variations are obviously pathogenic, but most are not. Clinicians must become familiar with the essentials of molecular genetic analysis, and molecular biologists must recognize that the phenotype, which is what matters to the patient, can never be perfectly predicted from the genotype. It is dangerous, therefore, to allow departments of clinical biochemistry, or molecular biology laboratories, to confirm or exclude diagnoses of clinical syndromes such as FH on the basis only of molecular genetic analyses. Similar considerations apply to most if not all other genetic diseases.

Uses of molecular genetic analysis

Nevertheless, and with all of these caveats, detection of a mutation in the gene, e.g. the LDL receptor can serve several purposes. It can, first of all, allow physician and patient to understand disease better in a particular patient and his or her family. Although there can be adverse psychological reactions to detection of a mutation, most patients and healthy family members prefer understanding the disease to being in the dark [25].

Second, the nature of the genetic variation can affect clinical decisions. Many base pair changes and amino acid substitutions are innocuous, and the protein works perfectly well. Other changes in gene structure are not. Proteins cannot function, as an extreme example, if stop codons in the gene have deleted important parts of the protein. There are several ways to establish whether a given variation in the gene is pathogenic or not. If many family members can be studied, it is possible to ascertain whether genetic variation and disease trait accompany each other (co-segregate) within the family. The variation is probably pathogenic if they do. Another option is a functional assay of some kind to test whether the genetic variation compromises protein function. In the case of the LDL receptor, function can be studied by flow cytometry, but the method requires several study subjects, and it is not suitable for analysis of individual patients [26]. A third option is comparison of the human gene with the corresponding gene in other animals to see whether the genetic variation changes a part of the protein that has been conserved through evolution. Conserved parts of the protein are likely to be important for protein function, and altered structure in those parts is therefore more probably pathogenic.

Third, molecular genetic analysis can be used to work out whether or not a family member has inherited the variation that renders them more susceptible to disease. They can then be counselled more appropriately than would otherwise be possible. While it is technically demanding to find the mutation in the index patient, once found it is fairly easy to look for it in family members.

The utility of screening of family members to detect carriers of a disease gene depends *inter alia* on whether the disease is inherited in a dominant or recessive manner. If it is inherited as a dominant trait, in which only one allele of the gene is abnormal, it makes sense to screen all first-degree relatives (parents, brothers, sisters and children). That is because, on average, half of them carry the mutation related to the disease in the index patient. Heterozygous FH is just one example of this kind of disease. Others are most of the disorders of myocardial function such as long QT syndrome, hypertrophic cardiomyopathy and arrythmogenic right ventricle.

If, on the other hand, the disease is inherited as a recessive trait, in which both alleles of the gene must be abnormal, it makes sense to limit genetic screening to brothers and sisters of the index patient, because they have a 25% risk of also having inherited the disease. It is generally not necessary to screen the other first-degree relatives (parents and children). Although each parent and each child carry one allele for the disease, the chance that they have inherited another disease allele is extremely small. That is because most recessive diseases are very rare, and very few people in any population are carriers of the abnormal allele. A wider genetic screening programme can be justified only if the recessive disease is not very rare in the population in question.

Molecular genetic analysis can be exploited in genetic counselling by which parents are given the information necessary to decide whether or not to request abortion of an affected fetus. With one exception, no dyslipidaemia causes disease that is serious enough (severe disability or death in childhood or early adulthood) to merit consideration of abortion. The exception is homozygous familial hypercholesterolaemia. Even in this situation, however, the case for abortion is not clear-cut, because children with homozygous FH can be treated, albeit imperfectly. Nevertheless, parents who are both heterozygous for FH face a difficult choice. On average, 25% of their children will be normolipidaemic, 50% will also have heterozygous FH, and 25% will have homozygous FH. There is a valid but not absolute medical argument for aborting a fetus that is homozygous for familial hypercholesterolaemia. There is no valid medical argument, however, for aborting a fetus that is heterozygous for the disease. When the parents have understood the genetic issue, they must be supported in the decision they make to have or not to have the fetus genotyped.

There are no other valid uses of molecular genetic analysis for diagnostic purposes, despite the plethora of commercially available genetic tests. Molecular genetic analysis should not be used for diagnostic purposes if the relationship of genotype (mutations) to phenotype (disease) is not adequately understood by the responsible physician, and it can be wise for the patient to purchase life insurance policies before he or she is examined for an inherited disease.

GENOTYPING IN RISK ASSESSMENT

A gene polymorphism could be a useful risk factor if its association with disease is sufficiently strong and consistent. It does not have to participate in the actual interaction between the many agents that ultimately cause disease. Since the mid-1980s, research has suggested numerous polymorphisms in various genes as risk factors. Prominent among them is the insertion/deletion polymorphism in the gene for angiotensin-converting enzyme (ACE). Cambien *et al.* [27] initially reported that the DD (deletion/deletion) genotype, which is associated with higher levels of circulating ACE than the ID and II genotypes, was significantly more frequent in patients with myocardial infarction than in controls, and they suggested that the polymorphism could be used in assessing risk of disease. Later studies, also fairly small, supported these initial findings, but the relationship between the ACE polymorphism and risk of myocardial infarction seemed to evaporate when it was examined in very large studies [28].

The importance of appropriate sample size and avoidance of excessive subgroup analysis has certainly been under-appreciated in case–control studies of genetic polymorphisms and disease [29], but there is another and possibly decisive issue. Genetic polymorphisms, like other risk factors, may be clinically important only in some populations or in some individuals [30]. It depends on context in the broadest sense: variation in other genes, age, sex, diet, physical environment, etc. The epidemiological and mathematical research that will be necessary to develop risk assessment models appropriate to population subgroups or individuals is only just getting started, however, and the inclusion of genetic polymorphisms in algorithms used for risk assessment is, at present, not adequately documented [4].

SUMMARY

The simplest and most useful way to assess long-term risk of cardiovascular disease in young people remains the calculation of the long-term consequences of maintaining current patterns of high-risk behaviour and failing to correct hypertension, dyslipidaemia, hyperglycaemia, etc. Inherited susceptibility to cardiovascular disease can be assessed by taking a family history and, in the rare cases of monogenetic disorders, by cautious use of molecular genetic analysis.

REFERENCES

1. Enos WF, Holmes RH, Beyer J. Coronary disease among United States soldiers killed in action in Korea. *JAMA* 1953; 152:1090–1093.
2. Wissler RW, Strong JP. Risk factors and progression of atherosclerosis in youth. PDAY Research Group. Pathological Determinants of Atherosclerosis in Youth. *Am J Pathol* 1998; 153:1023–1033.
3. Arad Y, Goodman KJ, Roth M, Newstein D, Guerci AD. Coronary calcification, coronary disease risk factors, C-reactive protein, and atherosclerotic cardiovascular disease events. The St. Francis Heart Study. *J Am Coll Cardiol* 2005; 46:158–165.

4. Lloyd-Jones DM, Larson MG, Leip EP *et al.*; Framingham Heart Study. Lifetime risk for developing congestive heart failure. *Circulation* 2002; 106:3068–3072.

5. Liese AD, Hense HW, Brenner H, Lowel H, Keil U. Assessing the impact of classical risk factors on myocardial infarction by rate advancement periods. *Am J Epidemiol* 2000; 152:884–888.

6. Graham I, Atar D, Borch-Johnsen K *et al.* Fourth Joint Task of European Society of Cardiology and other Societies on Cardiovascular Disease Prevention in Clinical Practice. European Guidelines on Cardiovascular Disease Prevention in Clinical Practice. *Eur J Cardiovasc Prev Rehabil* 2007;14(suppl 2).

7. Third Report of the National Cholesterol Education Program (NCEP). Expert Panel on Detection, Evaluation, and Treatment of High Blood Cholesterol in Adults (Adult Treatment Panel III) final report. *Circulation* 2002; 106:3143–3421.

8. Grundy SM. Coronary plaque as a replacement for age as a risk factor in global risk assessement. *Am J Cardiol* 2001; 88(suppl):E8–E11.

9. Stampfer MJ, Sacks FM, Salvini S, Willett WC, Hennekens CH. A prospective study of cholesterol, apolipoproteins, and the risk of myocardial infarction. *N Engl J Med* 1991; 325:373–381.

10. Kannel WB, Wilson PW. Efficacy of lipid profiles in prediction of coronary disease. *Am Heart J* 1992; 124:768–774.

11. Nam BH, Kannel WB, D'Agostino RB. Search for an optimal atherogenic lipid risk profile: from the Framingham Study. *Am J Cardiol* 2006; 97:372–375.

12. Walldius G, Jungner I, Holme I, Aastveit AH, Kolar W, Steiner E. High apolipoprotein B, low apolipoprotein A-I, and improvement in the prediction of fatal myocardial infarction (AMORIS study): a prospective study. *Lancet* 2001; 358:2026–2033.

13. Yusuf S, Hawken S, Ounpuu S *et al.* Effect of potentially modifiable risk factors associated with myocardial infarction in 52 countries (the INTERHEART study): case-control study. *Lancet* 2004; 364:937–952.

14. Baigent C, Keech A, Kearney PM *et al.* Efficacy and safety of cholesterol-lowering treatment: prospective meta-analysis of data from 90,056 participants in 14 randomised trials of statins. *Lancet* 2005; 366:1267–1278.

15. Sniderman AD, Furberg CD, Keech A *et al.* Apolipoproteins versus lipids as indices of coronary risk and as targets for statin treatment. *Lancet* 2003; 361:777–780.

16. Gotto AM Jr, Whitney E, Stein EA *et al.* Relation between baseline and on-treatment lipid parameters and first acute major coronary events in the Air Force/Texas Coronary Atherosclerosis Prevention Study (AFCAPS/TexCAPS). *Circulation* 2000; 101:477–484.

17. Barter PJ. Cardioprotective effects of high-density lipoproteins: the evidence strengthens. *Arterioscler Thromb Vasc Biol* 2005; 25:1305–1306.

18. Nissen SE, Tsunoda T, Tuzcu EM *et al.* Effect of recombinant ApoA-I Milano on coronary atherosclerosis in patients with acute coronary syndromes: a randomized controlled trial. *JAMA* 2003; 290:2292–2300.

19. Brousseau ME, Schaefer EJ, Wolfe ML *et al.* Effects of an inhibitor of cholesteryl ester transfer protein on HDL cholesterol. *N Engl J Med* 2004; 350:1505–1515.

20. Marenberg ME, Risch N, Berkman LF, Floderus B, de Faire U. Genetic susceptibility to death from coronary heart disease in a study of twins. *N Engl J Med* 1994; 330:1041–1046.

21. Zdravkovic S, Wienke A, Pedersen NL, Marenberg ME, Yashin AI, de Faire U. Heritability of death from coronary heart disease: a 36-year follow-up of 20, 966 Swedish twins. *J Intern Med* 2002; 252:247–254.

22. Brown MS, Goldstein JL. Familial hypercholesterolemia: defective binding of lipoproteins to cultured fibroblasts associated with impaired regulation of 3-hydroxy-3-methylglutaryl coenzyme: a reductase activity. *Proc Natl Acad Sci USA* 1974; 71:788–792.

23. Pimstone SN, Sun XM, du Souich C, Frohlich JJ, Hayden MR, Soutar AK. Phenotypic variation in heterozygous familial hypercholesterolemia: a comparison of Chinese patients with the same or similar mutations in the LDL receptor gene in China or Canada. *Arterioscler Thromb Vasc Biol* 1998; 18:309–315.

24. Damgaard D, Larsen ML, Nissen PH *et al.* The relationship of molecular genetic to clinical diagnosis of familial hypercholesterolemia in a Danish population. *Atherosclerosis* 2005; 180:155–160.

25. Andersen LK, Jensen HK, Juul S, Faergeman O. Patients' attitudes toward detection of heterozygous familial hypercholesterolemia. *Arch Intern Med* 1997; 157:553–560.

26. Raungaard B, Heath F, Brorholt-Petersen JU, Jensen HK, Faergeman O. Flow cytometry with a monoclonal antibody to the low density lipoprotein receptor compared with gene mutation detection in diagnosis of heterozygous familial hypercholesterolemia. *Clin Chem* 1998; 44:966–972.

27. Cambien F, Poirier O, Lecerf L *et al*. Deletion polymorphism in the gene for angiotensin-converting enzyme is a potent risk factor for myocardial infarction. *Nature* 1992; 359:641–644.

28. Agerholm-Larsen B, Nordestgaard BG, Tybjaerg-Hansen A. ACE gene polymorphism in cardiovascular disease: meta-analyses of small and large studies in whites. *Arterioscler Thromb Vasc Biol* 2000; 20:484–492.

29. Keavney B. Common genetic polymorphisms and coronary heart disease. *Semin Vasc Med* 2002; 2:233–241.

30. Schieffer B. ACE gene polymorphism and coronary artery disease: a question of persuasion or statistical confusion? *Arterioscler Thrombo Vasc Biol* 2000; 20:281–282.

5

Management of cardiovascular risk in the older person

C. W. Fan, R. A. Kenny

INTRODUCTION

CHANGING DEMOGRAPHY OF THE POPULATION

As part of the International Year of the Older Persons, Kinsella and Velkoff [1] published a report on 'The Aging World: 2001' which demonstrated the exponential rise in the elderly population worldwide: at a rate of 795 000 each month. Figure 5.1 shows how the age–sex profile will change in the next 50 years towards a greying world and a disproportionate increase in older women. This rapid growth will occur in both the developed and the developing world (Figure 5.2).

Although most developed countries are considered to be demographically the oldest, there are more old people in developing countries and this number is rising. More than half of the world's older people now live in the developing nations (51%, 249 million in year 2000). By 2030, it is projected that 71% (686 million) of older people will be in the developing nations.

THE GLOBAL BURDEN OF CARDIOVASCULAR DISEASE

Cardiovascular disease (CVD) is still one of the leading causes of death globally. The World Health Organization estimated in 2002 that 16.7 million people died from CVD [2]. This accounted for one-third of global deaths. Although the rate of CVD is declining in the developed world, it remains the primary killer amongst older people. Nearly 60% of all deaths in women and 50% of deaths in men aged 60 and over are attributed to CVD [3]. Although atherosclerosis is perceived as a disease of affluent industrialized countries, there is an emerging epidemic in developing countries [4]. Two-thirds of the global cardiovascular and three-quarters of stroke deaths occur in the developing nations [5]. As a disease burden, CVD is now more prevalent in India and China than in developed countries combined.

Statistics from a recent American Heart Association publication clearly demonstrate that CVD burden lies principally with the older person (Figure 5.3). While this condition affects one in three of middle-aged Americans, the prevalence is over 80% in those 75 and older. The scourge of this epidemic needs to be tackled.

Chie Wei Fan, MRCP(I), DME, Lecturer in Medical Gerontology (Trinity College), Falls and Blackout Clinic, St James's Hospital, Dublin, Ireland

Rose Anne Kenny, FRCP(I), FRCP, FESC, Head, Department of Medical Gerontology, Trinity College, Dublin, Director, Falls and Blackout Clinic, St James's Hospital, Dublin, Ireland

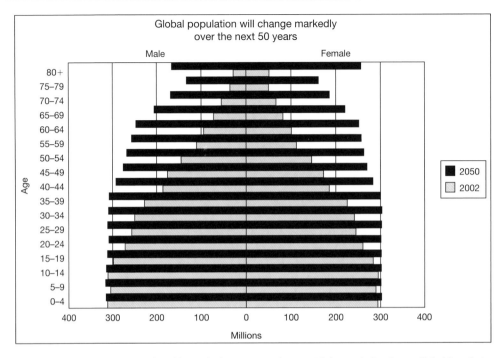

Figure 5.1 Age–sex structure of world population: 2002 and 2050. With permission from: *Global Population at a glance: 2002 and Beyond*. International population report, issued March 2004 by US Census Bureau (International Population Reports No. WP/02-1). US Government Printing Office, Washington DC, 2001.

Source: US Census Bureau, International Programs Center, International Data Base.

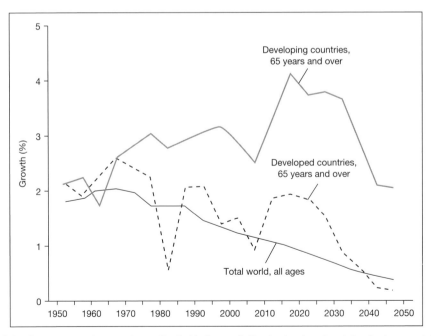

Figure 5.2 Average annual per cent growth of elderly population in developed and developing countries. With permission from reference [1].

Source: United Nations, 1990.

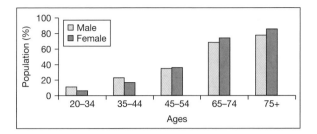

Figure 5.3   Prevalence of CVD in Americans age 20 and older by age and sex. NHANES: 1999–2002. Adapted with permission from: American Heart Association, Live and Learn, CDC/NCHS and NHLBI.

Table 5.1   Morphological and functional pathophysiological changes in the cardiovascular system with ageing

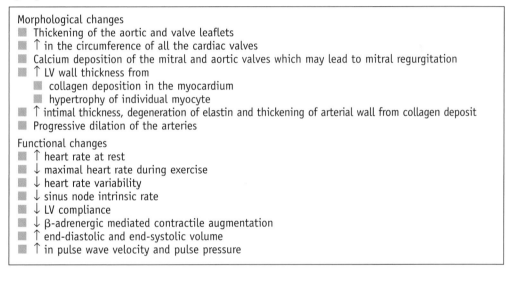

Morphological changes
- Thickening of the aortic and valve leaflets
- ↑ in the circumference of all the cardiac valves
- Calcium deposition of the mitral and aortic valves which may lead to mitral regurgitation
- ↑ LV wall thickness from
  - collagen deposition in the myocardium
  - hypertrophy of individual myocyte
- ↑ intimal thickness, degeneration of elastin and thickening of arterial wall from collagen deposit
- Progressive dilation of the arteries

Functional changes
- ↑ heart rate at rest
- ↓ maximal heart rate during exercise
- ↓ heart rate variability
- ↓ sinus node intrinsic rate
- ↓ LV compliance
- ↓ β-adrenergic mediated contractile augmentation
- ↑ end-diastolic and end-systolic volume
- ↑ in pulse wave velocity and pulse pressure

AGE-RELATED PATHOPHYSIOLOGY OF THE CARDIOVASCULAR SYSTEM

Both morphological and functional pathophysiological changes occur with ageing [6, 7] (Table 5.1). Left ventricular (LV) hypertrophy, diastolic dysfunction, aortic stiffness and conduction defects are characteristic features of the ageing heart.

LEFT VENTRICULAR HYPERTROPHY

LV wall thickness increases due to an accumulation of interstitial connective tissue and amyloid deposits. The consequent loss of myocytes is partly compensated for by hypertrophy of remaining myocytes. Increasing age, hypertension and aortic valve calcification are associated with increased LV mass [8]. LV hypertrophy alters cardiac function and flow dynamics [9]. The enlarged muscle mass reduces the number of coronary capillaries and the ability of the coronary arteries to dilate leaving the myocardium more susceptible to ischaemia and ventricular arrhythmia [10–12].

CARDIAC OUTPUT AND DIASTOLIC DYSFUNCTION

LV function is usually preserved in the absence of coronary heart disease (CHD) or hypertension. Diastolic dysfunction, however, is more prevalent because the ventricles become less compliant with hypertrophy. There is also a decline in the rate and volume of diastolic filling. The heart consequently relies on atrial contraction to maintain cardiac filling during diastole. Atrial fibrillation (AF) can therefore adversely affect cardiac output.

CARDIAC CONDUCTING SYSTEM

Age-related pathological changes in the cardiac conduction systems predispose to tachyarrhythmia and bradyarrhythmias. By 75 years, only 10% of cells in the sino-atrial node remain intact due to an increase in fibrous tissue deposition within the internodal tracts thereby predisposing the older person to AF and sino-atrial and ventricular arrhythmia. A prevalence study in the UK detected AF in 10% of those 75 years and older [13] (*see* Table 5.3). First degree atrioventricular (AV) block affects 1 in 1000 people over 40 years old [14]. This condition is benign and is also prevalent in 8% of trained athletes and medical students [15]. A study in centenarians found that they were more likely to have more first and second degree AV block compared to persons in their seventies (25% vs. 1%) [16]. Second and third degree AV blocks are more sinister and can result in dizziness, falls and syncope [17–19].

CORONARY STENOSIS

With advancing years, coronary atherosclerosis becomes more prevalent. Fifty per cent of elderly women and 80% of elderly men have obstructive coronary artery disease on postmortem [20]. In one post-mortem study of patients 90 years of age and over, 70% had one or more coronary arteries occluded [21].

AORTIC SCLEROSIS AND STENOSIS

Aortic sclerosis and stenosis also occur more commonly. Aortic valve sclerosis is present in 30% of individuals aged 65 and older and in 50% of those aged 85 and older. Aortic sclerosis is not a benign condition as the risk of overall cardiovascular mortality and myocardial infarction (MI) is increased [22, 23].

AORTIC STIFFNESS

During normal ventricular contraction, the pulse wave travels along the length of the aorta and is reflected from the periphery back to the heart during diastole. The reflected pressure augments blood pressure (BP) during diastole and aids coronary blood flow. Age-related structural changes within the arterial system cause a gradual stiffening of the vasculature and consequent increase in pressure wave velocity as it travels down the aorta. The reflected wave returns more rapidly to the heart during systole and augments systolic BP. This asynchrony of the reflected wave reduces coronary filling and exacerbates myocardial ischaemia.

   Aortic stiffness is associated with higher cardiac mortality in high-risk groups such as older hypertensives [24] and persons with end-stage renal failure [25]. Furthermore, subjects with essential hypertension and aortic stiffness are more likely to have primary coronary events [26] and fatal strokes [27]. Even among well-functioning older persons of 70–79 years, aortic stiffness is a risk factor for CHD and strokes [28].

   Aortic stiffness is evident from an increase in pulse pressure. The widened pulse pressure eventually progresses to isolated systolic hypertension which affects 30% of adults by the

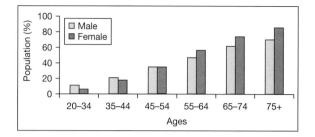

Figure 5.4 Prevalence of hypertension in Americans by age and sex. NHANES: 1999–2002. Adapted with permission from: American Heart Association, Live and Learn, CDC/NCHS and NHLBI.

time they reach 80 years [29]. A 10 mmHg increment in pulse pressure is associated with a 12% increase in CHD, heart failure and overall mortality [30].

RISK FACTORS

The following section focuses on cardiovascular risk factors pertinent to the older population.

HYPERTENSION

One in three adults in the US has hypertension [31]. The risk of hypertension rises with age in keeping with age-related changes in the vasculature. The prevalence increases exponentially from 34% of persons aged 45–54 to over 70% amongst those 75 years and older (Figure 5.4). The Third National Health and Nutrition Examination Study (NHANES) III survey showed an almost linear relationship between systolic/diastolic BP and age from adult life to age 65 [32]. Isolated systolic hypertension is the predominant hypertension in the older person [33]. The association between hypertension and CVD such as CHD, strokes, heart failure and renal failure is well-established. The risk of stroke increases exponentially above BP levels of 115/75 mmHg and doubles with every increment of 20/10 mmHg [34]. Almost two-thirds of stroke worldwide is attributed to sub-optimal control of BP.

Despite the high prevalence of hypertension in the older age group, a meta-analysis by Staessen *et al.* [35] showed that only 13% of subjects in the trials were 80 years and over. Studies which focused on older participants such as the Systolic Hypertension in the Elderly Programme (SHEP) [36], the Medical Research Council (MRC) working group on hypertension [37] and the European working group on systolic hypertension (Syst-Eur) [38] consistently showed that treatment of BP reduced stroke and coronary events. By controlling systolic hypertension, the SHEP study [36] reported a reduction in MI (27%), major cardiovascular events (32%) and all-cause mortality (13%). The MRC working group on hypertension [37] also reported reductions in stroke, coronary event and all cardiovascular events by 25%, 19% and 17%, respectively, by optimizing treatment of hypertension in older patients.

A recent meta-analysis by Lawes *et al.* [39], however, discovered that older people had attenuation of risk reduction with increasing age (50% risk reduction in those <60 years vs. 30% in those >70 years), the reason for which is unclear. However, given the higher stroke rates amongst older people, risk reduction in this group is still significant in absolute numbers.

BP lowering apart from stroke reduction has an added benefit of causing LV regression particularly when using angiotensin receptor or calcium channel blockers. LV regression is associated with reducing CHD events [40, 41].

The Seventh Report of the Joint National Committee on Prevention, Detection, Evaluation, and Treatment of High Blood Pressure (JNC 7) recommends the target BP of <149/90 mmHg or <130/80 mmHg for those with diabetes or kidney disease [34]. Despite the message of aggressive BP lowering, caution is important when managing the older patient. Frail older persons may not be able to tolerate the recommended target BP. Paradoxically, low BP in the elderly is associated with increased mortality within 3 years of diagnosis [42]. Gait and balance impairment are common findings amongst older persons. One in three community-dwelling older people fall at least once a year [43]. Orthostatic hypotension is a well-recognized cause of falls and syncope. Coupled with common comorbidity such as orthostatic hypotension (22–60%) [44, 45], carotid sinus hypersensitivity (39%) [46] and gait and balance impairment, excessive BP lowering may exacerbate the risk of falls. When monitoring BP in older persons, we recommend lying and standing BP measurement in order to capture orthostatic hypotension.

Hypertension is common amongst older people and should be managed with caution in this age group.

HYPERCHOLESTEROLAEMIA

Low-density lipoprotein (LDL) causes atherosclerosis. The association between raised LDL and CHD is recognized from several epidemiological studies [47–49]. The Framingham Heart Study found that the relative risk of developing symptomatic heart disease is increased 1.5 times in men and 2.3 times in women when the serum cholesterol is greater than 5.2 mmol/l [47]. Raised high-density lipoprotein cholesterol (HDL-c) concentration, on the other hand, confers protection against cardiovascular events in those over 65 years [49].

In population studies mean cholesterol levels fall with advancing years [50]: serum cholesterol is 5.0 mmol/l in the 71–74 age group and 4.6 mmol/l in persons over 85. The relationship of cholesterol level to mortality in older persons is also noteworthy. Two regional studies, in Honolulu [50] and Italy [51], reported that subjects at the lowest quartile of cholesterol level (2.1–4.3 mmol/l) had the highest age-adjusted mortality. Casiglia *et al.* [51] also found that all-cause mortality, in particular neoplastic mortality, increased when serum cholesterol fell below 5.1 mmol/l. Schatz *et al.* [50] suggested that the decline in serum cholesterol occurred before the diagnosis of inflammatory or neoplastic disease. Low serum cholesterol was also associated with low body mass index, weight loss and inflammatory markers which all point to poor health [52].

Many of the lipid-lowering studies included older subjects [49, 53–56]. For instance, in the Scandinavian Simvastatin Survival Study (4S) [53], in which a quarter of participants were over 65 years, there was a reduction in all-cause mortality (34%), major coronary events (34%) and requirement for revascularization procedures (41%) regardless of age. Furthermore, during long-term follow-up (8 years) survival was greater in the treatment group (88.5% vs. 84.1%) [57]. The Heart Protection Study, which recruited 20 536 UK adults aged between 40 and 80 years old, reported reductions in mortality from all-cause as well as first-ever cardiac event and revascularization by a quarter. The effects were present regardless of baseline LDL level and in all subgroups, including women and the elderly [58].

Another study, the Prospective Study of Pravastatin in the Elderly at Risk (PROSPER) trial [55], specifically recruited elderly subjects at risk of CHD. The inclusion criteria were subjects aged 70–82 with either pre-existing vascular disease or at least one major vascular risk factor (hypertension, cigarette smoking, or diabetes mellitus). Major coronary events were reduced by 19%, CHD mortality by 24% and transient ischaemic attacks by 25% at the conclusion of the study at 3 years. There was, however, no reduction in stroke. The investigator found a lower stroke rate, half of that predicted. The investigators suggested that the absence of benefit on stroke could be a consequence of a lack of statistical power and the short duration of the study. Stroke benefit from statin does not appear until after 3 years whereas coronary disease benefit appears earlier. Nevertheless, elderly people should be prescribed LDL-c lowering medications.

Low cholesterol in the older person is a marker of frailty and poor outcome. But as with younger persons, hypercholesterolaemia increases CVD. Lipid-lowering regimens in studies that recruited older subjects confirm that treatment lowers CVD burden and mortality.

Table 5.2 The traditional and new risk factors for predicting CVD

Traditional	New
Sex (men>women)	High-normal BP
Age	Metabolic syndrome
Family history of premature CVD	Diabetes mellitus; impaired glucose tolerance; impaired fasting glucose
Total cholesterol	Apolipoprotein B; apolipoprotein A-1
Hypertension	Triglyceride; triglyceride-rich lipoprotein remnants
Smoking	Homocysteine
Overweight/obesity	High-sensitivity CRP

Adapted with permission from reference [63].

SMOKING

Older people tend to smoke less than younger counterparts. UK data from 2003 showed a peak in those between 20 and 35 years old (*see* Figure 5.5) which declined thereafter. Fewer than one in five persons older than 60 years smoke in the UK (16% of men and 14% of women) [59]. This trend reflects the number of men and women over the age of 35 who give up smoking. Nevertheless smoking is a significant cardiovascular risk. In the Framingham Heart Study [60], the number of cigarettes smoked was proportional to the risk of stroke. Relative risk of stroke in heavy smokers (more than 40 cigarettes a day) was twice that of light smokers (fewer than 10 cigarettes a day). In the presence of hypertension, the SHEP trial, where subjects had a mean age of 72 years, also reported a 73% increased risk of CHD in current smokers compared with non-smokers [36].

Stroke risk, however, decreased significantly 2 years after cessation and reached the level of a non-smoker within 5 years of abstinence [60]. A 60-year-old smoker can gain at least 3 years of life expectancy by stopping [61]. Verbal advice when given by medical professions is the most effective intervention in smoking cessation. When Op Reimer *et al.* [62] examined smoking cessation as part of the European Action on Secondary Prevention through Intervention to Reduce Events (EUROASPIRE) survey, more than half of those aged 60 years and over stopped smoking after verbal advice. Therefore, smoking cessation should be strongly encouraged even with advancing years.

NEW RISK FACTORS

Reports of newer risk factors are emerging; it is the composite of traditional and newer risk factors that forms a global risk profile which allows better predictions than a single risk factor [63]. The newer risk factors are metabolic factors such as impaired glucose tolerance/impaired fasting glucose (IGT/IFG), plasma homocysteine level, thrombogenic/haemostatic factors (fibrinogen) and inflammatory markers [63]. For instance, the Framingham Offspring Study (subjects aged 31–73 years) showed that, compared with those with normal glucose tolerance, subjects with IGT/IFG were more likely to have subclinical coronary atherosclerosis [64]. Table 5.2 outlines the newer risk factors although some of the newer risk factors were studied in middle-aged subjects only.

HYPERHOMOCYSTEINAEMIA

Plasma total homocysteine level increases throughout life in both sexes and is consistent across various population groups [65–67]. From age 4 to 10 years, total homocysteine levels are similar between boys and girls. The levels diverge after age 10 and increase during adolescence. At age 4, the mean homocysteine level is 4.4 μmol/l. By 19 years old, boys have higher levels than girls (8.3 μmol/l vs. 6.9 μmol/l). At middle-age (forties), the mean values for men and women are 11 μmol/l and 9 μmol/l, respectively. After the menopause, the gender-related differences in homocysteine levels diminish [65].

Plasma homocysteine level is affected by diet and genetic factors. Deficiency in dietary folic acid and Vitamin B6 and B12 can result in a higher serum level. Elevated plasma homocysteine level (>14 μmol/l) is strongly associated with atherosclerotic and thromboembolic events [68–70].

People with high homocysteine levels are at increased risk of stroke [71, 72], heart disease, Alzheimer's disease (AD) [73], cognitive deficits [74], brain atrophy [75] and CVD mortality in elderly men and women [76]. The Framingham Heart Study investigators reported a doubled risk of dementia when plasma homocysteine level is greater than 14 μmol/l [77]. Cognitive decline associated with hyperhomocysteinaemia is more pronounced in persons aged 60 years and older [78]. For every 1 μmol/l increase in homocysteine level, the risk of MI and stroke increases 6–7-fold [79]. The risk is higher in the presence of hypertension.

Ford et al. [80] carried out a systematic review and meta-analysis on the role of homocysteine in CVD. The odds ratio for a 5-μmol/l increase in homocysteine concentration was up to 1.7 for CVD and up to 2.16 for stroke. Therefore, raised homocysteine concentration is associated with coronary heart and cerebrovascular disease.

C-REACTIVE PROTEIN, INTERLEUKIN 6 AND FIBRINOGEN

C-reactive protein (CRP), interleukin (IL)-6 and fibrinogen are useful markers for CVD pathology. The ageing process is associated with a 2–4-fold increase in serum inflammatory markers [81]. Elevated high-sensitive CRP (hs-CRP) is associated with increased coronary risk. In the Cardiovascular Health Study the 10-year cumulative CHD incidence was raised at 33% for men and 17% for women when hs-CRP levels were elevated [82]. Raised CRP and IL-6 were also associated with increased CVD risk amongst community-living older persons [83] and persons who were not previously diagnosed with CHD [84]. Lower CRP levels after statin treatment were associated with better clinical outcomes regardless of LDL levels [85].

Fibrinogen is a thrombogenic marker. In a meta-analysis, Danesh et al. [86] found that for each g/l increase in usual fibrinogen level, the age- and sex-adjusted mortality increased at least 2-fold for CHD, stroke and other vascular mortality. Raised fibrinogen was also associated with a 2-fold increase in non-vascular mortality. These findings were consistent across the age range from 40 to over 70 years old.

Homocysteine and inflammatory markers are emerging as useful predictors either alone or in combination with traditional risk factors for CVD in older persons.

UNDER-TREATMENT AND INVESTIGATIONS OF RISK FACTORS IN THE ELDERLY

There is a perception of under-investigation and under-treatment of risk factors in the older person. This is borne out by a recent US report which revealed that only 38% of men and 23% of women over 80 years old met target BP when on treatment [31]. Ghosh et al. [87] and Mendelson and Aronow [88] reported consistent under-treatment of cardiovascular risk factors in older persons in the US. The reason for this is unclear but it may be that physicians are wary of adverse events such as orthostatic hypotension in older persons.

The Prospective Registry of Acute Ischaemic Syndromes in the UK (PRAIS-UK) [89] also reported that younger patients were more likely to receive appropriate treatment for acute coronary syndrome. Older patients had significantly lower rates of angiography (36.4% vs. 5.0%) and revascularization (18.9% vs. 3.4%) following acute coronary syndrome.

Implementation of secondary prevention in the UK for cardiovascular risk factors is also deficient in older persons. Ramsay *et al.* [90] reported that older patients (74–85 years) were 60% less likely to receive a statin compared with younger patients. Another study found that two-thirds of older patients (aged 70 and over) with LV dysfunction on echocardiogram were not on angiotensin-converting enzyme inhibitors and only 41% with AF were prescribed antithrombotic therapy [91].

RISK STRATIFICATION AND CARDIOVASCULAR RISK SCORES

The two popular cardiovascular risk scores, the Framingham risk function [92] and the Systematic Coronary Risk Evaluation (SCORE) risk [93] are useful only for those aged under 79 (Framingham risk function) and under 65 (SCORE).

Framingham risk function [47] predicts the 10-year risk of a major coronary heart event in subjects up to 79 years. The equation is based on age (in 5-year age bands), sex, cigarette smoking status, diabetes status, and BP, cholesterol and HDL cholesterol levels only. However the risk function was derived from a homogeneous population. Consequently, population studies from Germany, China and Britain have found overestimations of coronary events using this risk function [92, 94–96]. Recalibration can adjust for these differences, especially if hard endpoints are used.

The SCORE risk project differentiates between high- and low-risk populations by country. The low-risk chart is used in Belgium, France, Greece, Italy, Luxembourg, Spain, Switzerland and Portugal while the high-risk chart applies to the remainder of participating European countries. Conroy *et al.* [93] calculated the 10-year risk of fatal CVD from the gender, age, smoking status, systolic BP and total from high-risk and low-risk countries. This was derived from 12 European cohort studies involving 250 000 patients' data with 3 million person-years' follow-up. The risk estimations were performed for only those aged under 65.

Given the prevalent cardiovascular risk factors and age-related pathophysiological changes, it may well be that risk stratification does not apply to older persons. One approach [13] is to consider older persons as automatically being in a high-risk category and stratify as such. Further studies of risk stratification in the oldest old are necessary.

CARDIOVASCULAR DISEASE IN THE ELDERLY

ACUTE CORONARY SYNDROME, STROKE AND HEART FAILURE

The presentation of CVD in the elderly can be atypical [97]; for example, cerebral vascular disease may present as falls, poor mobility or cognitive decline. Lack of physical activity and atypical clinical presentation (vague and poorly localized chest symptoms, tiredness, fatigue or breathlessness) could partly explain under-detection of CHD amongst older people. The tendency for under-investigation of older persons further contributes to low detection rates *in vivo* [98].

While the prevalence of smoking declines with age (Figure 5.5), acute coronary syndrome, stroke and heart failure occur with increasing frequency with age (Figures 5.6–5.8). Between 1987 and 2000 in the US, older persons (65+) accounted for two-thirds of MI in the US (Figure 5.6).

Stroke, symptomatic or silent, is predominantly a disease in those over 65 (Figure 5.7). A longitudinal study (Cardiovascular Health Study) in 65-year-olds found that 89% of the cerebral infarcts were asymptomatic [99]. The prevalence of silent cerebral infarcts increased with age and is associated with cognitive decline [100]. The prevalence of silent infarct in persons aged 55–64 years was 11%, 65–69 years (22%), 70–74 years (28%), 75–79 years (32%), 80–85 years (40%), and over 85 years (43%).

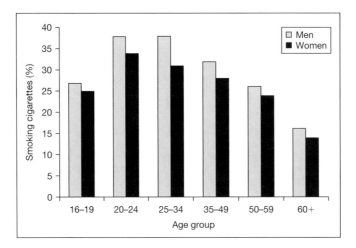

Figure 5.5 Prevalence of cigarette smoking by sex and age in 2003, Great Britain. With permission from reference [59].

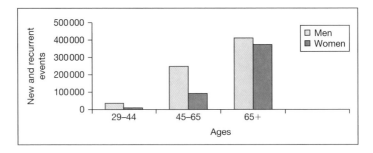

Figure 5.6 Myocardial infarction in Americans by age and sex. Adapted with permission from: American Heart Association, Live and Learn, CDC/NCHS and NHLBI.

The lifetime risk of developing heart failure is 1 in 9 in men and 1 in 6 in women without preceding MI [101]. The risk doubles to 1 in 5 in the presence of hypertension. Heart failure is a disease of the old and only affects 17% of patients younger than 65 [102]. The prevalence rises from 1% of persons in their fifties to 10% of those over 80 years [103]. Figure 5.8 shows the increasing prevalence of heart failure with age in the UK and US. Heart failure is a malignant condition where the annual mortality of those in the New York Heart Association classification of grades III and IV approaches 50% [104]. Diastolic heart failure is also common amongst older people. The Helsinki Ageing Study [105] found that up to 51% of patients aged 80 and older had preserved systolic function despite having symptomatic heart failure. Another UK community study revealed that diastolic heart failure affected 5.54% of patients aged 70 and older [106].

ATRIAL FIBRILLATION

AF, often a sequela of CHD, also increases with age and 5% of those aged 65 and older have this condition [107]. The lifetime risk of developing AF is 1 in 4 [108]. The American Heart Association statistics update in 2006 reported that the mean ages of men and women with AF were 66.8 years and 74.6, respectively [31]. Table 5.3 illustrates the prevalence rates across several regions in the UK and US.

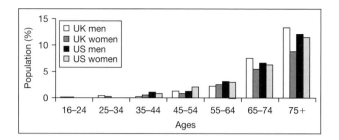

Figure 5.7 Prevalence of stroke in adults aged 20 and over by age, sex and region. Adapted with permission from: UK statistics: Coronary Heart Disease Statistics 2005 edition, British Heart Foundation Health Promotion Research Group; US Statistics: NHANES: 1999–2002, CDC/NCHS and NHLBI.

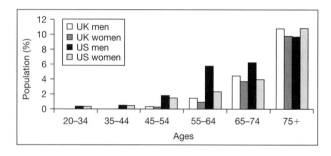

Figure 5.8 Prevalence of heart failure by age, sex and region. Adapted with permission from: UK statistics: Coronary Heart Disease Statistics 2005 edition, British Heart Foundation Health Promotion Research Group; US Statistics: NHANES: 1999–2002, CDC/NCHS and NHLBI.

END-STAGE RENAL DISEASE

End-stage renal disease is closely linked to hypertension and the incidence has doubled in the past 10 years. As the prevalence of hypertension increases with age, the group with the highest incidence and prevalence rates is those over 70 years old [31].

DEMENTIA

Cardiovascular risk factors (CVRF) are increasingly important in the investigation and diagnosis of dementia. The prevalence of dementia doubles every 5 years from age 65 [109, 110]. Figure 5.9 is an example of the prevalence in two population studies. It is estimated that 24.3 million people worldwide had dementia in 2005 and 4.6 million new cases are diagnosed every year [111].

The three main types of dementia are AD, vascular dementia (VaD) and Diffuse Lewy body dementia (DLB) and overlap between the three subtypes is common [112]. AD and VaD pathology coexists in 24–28% of cases [113, 114]. In fact, vascular lesions compound the severity of dementia in AD. Vascular pathology also contributes to cognitive decline in AD [115]. A major epidemiological study (the Nun study) [116, 117] found that persons with cerebral infarcts required 8 times less neurofibrillary tangles to achieve the same dementia severity when compared with those without infarcts.

The cardiovascular risk factors of dementia are diabetes mellitus, stroke disease, high cholesterol, thrombogenic factor, apoF4, high serum homocysteine, high fibrinogen levels,

Table 5.3   Prevalence of atrial fibrillation in adults aged 40 years and over as a percentage of population

Age	Over 40	50–59		60–69		75+		80+
		M	F	M	F	M	F	
Framingham [107]	–	0.5	–	1.8	–	–	–	8.8**
Feinberg [129]	2–3	–	–	5.9*	–	–	–	10.0
Renfrew Paisley [130]	–	0.72	0.29	1.02	0.74	–	–	–
Southern Northumberland [13]	–	–	–	4.7*	–	10.0	5.6	–
SAFE [131]	–	–	–	7.2*	–	–	–	–

*Aged 65 and over.

**Aged 80–89 years.

SAFE = Screening for Atrial Fibrillation in the Elderly (Birmingham).

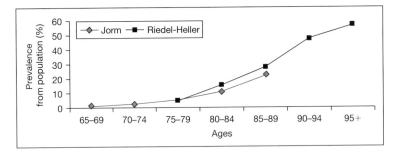

Figure 5.9   Prevalence of dementia from two population studies [109, 110].

hypertension, and hypotension. Luchsinger *et al.* [118] reported that the aggregation of multiple vascular risk factors (diabetes, hypertension, heart disease and current smoking) increases the risk of AD by more than 3 times. A longitudinal cohort study in the US found that subjects with prevalent CVD were 1.3 times more likely to develop dementia. Those with extensive peripheral atherosclerosis were at a higher risk (2.4 times) [119]. Furthermore, arterial stiffness [120] and raised fibrinogen levels [121] are also linked to cognitive decline. Those with cardiovascular risk factors in mid-life (40–44 years) were 20–40% more likely to develop dementia in late-life [122].

Neuropathology
Long-standing hypertension results in thickening of the vessel walls through lypolyalinosis in the media and the narrowing of the lumen of the blood vessels. The small perforating arteries in the brain that nourish the deep white matter are similarly affected. Any compromise to cerebral perfusion can result in small infarcts [123]. These infarcts are shown up as deep white matter hyperdensities (DWMH) under fluid-attenuated inversion recovery (FLAIR) sequences on magnetic resonance imaging (MRI). The volume of DWMH correlates with the degree of episodic hypotension [124]. Matsushita found that DWMH matched the degree of drop in systolic BP [125]. These hyperintensities are areas of underlying infarcts within the deep white matter [126]. Even in the absence of dementia, the burden of hyperintensity correlates with poorer attention and processing speed tasks during

neuropsychological testing amongst stroke survivors [127]. Neuro-imaging and neuro-pathological studies of cross-sectional design suggest that diffuse white matter changes, microvascular disease and hippocampal atrophy are the main predictors of dementia in vascular cognitive impairment [124, 128].

Hypoperfusion occurring in isolation or as a consequence of hypertension or atherosclerosis, may play a key role in dementia either as a trigger or accelerator of pathological or cognitive decline. In the effort to control cardiovascular risk factors, one needs to caution against excessive hypotension.

SUMMARY

In conclusion, the burden of CVD lies with the older population. This is a growing issue even in the developing world. It is therefore imperative that risk predictions and modifications of CHD in the older person be considered when we promote successful ageing. Clearly, there is a need to invest in services required to manage CVD in this population. There are pertinent issues such as comorbidity and frailty when we manage risk factors in the elderly. Episodic hypotension, as part of the CHD spectrum, may contribute to progressive cognitive dysfunction in the elderly. An interesting area of research is cardiovascular risk factors for dementia and the underlying mechanism and pathophysiology. An encouraging sign is that more studies are inclusive of older subjects. This trend will enable better risk predictions and management of CVD in older people.

REFERENCES

1. Kinsella K, Velkoff VA. An Aging World: 2001. U.S. Census Bureau, Series P95/01-1, US Government Printing Office, Washington, 2001, p 16.
2. International Cardiovascular Disease Statistics. American Heart Association [cited 8/2/2006]; Available from: http://www.americanheart.org/downloadable/heart/1140811583642International CVD.pdf
3. Murray CJ, Lopez AD. Mortality by cause for eight regions of the world: Global Burden of Disease Study. *Lancet* 1997; 349:1269–1276.
4. Reddy KS, Yusuf S. Emerging epidemic of cardiovascular disease in developing countries. *Circulation* 1998; 97:596–601.
5. Truelsen T, Bonita R, Jamrozik K. Surveillance of stroke: a global perspective. *Int J Epidemiol* 2001; 30:S11–S16.
6. Hickey P. Ageing Cardiovascular System [cited 25/1/2006]; Available from: http://www.jr2.ox.ac.uk/geratol/doccard.htm
7. Lye M, Donnellan C. Heart disease in the elderly. *Heart* 2000; 84:560–566.
8. Lindroos M, Kupari M, Valvanne J, Strandberg T, Heikkila J, Tilvis R. Factors associated with calcific aortic valve degeneration in the elderly. *Eur Heart J* 1994; 15:865–870.
9. Lindroos M, Kupari M, Heikkila J, Tilvis R. Predictors of left ventricular mass in old age: an echocardiographic, clinical and biochemical investigation of a random population sample. *Eur Heart J* 1994; 15:769–780.
10. Dellsperger KC, Marcus ML. Effects of left ventricular hypertrophy on the coronary circulation. *Am J Cardiol* 1990; 65:1504–1510.
11. Polese A, De Cesare N, Montorsi P *et al.* Upward shift of the lower range of coronary flow autoregulation in hypertensive patients with hypertrophy of the left ventricle. *Circulation* 1991; 83:845–853.
12. Singh JP, Johnston J, Sleight P, Bird R, Ryder K, Hart G. Left ventricular hypertrophy in hypertensive patients is associated with abnormal rate adaptation of QT interval. *J Am Coll Cardiol* 1997; 29:778–784.
13. Sudlow M, Thomson R, Thwaites B, Rodgers H, Kenny RA. Prevalence of atrial fibrillation and eligibility for anticoagulants in the community. *Lancet* 1998; 352:1167–1171.
14. Mymin D, Mathewson FA, Tate RB, Manfreda J. The natural history of primary first-degree atrioventricular heart block. *N Engl J Med* 1986; 315:1183–1187.
15. Bexton RS, Camm AJ. First degree atrioventricular block. *Eur Heart J* 1984; 5(suppl A):107–109.

16. Wakida Y, Okamoto Y, Iwa T *et al.* Arrhythmias in centenarians. *Pacing Clin Electrophysiol* 1994; 17(Pt 2):2217–2221.

17. Bexton RS, Camm AJ. Second degree atrioventricular block. *Eur Heart J* 1984; 5(suppl A):111–114.

18. Rowland E, Morgado F. Sino-atrial node dysfunction, atrioventricular block and intraventricular conduction disturbances. *Eur Heart J* 1992; 13(suppl H):130–135.

19. Seifer C, Kenny RA. The prevalence of falls in older persons paced for atrioventricular block and sick sinus syndrome. *Am J Geriatr Cardiol* 2003; 12:298–301; quiz 304–305.

20. Wenger NK. Cardiovascular Disease in the Octogenarian and Beyond. Martin Dunitz Ltd, London, 1999.

21. Waller BF, Roberts WC. Cardiovascular disease in the very elderly. Analysis of 40 necropsy patients aged 90 years or over. *Am J Cardiol* 1983; 51:403–421.

22. Otto CM, Lind BK, Kitzman DW, Gersh BJ, Siscovick DS. Association of aortic-valve sclerosis with cardiovascular mortality and morbidity in the elderly. *N Engl J Med* 1999; 341:142–147.

23. Lindroos M, Kupari M, Heikkila J, Tilvis R. Prevalence of aortic valve abnormalities in the elderly: an echocardiographic study of a random population sample. *J Am Coll Cardiol* 1993; 21:1220–1225.

24. Laurent S, Boutouyrie P, Asmar R *et al.* Aortic stiffness is an independent predictor of all-cause and cardiovascular mortality in hypertensive patients. *Hypertension* 2001; 37:1236–1241.

25. Covic A, Haydar AA, Bhamra-Ariza P, Gusbeth-Tatomir P, Goldsmith DJ. Aortic pulse wave velocity and arterial wave reflections predict the extent and severity of coronary artery disease in chronic kidney disease patients. *J Nephrol* 2005; 18:388–396.

26. Boutouyrie P, Tropeano AI, Asmar R *et al.* Aortic stiffness is an independent predictor of primary coronary events in hypertensive patients: a longitudinal study. *Hypertension* 2002; 39:10–15.

27. Laurent S, Katsahian S, Fassot C *et al.* Aortic stiffness is an independent predictor of fatal stroke in essential hypertension. *Stroke* 2003; 34:1203–1206.

28. Sutton-Tyrrell K, Najjar SS, Boudreau RM *et al.* Elevated aortic pulse wave velocity, a marker of arterial stiffness, predicts cardiovascular events in well-functioning older adults. *Circulation* 2005; 111:3384–3390.

29. Staessen J, Amery A, Fagard R. Isolated systolic hypertension in the elderly. *J Hypertens* 1990; 8:393–405.

30. Vaccarino V, Berger AK, Abramson J *et al.* Pulse pressure and risk of cardiovascular events in the systolic hypertension in the elderly program. *Am J Cardiol* 2001; 88:980–986.

31. Writing Group members, Thom T, Haase N *et al.* Heart disease and stroke statistics – 2006 update. A Report from the American Heart Association Statistics Committee and Stroke Statistics Subcommittee. *Circulation* 2006:CIRCULATIONAHA.105.171600.

32. Burt VL, Cutler JA, Higgins M *et al.* Trends in the prevalence, awareness, treatment, and control of hypertension in the adult US population: data from the health examination surveys, 1960 to 1991. *Hypertension* 1995; 26:60–69.

33. Ekpo EB, Ashworth IN, Fernando MU, White AD, Shah IU. Prevalence of mixed hypertension, isolated systolic hypertension and isolated diastolic hypertension in the elderly population in the community. *J Hum Hypertens* 1994; 8:39–43.

34. Chobanian AV, Bakris GL, Black HR *et al.* The Seventh Report of the Joint National Committee on Prevention, Detection, Evaluation, and Treatment of High Blood Pressure: The JNC 7 Report. *JAMA* 2003; 289:2560–2571.

35. Staessen JA, Gasowski J, Wang JG *et al.* Risks of untreated and treated isolated systolic hypertension in the elderly: meta-analysis of outcome trials. *Lancet* 2000; 355:865–872.

36. SHEP Cooperative Research Group. Prevention of stroke by antihypertensive drug treatment in older persons with isolated systolic hypertension. Final results of the Systolic Hypertension in the Elderly Program (SHEP). *JAMA* 1991; 265:3255–3264.

37. MRC Working Party. Medical Research Council trial of treatment of hypertension in older adults: principal results. *BMJ* 1992; 304:405–412.

38. Staessen JA, Fagard R, Thijs L *et al.* Randomised double-blind comparison of placebo and active treatment for older patients with isolated systolic hypertension. The Systolic Hypertension in Europe (Syst-Eur) Trial Investigators. *Lancet* 1997; 350:757–764.

39. Lawes CM, Bennett DA, Feigin VL, Rodgers A. Blood pressure and stroke: an overview of published reviews. *Stroke* 2004; 35:776–785.

40. Kloner RA, Sowers JR, DiBona GF, Gaffney M, Wein M. Effect of amlodipine on left ventricular mass in the Amlodipine Cardiovascular Community Trial. *J Cardiovasc Pharmacol* 1995; 26:471–476.

41. Devereux RB, Dahlof B, Gerdts E *et al*. Regression of hypertensive left ventricular hypertrophy by losartan compared with atenolol: the Losartan Intervention for Endpoint Reduction in Hypertension (LIFE) trial. *Circulation* 2004; 110:1456–1462.

42. Glynn RJ, Field TS, Rosner B, Hebert PR, Taylor JO, Hennekens CH. Evidence for a positive linear relation between blood pressure and mortality in elderly people. *Lancet* 1995; 345:825–829.

43. Blake AJ, Morgan K, Bendall MJ *et al*. Falls by elderly people at home: prevalence and associated factors. *Age Ageing* 1988; 17:365–372.

44. Luukinen H, Koski K, Laippala P, Kivela SL. Prognosis of diastolic and systolic orthostatic hypotension in older persons. *Arch Intern Med* 1999; 159:273–280.

45. Mulcahy R, Jackson SH, Richardson DA, Lee DR, Kenny RA. Circadian and orthostatic blood pressure is abnormal in the carotid sinus syndrome. *Am J Geriatr Cardiol* 2003; 12:288–292, 301.

46. McIntosh SJ, Lawson J, Kenny RA. Clinical characteristics of vasodepressor, cardioinhibitory, and mixed carotid sinus syndrome in the elderly. *Am J Med* 1993; 95:203–208.

47. Kannel WB, McGee D, Gordon T. A general cardiovascular risk profile: the Framingham Study. *Am J Cardiol* 1976; 38:46–51.

48. Keys A, Menotti A, Aravanis C *et al*. The seven countries study: 2,289 deaths in 15 years. *Prev Med* 1984; 13:141–154.

49. Psaty BM, Anderson M, Kronmal RA *et al*. The association between lipid levels and the risks of incident myocardial infarction, stroke, and total mortality: The Cardiovascular Health Study. *J Am Geriatr Soc* 2004; 52:1639–1647.

50. Schatz IJ, Masaki K, Yano K, Chen R, Rodriguez BL, Curb JD. Cholesterol and all-cause mortality in elderly people from the Honolulu Heart Program: a cohort study. *Lancet* 2001; 358:351–355.

51. Casiglia E, Mazza A, Tikhonoff V, Scarpa R, Schiavon L, Pessina AC. Total cholesterol and mortality in the elderly. *J Intern Med* 2003; 254:353–362.

52. Schalk BWM, Visser M, Deeg DJH, Bouter LM. Lower levels of serum albumin and total cholesterol and future decline in functional performance in older persons: the Longitudinal Aging Study Amsterdam. *Age Ageing* 2004; 33:266–272.

53. Miettinen TA, Pyörälä K, Olsson AG *et al*. Cholesterol-lowering therapy in women and elderly patients with myocardial infarction or angina pectoris: findings from the Scandinavian Simvastatin Survival Study (4S). *Circulation* 1997; 96:4211–4218.

54. MRC/BHF Heart Protection Study of cholesterol lowering with simvastatin in 20,536 high-risk individuals: a randomised placebo-controlled trial. *Lancet* 2002; 360:7–22.

55. Shepherd J, Blauw GJ, Murphy MB *et al*. Pravastatin in elderly individuals at risk of vascular disease (PROSPER): a randomised controlled trial. *Lancet* 2002; 360:1623–1630.

56. Sever PS, Dahlof B, Poulter NR *et al*. Prevention of coronary and stroke events with atorvastatin in hypertensive patients who have average or lower-than-average cholesterol concentrations, in the Anglo-Scandinavian Cardiac Outcomes Trial – Lipid Lowering Arm (ASCOT-LLA): a multicentre randomised controlled trial. *Lancet* 2003; 361:1149–1158.

57. Pedersen TR, Wilhelmsen L, Faergeman O *et al*. Follow-up study of patients randomized in the Scandinavian Simvastatin Survival Study (4S) of cholesterol lowering. *Am J Cardiol* 2000; 86:257–262.

58. Collins R, Armitage J, Parish S, Sleigh P, Peto R. MRC/BHF Heart Protection Study of cholesterol-lowering with simvastatin in 5,963 people with diabetes: a randomised placebo-controlled trial. *Lancet* 2003; 361:2005–2016.

59. Peterson S, Peto V, Scarborough PR, Rayner M. *Coronary Heart Disease Statistics*. British Heart Foundation 2005 [cited 1/2/2005]; Available from: http://www.heartstats.org/uploads/documents%5C2004pdf.pdf

60. Wolf PA, D'Agostino RB, Kannel WB, Bonita R, Belanger AJ. Cigarette smoking as a risk factor for stroke. The Framingham Study. *JAMA* 1988; 259:1025–1029.

61. Stampfer M. New insights from the British doctors study. *BMJ* 2004; 328:1507.

62. Op Reimer WS, de Swart E, De Bacquer D *et al*. Smoking behaviour in European patients with established coronary heart disease. *Eur Heart J* 2006; 27:35–41.

63. Fruchart J-C, Nierman MC, Stroes ESG, Kastelein JJP, Duriez P. New risk factors for atherosclerosis and patient risk assessment. *Circulation* 2004; 109(suppl 1):III-15–19.

64. Meigs JB, Larson MG, D'Agostino RB *et al*. Coronary artery calcification in type 2 diabetes and insulin resistance: the Framingham Offspring Study. *Diabetes Care* 2002; 25:1313–1319.

65. Selhub J, Jacques PF, Wilson PW, Rush D, Rosenberg IH. Vitamin status and intake as primary determinants of homocysteinemia in an elderly population. *JAMA* 1993; 270:2693–2698.

66. Must A, Jacques PF, Rogers G, Rosenberg IH, Selhub J. Serum total homocysteine concentrations in children and adolescents: results from the third National Health and Nutrition Examination Survey (NHANES III). *J Nutr* 2003; 133:2643–2649.

67. Fakhrzadeh H, Ghotbi S, Pourebrahim R *et al.* Total plasma homocysteine, folate, and vitamin B12 status in healthy Iranian adults: the Tehran homocysteine survey (2003–2004)/a cross–sectional population based study. *BMC Public Health* 2006; 6:29.

68. Boushey CJ, Beresford SA, Omenn GS, Motulsky AG. A quantitative assessment of plasma homocysteine as a risk factor for vascular disease. Probable benefits of increasing folic acid intakes. *JAMA* 1995; 274:1049–1057.

69. Danesh J, Lewington S. Plasma homocysteine and coronary heart disease: systematic review of published epidemiological studies. *J Cardiovasc Risk* 1998; 5:229–232.

70. Stein JH, McBride PE. Hyperhomocysteinemia and atherosclerotic vascular disease: pathophysiology, screening, and treatment. *Arch Intern Med* 1998; 158:1301–1306.

71. Bots ML, Launer LJ, Lindemans J, Hofman A, Grobbee DE. Homocysteine, atherosclerosis and prevalent cardiovascular disease in the elderly: The Rotterdam Study. *J Intern Med* 1997; 242:339–347.

72. Casas JP, Bautista LE, Smeeth L, Sharma P, Hingorani AD. Homocysteine and stroke: evidence on a causal link from mendelian randomisation. *Lancet* 2005; 365:224–232.

73. McIlroy SP, Dynan KB, Lawson JT, Patterson CC, Passmore AP. Moderately elevated plasma homocysteine, methylenetetrahydrofolate reductase genotype, and risk for stroke, vascular dementia, and alzheimer disease in Northern Ireland. *Stroke* 2002; 33:2351–2356.

74. Morris MS, Jacques PF, Rosenberg IH, Selhub J. Hyperhomocysteinemia associated with poor recall in the third National Health and Nutrition Examination Survey. *Am J Clin Nutr* 2001; 73:927–933.

75. den Heijer T, Vermeer SE, Clarke R *et al.* Homocysteine and brain atrophy on MRI of non-demented elderly. *Brain* 2002; 126:170–175.

76. Bostom AG, Rosenberg IH, Silbershatz H *et al.* Nonfasting plasma total homocysteine levels and stroke incidence in elderly persons: the Framingham Study. *Ann Intern Med* 1999; 131:352–355.

77. Seshadri S, Beiser A, Selhub J *et al.* Plasma homocysteine as a risk factor for dementia and Alzheimer's disease. *N Engl J Med* 2002; 346:476–483.

78. Elias MF, Sullivan LM, D'Agostino RB *et al.* Homocysteine and cognitive performance in the Framingham offspring study: age is important. *Am J Epidemiol* 2005; 162:644–653.

79. Bots ML, Launer LJ, Lindemans J *et al.* Homocysteine and short-term risk of myocardial infarction and stroke in the elderly: the Rotterdam Study. *Arch Intern Med* 1999; 159:38–44.

80. Ford ES, Smith SJ, Stroup DF, Steinberg KK, Mueller PW, Thacker SB. Homocyst(e)ine and cardiovascular disease: a systematic review of the evidence with special emphasis on case-control studies and nested case-control studies. *Int J Epidemiol* 2002; 31:59–70.

81. Krabbe KS, Pedersen M, Bruunsgaard H. Inflammatory mediators in the elderly. *Exp Gerontol* 2004; 39:687–699.

82. Cushman M, Arnold AM, Psaty BM *et al.* C-reactive protein and the 10-year incidence of coronary heart disease in older men and women: the cardiovascular health study. *Circulation* 2005; 112:25–31.

83. Harris TB, Ferrucci L, Tracy RP *et al.* Associations of elevated interleukin-6 and C-reactive protein levels with mortality in the elderly. *Am J Med* 1999; 106:506–512.

84. Vasan RS, Sullivan LM, Roubenoff R *et al.* Inflammatory markers and risk of heart failure in elderly subjects without prior myocardial infarction: The Framingham Heart Study. *Circulation* 2003; 107:1486–1491.

85. Ridker PM, Cannon CP, Morrow D *et al.* C-reactive protein levels and outcomes after statin therapy. *N Engl J Med* 2005; 352:20–28.

86. Danesh J, Lewington S, Thompson SG *et al.* Plasma fibrinogen level and the risk of major cardiovascular diseases and nonvascular mortality: an individual participant meta-analysis. *JAMA* 2005; 294:1799–1809.

87. Ghosh S, Ziesmer V, Aronow WS. Underutilization of aspirin, beta blockers, angiotensin-converting enzyme inhibitors, and lipid-lowering drugs and overutilization of calcium channel blockers in older persons with coronary artery disease in an academic nursing home. *J Gerontol A Biol Sci Med Sci* 2002; 57:M398–M400.

88. Mendelson G, Aronow WS. Underutilization of measurement of serum low-density lipoprotein cholesterol levels and of lipid-lowering therapy in older patients with manifest atherosclerotic disease. *J Am Geriatr Soc* 1998; 46:1128–1131.

89. Collinson J, Bakhai A, Flather MD, Fox KA. The management and investigation of elderly patients with acute coronary syndromes without ST elevation: an evidence-based approach? Results of the Prospective Registry of Acute Ischaemic Syndromes in the United Kingdom (PRAIS-UK). *Age Ageing* 2005; 34:61–66.

90. Ramsay SE, Morris RW, Papacosta O, Lennon LT, Thomas MC, Whincup PH. Secondary prevention of coronary heart disease in older British men: extent of inequalities before and after implementation of the National Service Framework. *J Public Health (Oxf)* 2005; 27:338–343.

91. Ho SF, O'Mahony MS, Steward JA, Burr ML, Buchalter M. Left ventricular systolic dysfunction and atrial fibrillation in older people in the community – a need for screening? *Age Ageing* 2004; 33:488–492.

92. D'Agostino RB Sr, Grundy S, Sullivan LM, Wilson P. Validation of the Framingham coronary heart disease prediction scores: results of a multiple ethnic groups investigation. *JAMA* 2001; 286:180–187.

93. Conroy RM, Pyörälä K, Fitzgerald AP *et al.* Estimation of ten-year risk of fatal cardiovascular disease in Europe: the SCORE project. *Eur Heart J* 2003; 24:987–1003.

94. Hense HW, Schulte H, Lowel H, Assmann G, Keil U. Framingham risk function overestimates risk of coronary heart disease in men and women from Germany – results from the MONICA Augsburg and the PROCAM cohorts. *Eur Heart J* 2003; 24:937–945.

95. Liu J, Hong Y, D'Agostino RB Sr *et al.* Predictive value for the Chinese population of the Framingham CHD risk assessment tool compared with the Chinese Multi-Provincial Cohort Study. *JAMA* 2004; 291:2591–2599.

96. Brindle P, Emberson J, Lampe F *et al.* Predictive accuracy of the Framingham coronary risk score in British men: prospective cohort study. *BMJ* 2003; 327:1267.

97. Williams MA, Fleg JL, Ades PA *et al.* Secondary prevention of coronary heart disease in the elderly (with emphasis on patients > or =75 years of age): an American Heart Association scientific statement from the Council on Clinical Cardiology Subcommittee on Exercise, Cardiac Rehabilitation, and Prevention. *Circulation* 2002; 105:1735–1743.

98. Collinson J, Bakhai A, Flather MD, Fox KA. The management and investigation of elderly patients with acute coronary syndromes without ST elevation: an evidence-based approach? Results of the Prospective Registry of Acute Ischaemic Syndromes in the United Kingdom (PRAIS-UK). *Age Ageing* 2005; 34:61–66.

99. Longstreth WT Jr, Bernick C, Manolio TA, Bryan N, Jungreis CA, Price TR. Lacunar infarcts defined by magnetic resonance imaging of 3660 elderly people: the Cardiovascular Health Study. *Arch Neurol* 1998; 55:1217–1225.

100. Mosley TH Jr, Knopman DS, Catellier DJ *et al.* Cerebral MRI findings and cognitive functioning: the Atherosclerosis Risk in Communities study. *Neurology* 2005; 64:2056–2062.

101. Lloyd-Jones DM, Larson MG, Leip EP *et al.* Lifetime risk for developing congestive heart failure: The Framingham Heart Study. *Circulation* 2002; 106:3068–3072.

102. Mair FS, Crowley TS, Bundred PE. Prevalence, aetiology and management of heart failure in general practice. *Br J Gen Pract* 1996; 46:77–79.

103. Kannel WB, Belanger AJ. Epidemiology of heart failure. *Am Heart J* 1991; 121(Pt 1):951–957.

104. Pitt B, Zannad F, Remme WJ *et al.* The effect of spironolactone on morbidity and mortality in patients with severe heart failure. *N Engl J Med* 1999; 341:709–717.

105. Kupari M, Lindroos M, Iivanainen AM, Heikkila J, Tilvis R. Congestive heart failure in old age: prevalence, mechanisms and 4-year prognosis in the Helsinki Ageing Study. *J Intern Med* 1997; 241:387–394.

106. O'Mahony MS, Sim MFV, Ho SF, Steward JA, Buchalter M, Burr M. Diastolic heart failure in older people. *Age Ageing* 2003; 32:519–524.

107. Wolf PA, Abbott RD, Kannel WB. Atrial fibrillation: a major contributor to stroke in the elderly. The Framingham Study. *Arch Intern Med* 1987; 147:1561–1564.

108. Lloyd-Jones DM, Wang TJ, Leip EP *et al.* Lifetime risk for development of atrial fibrillation: The Framingham Heart Study. *Circulation* 2004; 110:1042–1046.

109. Jorm AF, Korten AE, Henderson AS. The prevalence of dementia: a quantitative integration of the literature. *Acta Psychiatr Scand* 1987; 76:465–479.

110. Riedel-Heller SG, Busse A, Aurich C, Matschinger H, Angermeyer MC. Prevalence of dementia according to DSM-III-R and ICD-10: results of the Leipzig longitudinal study of the aged (LEILA75+) Part 1. *Br J Psychiatr* 2001; 179:250–254.

111. Ferri CP, Prince M, Brayne C *et al.* Global prevalence of dementia: a Delphi consensus study. *Lancet* 2005; 366:2112–2117.

112. Langa KM, Foster NL, Larson EB. Mixed dementia: emerging concepts and therapeutic implications. *JAMA* 2004; 292:2901–2908.

113. Gearing M, Mirra SS, Hedreen JC, Sumi SM, Hansen LA, Heyman A. The consortium to establish a registry for Alzheimer's disease (CERAD). Part X. Neuropathology confirmation of the clinical diagnosis of Alzheimer's disease. *Neurology* 1995; 45:461–466.

114. Massoud F, Devi G, Stern Y *et al.* A clinicopathological comparison of community-based and clinic-based cohorts of patients with dementia. *Arch Neurol* 1999; 56:1368–1373.

115. Riekse RG, Leverenz JB, McCormick W *et al.* Effect of vascular lesions on cognition in Alzheimer's disease: a community-based study. *J Am Geriatr Soc* 2004; 52:1442–1448.

116. Snowdon DA, Greiner LH, Mortimer JA, Riley KP, Greiner PA, Markesbery WR. Brain infarction and the clinical expression of Alzheimer disease: The Nun Study. *JAMA* 1997; 277:813–817.

117. Snowdon DA. Healthy aging and dementia: findings from the Nun Study. *Ann Intern Med* 2003; 139 (Part 2):450–454.

118. Luchsinger JA, Reitz C, Honig LS, Tang MX, Shea S, Mayeux R. Aggregation of vascular risk factors and risk of incident Alzheimer disease. *Neurology* 2005; 65:545–551.

119. Newman AB, Fitzpatrick AL, Lopez O *et al.* Dementia and Alzheimer's disease incidence in relationship to cardiovascular disease in the Cardiovascular Health Study cohort. *J Am Geriatr Soc* 2005; 53:1101–1107.

120. Hanon O, Haulon S, Lenoir H *et al.* Relationship between arterial stiffness and cognitive function in elderly subjects with complaints of memory loss. *Stroke* 2005; 36:2193–2197.

121. van Oijen M, Witteman JC, Hofman A, Koudstaal PJ, Breteler MM. Fibrinogen is associated with an increased risk of Alzheimer disease and vascular dementia. *Stroke* 2005; 36:2637–2641.

122. Whitmer RA, Sidney S, Selby J, Johnston SC, Yaffe K. Midlife cardiovascular risk factors and risk of dementia in late life. *Neurology* 2005; 64:277–281.

123. O'Brien JT, Erkinjuntti T, Reisberg B *et al.* Vascular cognitive impairment. *Lancet Neurol* 2003; 2:89–98.

124. Ballard C, O'Brien J, Barber B *et al.* Neurocardiovascular instability, hypotensive episodes, and MRI lesions in neurodegenerative dementia. *Ann NY Acad Sci* 2000; 903:442–445.

125. Matsushita K, Kuriyama Y, Nagatsuka K, Nakamura M, Sawada T, Omae T. Periventricular white matter lucency and cerebral blood flow autoregulation in hypertensive patients. *Hypertension* 1994; 23:565–568.

126. Brant-Zawadzki M, Atkinson D, Detrick M, Bradley WG, Scidmore G. Fluid-attenuated inversion recovery (FLAIR) for assessment of cerebral infarction: initial clinical experience in 50 patients. *Stroke* 1996; 27:1187–1191.

127. Burton EJ, Kenny RA, O'Brien J *et al.* White matter hyperintensities are associated with impairment of memory, attention, and global cognitive performance in older stroke patients. *Stroke* 2004; 35:1270–1275.

128. Esiri MM, Wilcock GK, Morris JH. Neuropathological assessment of the lesions of significance in vascular dementia. *J Neurol Neurosurg Psychiatr* 1997; 63:749–753.

129. Feinberg WM, Blackshear JL, Laupacis A, Kronmal R, Hart RG. Prevalence, age distribution, and gender of patients with atrial fibrillation. Analysis and implications. *Arch Intern Med* 1995; 155:469–473.

130. Stewart S, Hart CL, Hole DJ, McMurray JJV. Population prevalence, incidence, and predictors of atrial fibrillation in the Renfrew/Paisley study. *Heart* 2001; 86:516–521.

131. Swancutt D, Hobbs R, Fitzmaurice D *et al.* A randomised controlled trial and cost effectiveness study of systematic screening (targeted and total population screening) versus routine practice for the detection of atrial fibrillation in the over 65s: (SAFE) [ISRCTN19633732]. *BMC Cardiovasc Disord* 2004; 4:12.

6

Overweight, physical inactivity, insulin resistance, impaired glucose tolerance, diabetes, the metabolic syndrome and cardiovascular risk

G. Hu, T. A. Lakka, H.-M. Lakka, J. Tuomilehto

INTRODUCTION

Cardiovascular disease (CVD), especially from coronary heart disease (CHD) and stroke, is the leading killer in western societies and its prevalence is also increasing dramatically in developing nations [1, 2]. Preliminary mortality data show that CVD as the underlying cause of death accounted for 37.3% of all 2 440 000 deaths in 2003 or 1 of every 2.7 deaths in the US [3]. Cardiovascular disease as an underlying or contributing cause of death (1 408 000 deaths in 2002) was about 58% of all deaths that year [3]. High blood pressure, smoking, dyslipidaemia, overweight or obesity, physical inactivity, diabetes, chronic inflammation, haemostatic factors, psychosocial factors, perinatal conditions and several dietary factors are the main risk factors for CVD [3–5]. In this chapter, we summarize the current evidence regarding the role of overweight, physical inactivity, insulin resistance, impaired glucose tolerance, diabetes, and the metabolic syndrome in the development of CVD.

OVERWEIGHT, OBESITY AND CARDIOVASCULAR DISEASES

Overweight and obesity are important lifestyle-related public health problems in the world [6, 7]. Two in three adults in the US are currently classified as overweight (body mass index [BMI] 25.0–29.9 kg/m^2) or obese (BMI $\geq$30 kg/m^2), compared with fewer than one in four adults in the early 1960s [8, 9]. This trend is similar for all age, gender and race groups [9]. More than one-half of the adults in most European and other developed countries are overweight or obese, and the prevalence of obesity is increasing rapidly in these countries, and is becoming a problem also in developing countries [10]. Overweight in childhood and adolescence has more than doubled over the past decades for instance in the US [11], some European countries, Japan and urban China [10, 12].

To what extent is obesity an independent risk factor for CVD in its own right, and to what extent are its effects mediated through effects on blood pressure, lipids, glucose intolerance

Gang Hu, MD, PhD, Senior Researcher and Docent, Department of Epidemiology and Health Promotion, National Public Health Institute, Helsinki, Department of Public Health University of Helsinki, Helsinki, Finland

Timo A. Lakka, MD, PhD, Professor of Medical Physiology, Institute of Biomedicine, Department of Physiology, University of Kuopio, Kuopio Research Institute of Exercise Medicine, Kuopio, Finland

Hanna-Maaria Lakka, MD, PhD, Assistant Professor, Department of Public Health and Clinical Nutrition, University of Kuopio, Department of Epidemiology and Health Promotion, National Public Health Institute, Helsinki, Finland

Jaakko Tuomilehto, MD, MPolSc, PhD, Professor of Public Health, Department of Public Health, University of Helsinki, Helsinki; South Ostrobothnia Central Hospital, Seinajoki, Finland

and other risk factors? In general, after adjusting for other factors, the residual effect of obesity *per se* seems to be small. To the pragmatist, this may not matter very much; if reducing weight improves health, whether the effect is direct or indirect is not of practical importance to the subject concerned.

OVERWEIGHT, OBESITY AND CARDIOVASCULAR MORTALITY

Overweight and obesity are currently recognized as important risk factors for atherosclerotic CVD and premature mortality [7, 13]. Prospective epidemiological studies have shown that cardiovascular and total mortality increase throughout the range of overweight and obesity. Overweight and obesity predict cardiovascular mortality in both men [14–18] and women [15–20] (Table 6.1). Obesity also markedly decreases life expectancy, particularly in young adults [21]. The associations of overweight and obesity with cardiovascular and overall mortality may even be stronger in healthy non-smoking individuals [16, 19, 20]. There is some evidence that the risk of CVD starts to increase from BMI levels of as low as 22–23 kg/m^2 [14, 19, 22, 23], which suggests that the optimal BMI may be in the middle of the range of values currently considered as normal weight. Overweight and obesity increase cardiovascular and total mortality in adults, and the relative risk appears to be higher among younger individuals [15, 16]. Because mortality rises dramatically with age, however, the absolute excess risk of CVD associated with overweight and obesity increases rather than decreases with age. The association of overweight and obesity with cardiovascular and total mortality has been observed in all ethnic groups, although in the US the relative risk was greater for Caucasians compared with African-Americans [16].

OVERWEIGHT, OBESITY AND CORONARY HEART DISEASE

Prospective epidemiological studies have consistently shown that overweight and obesity are associated with an increased risk of CHD. Overweight and obesity predict CHD in both men and women [22–29]. Abdominal obesity has been found to be a stronger risk factor for CHD than overall obesity in men and women and may provide additional information beyond overall obesity in the prediction of CHD [26, 27, 30–34]. While the relative risk of CHD associated with obesity appears to decline with increasing age, abdominal obesity remains a strong and independent predictor of CVD in men of all age groups, including the elderly [25, 30, 35].

OVERWEIGHT, OBESITY AND STROKE

Prospective epidemiological studies have reported that obesity is associated with an increased risk of total stroke in men and women [36–41]. Abdominal obesity has been more closely associated with the risk of stroke than has overall obesity, and the increased risk appears to be independent of overall obesity [38, 42, 43]. The association between abdominal obesity and the risk of ischaemic stroke was evident in all ethnic groups, including Whites, Blacks and Hispanics [38]. Obesity has been associated with an increased incidence of ischaemic stroke [36–41], whereas the association with haemorrhagic stroke remains unclear. Some studies have shown an increased risk of haemorrhagic stroke among the lean [36, 39, 41], but other studies have found no association [40] or an increased risk with increasing BMI [37].

WEIGHT GAIN AND CARDIOVASCULAR DISEASES

Most people are not overweight when growth ends around 20 years of age, and excess body fat primarily accrues in subsequent decades [6]. In men, much of the weight increase takes place in the twenties and the thirties, while in women it is 10–15 years later and especially

Table 6.1 Hazard ratios for risk of CVD according to different levels of body mass index by sex, the FINMONICA study

| | Number of events | | Person-years | | Hazard ratios (95% CIs)* | | | | | |
| | | | | | Men | | | Women | | |
Body mass index	Men	Women	Men	Women	Model 1	Model 2	Model 3	Model 1	Model 2	Model 3
<20	4	6	1336	5569	1.10 (0.40–2.98)	0.88 (0.32–2.40)	1.18 (0.43–1.61)	1.24 (0.54–2.87)	1.11 (0.48–2.56)	1.20 (0.52–2.79)
20–24.9	98	68	27 429	40 526	1.00	1.00	1.00	1.00	1.00	1.00
25–29.9	262	104	36 812	29 369	1.36 (1.08–1.72)	1.48 (1.17–1.87)	1.27 (1.00–1.61)	1.23 (0.90–1.68)	1.26 (0.92–1.72)	1.09 (0.79–1.50)
≥30	159	117	12 972	16 350	2.08 (1.61–2.67)	2.12 (1.64–2.74)	1.60 (1.23–2.09)	2.04 (1.50–2.78)	1.99 (1.45–2.73)	1.49 (1.07–2.08)
P for trend					<0.001	<0.001	0.006	<0.001	<0.001	0.06

*Model 1: adjusted for age and study year; model 2: additionally adjusted for education, smoking, and physical activity; model 3: adjusted also for systolic blood pressure, total and HDL cholesterol, and diabetes at baseline.

Reproduced with permission from Oxford University Press [18].

after the menopause. Weight gain among men and women during early and middle adulthood has been associated with a significantly increased risk of CVD in a dose–response fashion [6, 22, 25, 44, 45]. Men and women with even a modest weight gain of 5–10 kg during early and middle adulthood are at increased risk of CHD, type 2 diabetes and hypertension as compared with individuals who maintain their weight within 2 kg of their weight at 18–20 years of age. Also, non-smoking women who experienced a weight gain of more than 10 kg since the age of 18 years had higher premature cardiovascular mortality than those who maintained their weight within 4 kg of their weight [19]. The increased risk of CHD during adulthood associated with weight gain is evident at any level of BMI at the age of 18 years [19].

WEIGHT LOSS AND CARDIOVASCULAR DISEASES

Epidemiological prospective studies and clinical trials have shown that even modest weight reductions of 5–10%, due to either an increase in physical activity or a decrease in energy intake or both, can substantially lower blood pressure [46]; improve blood lipid profile [46], insulin sensitivity [46] and glucose tolerance [46]; and decrease the incidence of type 2 diabetes [47, 48] and hypertension [45] among overweight individuals. In prospective epidemiological studies, intentional weight loss has been associated with a reduction or no change in cardiovascular and total mortality [49, 50], while unintentional weight loss, likely reflecting existing disease, has been associated with increased premature mortality [50]. Although clinical trials have not specifically examined the effect of weight reduction on the incidence of clinical manifestation of CVD, weight loss is likely to be important in the prevention and treatment of CVD, because it improves many cardiovascular risk factors [46].

WEIGHT FLUCTUATION AND CARDIOVASCULAR DISEASES

Information on the association between weight fluctuation and the risk of CVD is limited and inconsistent. Whereas some studies have observed that a large weight variability is associated with an increased risk of cardiovascular and total mortality, especially at the lower end of the body weight distribution [51], other studies suggest that weight variability does not predict mortality independent of weight loss or weight gain [52]. Involuntary weight fluctuation may indicate the presence of subclinical disease, especially in the elderly.

OVERWEIGHT, OBESITY AND CARDIOVASCULAR MORTALITY IN PATIENTS WITH TYPE 2 DIABETES

Only a few prospective studies have evaluated the association between obesity and cardiovascular mortality among diabetic patients, and the results are controversial. The results from the United Kingdom Prospective Diabetes Study indicated that high levels of BMI and waist-to-hip ratio were not major risk factors for CHD among diabetic patients [53]. A direct association between BMI and mortality among men with diabetes was found in the Aerobics Center Longitudinal Study, however, this association became non-significant when fitness was accounted for [54]. We recently found that diabetic patients with obesity, defined as the highest tertile of BMI, had a higher risk of total and cardiovascular mortality than those in the lowest tertile of BMI after controlling for many other potential risk factors [55].

PHYSICAL ACTIVITY AND CARDIOVASCULAR DISEASES

Sedentary lifestyle is currently recognized as another of the major risk factors for atherosclerotic CVD [56, 57]. More than one-half of the adults in the US do not engage in physical activity at the level currently recommended for health promotion, e.g. 30 min or more of moderate-intensity physical activity on most days of the week [57–59]. What is even more alarming is that almost two-thirds of children 9–13 years of age do not participate in any organized physical activity during their leisure time and almost one in four children of this age do not engage in any leisure time physical activity [60].

PHYSICAL ACTIVITY AND CARDIOVASCULAR MORTALITY

Prospective epidemiological studies have consistently shown that regular physical activity and cardiorespiratory fitness prevent CVD and premature cardiovascular mortality in men and women (Table 6.2) [20, 61–65]. Moreover, an increase in physical activity and an improvement in cardiorespiratory fitness have been associated with reduced cardiovascular and total mortality [66–69]. The association between physical activity and cardiovascular mortality is independent of conventional cardiovascular risk factors and graded; the risk is lowest in the most active individuals. The protective effect of physical activity is strong; most physically active individuals usually have about half the cardiovascular mortality compared with that in the least active people. Exercise or sports in young adulthood only may not prevent premature cardiovascular mortality in later years, which emphasizes the importance of lifelong engagement in physical activity [70].

PHYSICAL ACTIVITY AND CORONARY HEART DISEASE

The epidemiological evidence on the role of regular physical activity in the prevention of atherosclerotic CVD is strongest for CHD [57]. Regular physical activity, an increase in the level of physical activity, and cardiorespiratory fitness prevent CHD in men and women [29, 70–77]. Moderate-intensity aerobic exercise such as walking may be as effective as more vigorous exercise in the prevention of CHD [69, 71–75]. However, some studies suggest that vigorous exercise confers further protection and that the risk decreases in a dose-dependent fashion with increasing intensity of regular exercise [75]. Resistance training may also reduce the risk of CHD [75]. The accumulation of shorter daily sessions of physical activity may be as effective as longer, continuous exercise bouts [76].

PHYSICAL ACTIVITY AND STROKE

There is evidence that regular physical activity and cardiorespiratory fitness prevent ischaemic stroke in both men and women [78–85]. However, the association between physical activity and the risk of haemorrhagic stroke is inconsistent [79, 83, 85, 86]. The protective effect of regular physical activity on the risk of subarachnoid haemorrhagic or intracerebral haemorrhagic stroke can be found in some [79, 85] but not in all studies [83, 86]. Moreover, the association between physical activity and stroke is slightly weaker and less consistent than that with CHD [57, 87]. Regular exercise has been observed to protect against ischaemic stroke in different ethnic groups, including Whites, Blacks, and Hispanics [88]. There is some evidence that regular physical activity reduces the risk of stroke in a dose–response manner [78, 83, 88]. Whereas some studies have found that moderate-intensity physical activity, such as walking, is as effective as vigorous exercise in the prevention of ischaemic stroke [78], other studies suggest that more vigorous exercise confers some further protection [83, 88]. The American Heart Association has recently emphasized the importance of regular physical activity for the prevention of ischaemic stroke [87].

PHYSICAL ACTIVITY AND CARDIOVASCULAR DISEASE IN PATIENTS WITH TYPE 2 DIABETES

Several studies have found that regular leisure time physical activity, moderate or high occupational physical activity, and daily walking or cycling to and from work are independently

Table 6.2 Hazard ratios of CVD according to different levels of physical activity by sex, the FINMONICA study

| Physical activity | Number of events | | Person-years | | Hazard ratios (95% CIs)* | | | | | |
| | | | | | Men | | | Women | | |
	Men	Women	Men	Women	Model 1	Model 2	Model 3	Model 1	Model 2	Model 3
Low	105	77	8235	12686	1.00	1.00	1.00	1.00	1.00	1.00
Moderate	268	145	35695	43017	0.57	0.69	0.72	0.62	0.69	0.73
					(0.46–0.72)	(0.55–0.87)	(0.57–0.91)	(0.47–0.81)	(0.52–0.91)	(0.55–0.97)
High	150	73	34618	36111	0.52	0.64	0.68	0.51	0.60	0.64
					(0.40–0.67)	(0.50–0.84)	(0.52–0.88)	(0.37–0.71)	(0.43–0.83)	(0.45–0.89)
P for trend					<0.001	0.002	0.007	<0.001	0.006	0.02

*Model 1: adjusted for age and study year; model 2: additionally adjusted for education, smoking, and body mass index (in the continuous form); model 3: adjusted also for systolic blood pressure, total and HDL cholesterol, and diabetes at baseline.

Reproduced with permission from Oxford University Press [18].

and significantly associated with a reduced risk of cardiovascular and total mortality among men and women with diabetes (Table 6.3) [55, 89–93]. Walking has a similar inverse association with the risk of cardiovascular and total mortality to vigorous leisure time physical activity [89–92]. The protective benefits of physical activity were consistent regardless of BMI, blood pressure or cholesterol levels, or whether or not the person smoked [55]. Physical fitness had a strong and independent inverse association with total mortality in men with type 2 diabetes, and this association was seen in all BMI and body fatness groups [54, 94].

PHYSICAL ACTIVITY AND CARDIOVASCULAR DISEASE IN PATIENTS WITH CORONARY HEART DISEASE

Regular physical activity is also beneficial in the treatment of patients with CHD. Meta-analyses have confirmed that comprehensive exercise-based cardiac rehabilitation reduces total and cardiovascular mortality after myocardial infarction [95–97]. Cardiac rehabilitation programmes consisting of initially supervised exercise training of 2–6 months followed by unsupervised physical activity reduced total mortality by 27% and cardiovascular mortality by 31% in patients who had sustained a myocardial infarction, had angina pectoris or coronary artery disease identified by angiography, or had undergone coronary artery bypass grafting or percutaneous transluminal coronary angioplasty [97]. However, physical activity did not reduce the risk of recurrent non-fatal myocardial infarction [97].

Strenuous exercise can trigger myocardial infarction and sudden cardiac death, particularly in habitually sedentary people [98, 99], but the absolute risk of myocardial infarction or sudden cardiac death during any particular episode of vigorous exertion is extremely low [98, 99]. Moreover, it is important to recognize that regular physical activity effectively reduces the occurrence of myocardial infarction and sudden cardiac death associated with an episode of vigorous exertion [98, 99]. Due to the potential albeit low cardiac risks of strenuous exercise, the current recommendations of regular moderate-intensity physical activity appear to be well justified [56, 57].

INSULIN RESISTANCE OR THE METABOLIC SYNDROME AND CARDIOVASCULAR DISEASES

The concept of the metabolic syndrome, also known as insulin resistance, was introduced by Reaven [100] in 1988. It is characterized by the clustering of a number of metabolic abnormalities including impaired glucose tolerance, elevated triglycerides with decreased levels of high-density lipoprotein (HDL) cholesterol, raised blood pressure and central obesity. The key role of central obesity has been emphasized recently, and indeed the very existence of a discrete 'syndrome' has been challenged. Sorting out the possible independent effects of biologically inter-related components is a statistical challenge. From a practical point of view, the identification of one component should trigger a search for the others and a combined management strategy to deal with each, with a strong emphasis on physical activity and weight control.

INSULIN RESISTANCE AND CORONARY HEART DISEASE OR CARDIOVASCULAR MORTALITY

Hyperinsulinaemia, or insulin resistance has been shown to be associated with a cluster of cardiovascular risk factors, including hypertension, dyslipidaemia, obesity and glucose intolerance [101]. Any one or combination of them may increase the risk of CHD. However, the association of hyperinsulinaemia *per se* with CVD has been debated until recently. An association between elevated plasma insulin, fasting or after oral glucose load, with the risk of CHD or atherosclerotic CVD, has been found in many [102–110], but not in all [111–114], prospective studies. Among those studies showing the positive association between plasma insulin and

Table 6.3 Hazard ratios of cardiovascular mortality according to occupational, commuting and leisure time physical activity among subjects with type 2 diabetes, the FINMONICA study

	Deaths, n	Person-years	Hazard ratios (95% CIs)*			
			Model 1 (n = 3316)	Model 2 (n = 3316)	Model 3 (n = 3316)	Model 4 (n = 2596)
Occupation physical activity						
Light	517	25 549	1.00	1.00	1.00	1.00
Moderate	161	13 216	0.80 (0.67–0.96)	0.84 (0.70–1.01)	0.91 (0.75–1.10)	0.94 (0.74–1.18)
Active	225	22 305	0.58 (0.48–0.68)	0.59 (0.50–0.69)	0.60 (0.50–0.71)	0.69 (0.57–0.85)
P for trend			<0.001	<0.001	<0.001	0.001
Walking or cycling to and from work						
0 min	609	33 530	1.00	1.00	1.00	1.00
1–29 min	165	15 581	0.78 (0.65–0.92)	0.81 (0.67–0.96)	0.89 (0.75–1.07)	0.97 (0.79–1.20)
≥30 min	129	11 959	0.69 (0.57–0.84)	0.74 (0.61–0.90)	0.86 (0.70–1.06)	0.94 (0.74–1.19)
P for trend			<0.001	0.002	0.27	0.87
Leisure time physical activity						
Low	480	27 974	1.00	1.00	1.00	1.00
Moderate	381	28 072	0.83 (0.72–0.95)	0.85 (0.74–0.98)	0.83 (0.72–0.95)	0.84 (0.71–0.99)
High	42	5024	0.63 (0.46–0.87)	0.70 (0.51–0.96)	0.67 (0.49–0.93)	0.69 (0.49–0.99)
P for trend			0.002	0.016	0.005	0.038

*Model 1: adjusted for age, sex and study year; model 2: additionally adjusted for BMI, systolic blood pressure, cholesterol and smoking; model 3: adjusted also for other two physical activities; model 4: model 3 and excluding subjects who at baseline were diagnosed with CHD, stroke and heart failure, who may have been physically inactive because of severe disease or disability at baseline, or who died during the first two years of follow-up.

Reproduced with permission from Lippincott Williams & Wilkins [93].

Table 6.4 Meta-analyses of the association of fasting insulin, HOMA-IR and 2-h insulin (the highest quartile vs. quartiles 1–3) with cardiovascular mortality by sex, the DECODE study

	Overall hazard ratios (95% CIs)		
	Fasting insulin	HOMA-IR	2-h insulin*
Men			
Model 1**	1.58 (1.26–1.97)	1.59 (1.27–1.98)	1.28 (0.99–1.66)
Model 2***	1.53 (1.19–1.97)	1.53 (1.20–1.97)	1.07 (0.79–1.45)
Model 3 (10 studies)****	1.54 (1.16–2.03)	1.58 (1.20–2.09)	0.85 (0.60–1.21)
Non-specific insulin assay (7 studies)			
Model 1	1.46 (1.12–1.92)	1.43 (1.09–1.87)	1.19 (0.89–1.61)
Model 2	1.37 (1.01–1.87)	1.34 (0.98–1.81)	0.99 (0.70–1.40)
Specific insulin assay (4 studies)			
Model 1	1.82 (1.25–2.66)	1.94 (1.33–2.82)	1.59 (0.95–2.68)
Model 2	1.89 (1.24–2.88)	1.99 (1.31–3.04)	1.42 (0.75–2.69)
*Women (7 studies)*****			
Model 1	2.64 (1.54–4.51)	2.40 (1.37–4.20)	1.87 (0.87–4.02)
Model 2	2.72 (1.51–4.89)	2.41 (1.32–4.39)	1.28 (0.52–3.15)
Model 3	2.66 (1.45–4.90)	2.35 (1.27–4.37)	1.36 (0.53–3.45)

*2-h insulin data were not available from the Cremona Study; in the Hoorn Study 2-h insulin data were available only from a subsample of 472 subjects (230 men, and 242 women).

**Adjustment for age and smoking.

***Model 1 plus additional adjustment for body mass index, systolic blood pressure, fasting glucose (except in HOMA-IR analyses), 2-h glucose and total cholesterol.

****Model 2 plus additional adjustment for HDL cholesterol, and triglycerides; Helsinki Policemen Study excluded.

*****Only those studies in which the number of cardiovascular deaths was at least 4.

Reproduced with kind permission of Springer Science and Business Media [110].

CVD, the effect of adjustment for other risk factors has varied; in several studies the association has still remained statistically significant, although attenuated [102–105, 107, 109, 110], whereas in other studies it has become non-significant [106, 108]. The data on the association between hyperinsulinaemia and cardiovascular risk in women are scarce and conflicting. Some, [106, 109] but not all, studies [103, 107, 111, 112] have shown a significant association between hyperinsulinaemia and cardiovascular risk in women. In the Diabetes Epidemiology: Collaborative analysis Of Diagnostic criteria in Europe (DECODE) Study involving European men and women, we found that hyperinsulinaemia, defined by the highest quartile cut-off for fasting insulin or the score of homeostasis model assessment of insulin resistance (HOMA-IR), was significantly associated with cardiovascular mortality in both non-diabetic European men and women independently of other risk factors (Table 6.4) [110].

INSULIN RESISTANCE AND STROKE

Only a few prospective cohort studies have assessed the association between insulin resistance and stroke risk, and the results have varied, including a J-shaped [115] or direct association [108, 116, 117]. After adjustment for other risk factors, one study [117] but not other studies [108, 115, 116] showed a significant association.

Table 6.5 Meta-analyses of the association of the metabolic syndrome with the risk of all-cause and cardiovascular mortality* in 7 DECODE study cohorts** by sex [131]

Definition of the metabolic syndrome	Number of subjects		All-cause mortality		CVD mortality	
	Men n = 4339	Women n = 5183	Men n = 418	Women n = 255	Men n = 161	Women n = 63
Any ≥2 of the components***	1525****	1488	1.39 (1.15–1.68)	1.23 (0.96–1.57)	1.75 (1.28–2.39)	1.56 (0.93–2.60)
Any ≥3 of the components	543	534	1.47 (1.15–1.89)	1.41 (1.03–1.92)	1.74 (1.19–2.55)	2.17 (1.13–4.19)
Hyperinsulinaemia plus any ≥2 of the other components	677	727	1.44 (1.17–1.84)	1.38 (1.02–1.87)	2.26 (1.61–3.17)	2.78 (1.57–4.94)
Hyperinsulinaemia plus any ≥3 of the other components	331	330	1.43 (1.06–1.94)	1.49 (1.02–2.31)	1.98 (1.27–3.10)	2.74 (1.21–6.20)

*Data are given as hazard ratios (95% CI), adjusted for age, cholesterol and smoking. The modified WHO definition of the metabolic syndrome is indicated by bold type.

**FINMONICA, Northern Sweden MONICA, Hoorn Study, Newcastle Study, Goodinge Study, Ely Study and Cremona Study.

***These components of the metabolic syndrome include: obesity, dyslipidaemia, impaired glucose tolerance or impaired fasting glycaemia, and hypertension.

****Number of individuals who fulfilled the definition.

THE METABOLIC SYNDROME AND CARDIOVASCULAR MORTALITY

According to the Guidelines 2007, the term 'metabolic syndrome' refers to the combination of several factors that tend to cluster together – central obesity, hypertension, low HDL cholesterol, raised triglycerides and raised blood sugar – to increase the risk of diabetes and CVD. The concept of the metabolic syndrome was introduced by Reaven [100] in 1988 as described earlier. Subsequently, several new components to the syndrome, such as microalbuminuria, hyperuricaemia, abnormalities in haemostatic factors, inflammation, and poor cardiorespiratory fitness have been suggested [118–123]. There are five definitions of the metabolic syndrome that have been recommended by the World Health Organization (WHO) [100], the European Group for Study of Insulin Resistance (EGIR) [124], the National Cholesterol Education Program (NCEP) Expert Panel [125, 126], the American Association of Clinical Endocrinologists [127, 128], and the International Diabetes Federation [129] since 1998.

A recent report based on the Third National Health and Nutrition Examination Study (NHANES-III) survey estimated that approximately 24% of US adults had the metabolic syndrome [130]. In the DECODE Study involving European men and women, the age-standardized prevalence of the metabolic syndrome was 15.7% in non-diabetic men and 14.2% in non-diabetic-women [131]. The prevalence of the metabolic syndrome in Asian populations is lower than US and European populations, but increased significantly when using modified Asian criteria for obesity. The prevalence of the metabolic syndrome using modified Asian criteria for abdominal obesity with waist circumference (>90 cm in men and >80 cm in women) was 20.9% in men and 15.5% in women in Singapore National Health [132], and 22.1% in men and 27.8% in women in the Korean National Health and Nutrition Survey [133]. The data from the InterASIA Study in a nationally representative sample of 15 540 Chinese adults aged 35–74 years in 2000–1 indicated that the age-standardized prevalence of the metabolic syndrome was 9.8% or 24 million in men and 17.8% or 41 million in women [134].

Results from prospective epidemiological studies have consistently shown that the presence of the metabolic syndrome using different definitions is associated with a significantly increased risk of cardiovascular mortality [131, 135–142]. The metabolic syndrome predicts cardiovascular mortality in both men [131, 136, 138, 140–142] and women [131, 138, 140, 142]. In the DECODE study, non-diabetic men and women with the metabolic syndrome had an increased risk of death from all causes as well as CVD (Table 6.5) [131].

THE METABOLIC SYNDROME AND CORONARY HEART DISEASE

Most [136, 138, 141–146], but not all, [137, 147] prospective epidemiological studies have shown that the presence of metabolic syndrome using different definitions is associated with a significantly increased risk of CHD. The epidemiological evidence on the effect estimates of the relative risk associated with the metabolic syndrome is stronger for CHD than for atherosclerotic CVD [148]. In a recent meta-analysis, Ford [148] found that for studies using the most exact WHO definition of the metabolic syndrome, the fixed-effects estimates of relative risk were 1.93 for CVD and 2.60 for CHD.

THE METABOLIC SYNDROME AND STROKE

Many prospective epidemiological studies have assessed the association between the metabolic syndrome and the risk of stroke [137, 144–146, 149, 150]. Some [144, 146, 149, 150], but not all, [137, 145] studies have found that the metabolic syndrome is associated with an increased risk of stroke. The majority of studies were carried out in male populations or in men and women combined [137, 145, 146, 150], but only two studies reported results for men and women separately [144, 149].

IMPAIRED GLUCOSE TOLERANCE AND CARDIOVASCULAR DISEASES

Impaired glucose tolerance was first defined by the WHO expert committee on diabetes mellitus in 1980 [151]. It was defined as a metabolic state between normal and diabetes mellitus. New diagnostic criteria for diabetes mellitus were approved by the American Diabetes Association in 1997 and the WHO in 1999 [100, 152]. Subjects not previously diagnosed as diabetic are classified according to the following criteria: (1) 2-h plasma glucose criteria alone: 2-h plasma glucose ≥11.1 mmol/l for diabetes, 7.8–11.0 mmol/l for impaired glucose tolerance and <7.8 mmol/l for normal glucose tolerance; and (2) fasting plasma glucose criteria alone: fasting plasma glucose ≥7.0 mmol/l for diabetes, 6.1–6.9 mmol/l for impaired fasting glycaemia and <6.1 mmol/l for normal fasting glucose. In 2003, the American Diabetes Association Expert Committee recommended that the glucose level for impaired fasting glucose be lowered from 6.1 mmol/l to 5.6 mmol/l [153]. A major difference in the application of these diagnostic criteria for diabetes and glucose intolerance exists since the American Diabetes Association recommends the use of fasting plasma glucose alone whereas the WHO consultation emphasizes the primary use of 2-h plasma glucose together with fasting plasma glucose.

IMPAIRED GLUCOSE TOLERANCE AND CORONARY HEART DISEASE
OR CARDIOVASCULAR MORTALITY

The nature of the relationship between impaired glucose tolerance and impaired fasting glycaemia and cardiovascular mortality has been investigated since 1998, but until recently it has remained relatively poorly defined. A major part of the reason for this has been the limited statistical power of most studies. In the Japanese Funagata Diabetes Study, survival analysis concluded that impaired glucose tolerance, but not impaired fasting glycaemia, was a risk factor for CVD [154]. A recent Finnish study found that baseline impaired glucose tolerance was an independent risk predictor for incidence of CHD and premature death from CVD and all causes, which was not confounded by the development of clinically diagnosed diabetes during the follow-up [155]. Another American study indicated that women with impaired fasting glucose according to the 1997 definition (fasting glucose level from 6.1 to 6.9 mmol/l) had an approximately 40% increased risk for CHD outcomes, independent of traditional cardiac risk factors and additional components of the metabolic syndrome, but were at no increased risk for stroke [156]. Women with impaired fasting glucose according to the expanded 2003 definition (fasting glucose level 5.6–6.9 mmol/l) did not have a statistically significantly increased risk for any cardiovascular outcome compared with women with normal fasting glucose levels. However, this study did not measure 2-h plasma glucose [156]. A meta-regression analysis of the association between plasma glucose levels and cardiovascular events from 38 studies showed a pooled relative risk of CVD of 1.27 (95% confidence interval [CI], 1.13–1.43) comparing the top and bottom categories of glycaemia from studies measuring fasting blood glucose level and a relative risk of 1.27 (95% CI 1.09–1.48) from studies measuring post-challenge blood glucose level. However, this analysis did not include fasting and 2-h glucose in the same model [157].

The most convincing evidence of an increased risk of CHD related to abnormal glucose tolerance was provided by the DECODE study (Table 6.6). In this project, individual data from more than 10 prospective cohort studies including more than 22 000 subjects were analysed jointly [158, 159]. Death rates from all causes, CVD and CHD were significantly higher in subjects with impaired glucose tolerance, whereas there was no difference in mortality between subjects with impaired fasting glycaemia and those with normal fasting glucose. The largest absolute number of excess cardiovascular deaths was observed in subjects with impaired glucose tolerance especially those with impaired glucose tolerance but normal fasting glucose [158, 159].

IMPAIRED GLUCOSE TOLERANCE AND STROKE

Few prospective epidemiological studies have assessed the association between impaired glucose tolerance or impaired fasting glycaemia and the risk of stroke, and no significant association has been found [156, 159].

DIABETES AND CARDIOVASCULAR DISEASES

Diabetes is one of the fastest growing public health problems in both developing and developed countries due to increasing prevalence of obesity and sedentary behaviours [160, 161]. Much of the burden of diabetes is attributable to microvascular and macrovascular complications, such as retinopathy, nephropathy, CHD, and stroke. Cardiovascular disease accounts for more than 70% of total mortality among patients with type 2 diabetes [162].

DIABETES AND CORONARY HEART DISEASE OR CARDIOVASCULAR MORTALITY

The most common cause of diabetes-related morbidity and mortality is CVD [162]. For example, patients with type 2 diabetes have a 2–4 times higher risk of cardiovascular mortality than those without diabetes [163]. Several studies assessed the association of CHD with both fasting plasma glucose and 2-h plasma glucose. Based on longitudinal studies in Mauritius, Fiji and Nauru, Shaw et al. [164] reported that in people with isolated post-challenge hyperglycaemia cardiovascular mortality was doubled compared with that in non-diabetic

Table 6.6 Adjusted hazard ratios (95% CIs) for death from CVD, CHD, stroke and all-cause when both the fasting and the 2-h glucose classes were in the same model, the DECODE study

| | Plasma glucose categories (mmol/l), subjects not known as diabetic | | | | | | |
| | Fasting glucose criteria* | | | 2-h glucose criteria** | | | |
	Impaired fasting glycaemia (6.1–6.9)	Diabetes ≥7.0	χ² (P-value)***	Impaired glucose tolerance (7.8–11.0)	Diabetes ≥11.1	χ² (P-value)****	Known diabetes*
CVD mortality	1.01 (0.84–1.22)	1.20 (0.88–1.64)	1.34 (>0.10)	1.32 (1.12–1.56)	1.40 (1.02–1.92)	12.09 (<0.005)	1.96 (1.62–2.37)
CHD mortality	1.01 (0.77–1.31)	1.09 (0.71–1.67)	0.15 (>0.10)	1.27 (1.01–1.58)	1.56 (1.03–2.36)	6.81 (<0.05)	1.94 (1.51–2.50)
Stroke mortality	1.00 (0.66–1.51)	1.64 (0.88–3.07)	2.35 (>0.10)	1.21 (0.84–1.74)	1.29 (0.66–2.54)	1.23 (>0.10)	1.73 (1.12–2.68)
All-cause mortality	1.03 (0.93–1.14)	1.21 (1.01–1.44)	4.32 (>0.10)	1.37 (1.25–1.51)	1.73 (1.45–2.06)	61.35 (<0.001)	1.82 (1.60–2.06)

Adjusted for age, sex, centre, total cholesterol, body mass index, systolic blood pressure and smoking.

*Using fasting plasma glucose <6.1 mmol/l as reference group.

**Using 2-h post-load plasma glucose <7.8 mmol/l as reference group.

***Compared with the models with only the 2-h glucose criteria, 2df.

****Compared with the models with only the fasting glucose criteria, 2df.

persons, but no significant increase in mortality was associated with isolated fasting hyper-glycaemia (fasting plasma glucose ≥7.0 mmol/l and 2-h plasma glucose <11.1 mmol/l) [164]. In the Cardiovascular Health Study, including 4515 subjects aged >65 years, the rela-tive risk of CHD was higher in individuals with abnormal glucose (including impaired glu-cose tolerance, impaired fasting glucose, and newly diagnosed diabetes by both American Diabetes Association and WHO criteria) than in those with normal glucose. However, American Diabetes Association criteria based on fasting plasma glucose were less sensitive than the WHO criteria for predicting CHD among individuals with abnormal glucose [165]. A recent analysis of the US Second National Health and Nutrition Survey data, including 3092 adults aged 30–74 years, found a graded mortality associated with abnormal glucose tolerance ranging from a 40% greater risk in adults with impaired glucose tolerance to a 80% greater risk in adults with newly diagnosed diabetes [166].

In the DECODE study, multivariate Cox proportional hazard analyses showed that ele-vated 2-h plasma glucose was an independent predictor of mortality from all causes, CVD and CHD but elevated fasting plasma glucose alone was not (Table 6.6) [158, 159]. A high 2-h plasma glucose was found to be associated with an increased risk of death, independent of the level of fasting plasma glucose, whereas increased mortality in people with elevated fasting plasma glucose was largely due to the simultaneous elevation of 2-h plasma glucose. Thus, the DECODE study unequivocally confirmed that post-load hyperglycaemia independently increases cardiovascular morbidity and mortality and is a better predictor for CVD than high fasting plasma glucose.

In addition, several studies compared the magnitude of the risk of prior history of type 2 diabetes and myocardial infarction on subsequent CHD mortality [167–172]. The analyses from a Finnish cohort study including both men and women [167] and from the Nurses' Health Study [169] found that the risk of CHD among diabetic patients without prior myocardial infarction was similar to that in non-diabetic subjects with prior myocardial infarction. The analyses from our study and the Framingham Study indicated that in men prior myocardial infarction signifies a higher risk for CHD mortality than prior diabetes [170, 173, 174]. However, this is reversed in women, with prior diabetes being associated with greater risk for CHD mortality [170, 173, 174].

DIABETES AND STROKE

The results of prospective epidemiological studies on the independent association of type 2 diabetes and hyperglycaemia with the risk of stroke have been inconsistent. Some [116, 163, 175–180], but not all, studies [181–183] have identified type 2 diabetes or hyperglycaemia as an independent risk factor for stroke. Most of the previous studies have focused on ischaemic stroke alone [116, 177, 178, 180, 182, 183] because type 2 diabetes is not a prominent risk factor for haemorrhagic stoke [184].

GENDER DIFFERENCE IN CARDIOVASCULAR MORTALITY RELATED TO DIABETES

Among the middle-aged general population, men have 2–5 times higher risk of CHD than women [185–187]. The Framingham Study was the first one to point out that women with diabetes seem to lose their relative protection against CHD compared with men [188]. The reason for the higher relative risk of CHD in diabetic women than diabetic men is still unclear. The 14-year follow-up of the Rancho Bernardo study showed that the multivariate-adjusted relative hazards of death from CHD in diabetic compared with non-diabetic sub-jects was 3.3 in women and 1.9 in men [189]. A review about the impact of gender on the occurrence of atherosclerotic vascular disease in type 2 diabetes mellitus reported the over-all relative risk for gender (men vs. women) in CHD mortality as 1.46 (95% CI 1.21–1.95) in diabetic and 2.29 (2.05–2.55) in non-diabetic subjects [190]. The result from the DECODE study showed that screen-detected diabetic women had higher relative risks for cardiovascular mortality death than such men [191].

SUMMARY

Overweight or obesity, sedentary lifestyle, impaired glucose tolerance, diabetes, and the metabolic syndrome are major public health, clinical, and economic problems in modern societies, and each one or any combination of them may increase the risk of CHD and stroke. It is apparent that regular moderate-intensity physical activity, a healthy diet, and avoiding unhealthy weight gain are effective and safe ways to prevent and treat CVD and to prevent premature cardiovascular and total mortality in all population groups. Clinical trials have shown that lifestyle intervention is highly effective in preventing progression to overt type 2 diabetes in people with impaired glucose tolerance and the metabolic syndrome. Physical activity is an efficient tool also in the prevention of CVD events in type 2 diabetic patients. To combat the epidemic of overweight and to improve cardiovascular health at a population level, it is important to develop strategies to increase habitual physical activity and to prevent obesity in collaboration with communities.

REFERENCES

1. Murray CJ, Lopez AD. Mortality by cause for eight regions of the world: Global Burden of Disease Study. *Lancet* 1997; 349:1269–1276.
2. World Health Organization. Diet, nutrition, and the prevention of chronic diseases. WHO Technical Report Series 916. World Health Organization, Geneva, 2003.
3. Thom T, Haase N, Rosamond W *et al*. Heart disease and stroke statistics – 2006 update: a report from the American Heart Association Statistics Committee and Stroke Statistics Subcommittee. *Circulation* 2006; 113:e85–e151.
4. WHO Scientific Group. Cardiovascular disease risk factors: new areas for research. World Health Organization, Geneva, 1994.
5. Willett WC. Diet and health: what should we eat? *Science* 1994; 264:532–537.
6. Willett WC, Dietz WH, Colditz GA. Guidelines for healthy weight. *N Engl J Med* 1999; 341:427–434.
7. World Health Organization. Obesity: prevention and managing the global epidemic. WHO Technical Report Series 894. World Health Organization, Geneva, 2000.
8. Kuczmarski RJ, Flegal KM, Campbell SM, Johnson CL. Increasing prevalence of overweight among US adults. The National Health and Nutrition Examination Surveys, 1960 to 1991. *JAMA* 1994; 272:205–211.
9. Flegal KM, Carroll MD, Ogden CL, Johnson CL. Prevalence and trends in obesity among US adults, 1999–2000. *JAMA* 2002; 288:1723–1727.
10. Villa-Caballero L, Nava-Ocampo AA, Frati-Munari A, Ponce-Monter H. Oxidative stress, acute and regular exercise: are they really harmful in the diabetic patient? *Med Hypotheses* 2000; 55:43–46.
11. Ogden CL, Flegal KM, Carroll MD, Johnson CL. Prevalence and trends in overweight among US children and adolescents, 1999–2000. *JAMA* 2002; 288:1728–1732.
12. Li L, Rao K, Kong L *et al*. A description on the Chinese national nutrition and health survey in 2002. *Chin J Epidemiol* 2005; 26:474–484.
13. National Task Force on the Prevention and Treatment of Obesity. Overweight, obesity, and health risk. *Arch Intern Med* 2000; 160:898–904.
14. Lee IM, Manson JE, Hennekens CH, Paffenbarger RS Jr. Body weight and mortality. A 27-year follow-up of middle-aged men. *JAMA* 1993; 270:2823–2828.
15. Stevens J, Cai J, Pamuk ER, Williamson DF, Thun MJ, Wood JL. The effect of age on the association between body-mass index and mortality. *N Engl J Med* 1998; 338:1–7.
16. Calle EE, Thun MJ, Petrelli JM, Rodriguez C, Heath CW Jr. Body-mass index and mortality in a prospective cohort of U.S. adults. *N Engl J Med* 1999; 341:1097–1105.
17. Hu G, Tuomilehto J, Silventoinen K, Barengo NC, Peltonen M, Jousilahti P. The effects of physical activity and body mass index on cardiovascular, cancer and all-cause mortality among 47 212 middle-aged Finnish men and women. *Int J Obes Relat Metab Disord* 2005; 29:894–902.

18. Hu G, Tuomilehto J, Silventoinen K, Barengo N, Jousilahti P. Joint effects of physical activity, body mass index, waist circumference and waist-to-hip ratio with the risk of cardiovascular disease among middle-aged Finnish men and women. *Eur Heart J* 2004; 25:2212–2219.
19. Manson JE, Willett WC, Stampfer MJ *et al*. Body weight and mortality among women. *N Engl J Med* 1995; 333:677–685.
20. Hu FB, Willett WC, Li T, Stampfer MJ, Colditz GA, Manson JE. Adiposity as compared with physical activity in predicting mortality among women. *N Engl J Med* 2004; 351:2694–2703.
21. Fontaine KR, Redden DT, Wang C, Westfall AO, Allison DB. Years of life lost due to obesity. *JAMA* 2003; 289:187–193.
22. Willett WC, Manson JE, Stampfer MJ *et al*. Weight, weight change, and coronary heart disease in women. Risk within the 'normal' weight range. *JAMA* 1995; 273:461–465.
23. Field AE, Coakley EH, Must A *et al*. Impact of overweight on the risk of developing common chronic diseases during a 10-year period. *Arch Intern Med* 2001; 161:1581–1586.
24. Manson JE, Colditz GA, Stampfer MJ *et al*. A prospective study of obesity and risk of coronary heart disease in women. *N Engl J Med* 1990; 322:882–889.
25. Rimm EB, Stampfer MJ, Giovannucci E *et al*. Body size and fat distribution as predictors of coronary heart disease among middle-aged and older US men. *Am J Epidemiol* 1995; 141:1117–1127.
26. Rexrode KM, Carey VJ, Hennekens CH *et al*. Abdominal adiposity and coronary heart disease in women. *JAMA* 1998; 280:1843–1848.
27. Folsom AR, Kushi LH, Anderson KE *et al*. Associations of general and abdominal obesity with multiple health outcomes in older women: the Iowa Women's Health Study. *Arch Intern Med* 2000; 160:2117–2128.
28. Rexrode KM, Buring JE, Manson JE. Abdominal and total adiposity and risk of coronary heart disease in men. *Int J Obes Relat Metab Disord* 2001; 25:1047–1056.
29. Li TY, Rana JS, Manson JE *et al*. Obesity as compared with physical activity in predicting risk of coronary heart disease in women. *Circulation* 2006; 113:499–506.
30. Larsson B, Svardsudd K, Welin L, Wilhelmsen L, Bjorntorp P, Tibblin G. Abdominal adipose tissue distribution, obesity, and risk of cardiovascular disease and death: 13 year follow up of participants in the study of men born in 1913. *Br Med J* 1984; 288:1401–1404.
31. Casassus P, Fontbonne A, Thibult N *et al*. Upper-body fat distribution: a hyperinsulinemia-independent predictor of coronary heart disease mortality. The Paris Prospective Study. *Arterioscler Thromb* 1992; 12:1387–1392.
32. Folsom AR, Kaye SA, Sellers TA *et al*. Body fat distribution and 5-year risk of death in older women. *JAMA* 1993; 269:483–487.
33. Fujimoto WY, Bergstrom RW, Boyko EJ *et al*. Visceral adiposity and incident coronary heart disease in Japanese-American men. The 10-year follow-up results of the Seattle Japanese-American Community Diabetes Study. *Diabetes Care* 1999; 22:1808–1812.
34. Lakka HM, Lakka TA, Tuomilehto J, Salonen JT. Abdominal obesity is associated with increased risk of acute coronary events in men. *Eur Heart J* 2002; 23:706–713.
35. Baik I, Ascherio A, Rimm EB *et al*. Adiposity and mortality in men. *Am J Epidemiol* 2000; 152:264–271.
36. Rexrode KM, Hennekens CH, Willett WC *et al*. A prospective study of body mass index, weight change, and risk of stroke in women. *JAMA* 1997; 277:1539–1545.
37. Kurth T, Gaziano JM, Berger K *et al*. Body mass index and the risk of stroke in men. *Arch Intern Med* 2002; 162:2557–2562.
38. Suk SH, Sacco RL, Boden-Albala B *et al*. Abdominal obesity and risk of ischemic stroke: the Northern Manhattan Stroke Study. *Stroke* 2003; 34:1586–1592.
39. Song YM, Sung J, Davey Smith G, Ebrahim S. Body mass index and ischemic and hemorrhagic stroke: a prospective study in Korean men. *Stroke* 2004; 35:831–836.
40. Jood K, Jern C, Wilhelmsen L, Rosengren A. Body mass index in mid-life is associated with a first stroke in men: a prospective population study over 28 years. *Stroke* 2004; 35:2764–2769.
41. Kurth T, Gaziano JM, Rexrode KM *et al*. Prospective study of body mass index and risk of stroke in apparently healthy women. *Circulation* 2005; 111:1992–1998.
42. Welin L, Svardsudd K, Wilhelmsen L, Larsson B, Tibblin G. Analysis of risk factors for stroke in a cohort of men born in 1913. *N Engl J Med* 1987; 317:521–526.
43. Walker SP, Rimm EB, Ascherio A, Kawachi I, Stampfer MJ, Willett WC. Body size and fat distribution as predictors of stroke among US men. *Am J Epidemiol* 1996; 144:1143–1150.
44. Colditz GA, Willett WC, Rotnitzky A, Manson JE. Weight gain as a risk factor for clinical diabetes mellitus in women. *Ann Intern Med* 1995; 122:481–486.

45. Huang Z, Willett WC, Manson JE *et al*. Body weight, weight change, and risk for hypertension in women. *Ann Intern Med* 1998; 128:81–88.

46. Lee IM, Blair SN, Allison DB *et al*. Epidemiologic data on the relationships of caloric intake, energy balance, and weight gain over the life span with longevity and morbidity. *J Gerontol A Biol Sci Med Sci* 2001; 56(spec no 1):7–19.

47. Tuomilehto J, Lindstrom J, Eriksson JG *et al*. Prevention of type 2 diabetes mellitus by changes in lifestyle among subjects with impaired glucose tolerance. *N Engl J Med* 2001; 344:1343–1350.

48. Knowler WC, Barrett-Connor E, Fowler SE *et al*. Reduction in the incidence of type 2 diabetes with lifestyle intervention or metformin. *N Engl J Med* 2002; 346:393–403.

49. Williamson DF, Pamuk E, Thun M, Flanders D, Byers T, Heath C. Prospective study of intentional weight loss and mortality in never-smoking overweight US white women aged 40–64 years. *Am J Epidemiol* 1995; 141:1128–1141.

50. French SA, Folsom AR, Jeffery RW, Williamson DF. Prospective study of intentionality of weight loss and mortality in older women: the Iowa Women's Health Study. *Am J Epidemiol* 1999; 149:504–514.

51. Blair SN, Shaten J, Brownell K, Collins G, Lissner L. Body weight change, all-cause mortality, and cause-specific mortality in the Multiple Risk Factor Intervention Trial. *Ann Intern Med* 1993; 119:749–757.

52. Dyer AR, Stamler J, Greenland P. Associations of weight change and weight variability with cardiovascular and all-cause mortality in the Chicago Western Electric Company Study. *Am J Epidemiol* 2000; 152:324–333.

53. Turner RC, Millns H, Neil HA *et al*. Risk factors for coronary artery disease in non-insulin dependent diabetes mellitus: United Kingdom Prospective Diabetes Study (UKPDS: 23). *BMJ* 1998; 316:823–828.

54. Church TS, Cheng YJ, Earnest CP *et al*. Exercise capacity and body composition as predictors of mortality among men with diabetes. *Diabetes Care* 2004; 27:83–88.

55. Hu G, Jousilahti P, Barengo NC, Qiao Q, Lakka TA, Tuomilehto J. Physical activity, cardiovascular risk factors, and mortality among Finnish adults with diabetes. *Diabetes Care* 2005; 28:799–805.

56. Pate RR, Pratt M, Blair SN *et al*. Physical activity and public health. A recommendation from the Centers for Disease Control and Prevention and the American College of Sports Medicine. *JAMA* 1995; 273:402–407.

57. Thompson PD, Buchner D, Pina IL *et al*. Exercise and physical activity in the prevention and treatment of atherosclerotic cardiovascular disease: a statement from the Council on Clinical Cardiology (Subcommittee on Exercise, Rehabilitation, and Prevention) and the Council on Nutrition, Physical Activity, and Metabolism (Subcommittee on Physical Activity). *Circulation* 2003; 107:3109–3116.

58. Physical activity and cardiovascular health. NIH consensus development panel on physical activity and cardiovascular health. *JAMA* 1996; 276:241–246.

59. Macero CA, Jones DA, Yore MM *et al*. Prevalence of physical activity, including lifestyle activities among adults – United States, 2000–2001. *MMWR Morb Mortal Wkly Rep* 2003; 52:764–769.

60. Centers for Disease Control and Prevention: Physical activity levels among children aged 9–13 years – United States, 2002. *MMWR Morb Mortal Wkly Rep* 2003; 52:785–788.

61. Paffenbarger RS Jr, Hyde RT, Wing AL, Hsieh CC. Physical activity, all-cause mortality, and longevity of college alumni. *N Engl J Med* 1986; 314:605–613.

62. Blair SN, Kohl HW 3rd, Paffenbarger RS Jr, Clark DG, Cooper KH, Gibbons LW. Physical fitness and all-cause mortality. A prospective study of healthy men and women. *JAMA* 1989; 262:2395–2401.

63. Sandvik L, Erikssen J, Thaulow E, Erikssen G, Mundal R, Rodahl K. Physical fitness as a predictor of mortality among healthy, middle-aged Norwegian men. *N Engl J Med* 1993; 328:533–537.

64. Blair SN, Kampert JB, Kohl HW 3rd *et al*. Influences of cardiorespiratory fitness and other precursors on cardiovascular disease and all-cause mortality in men and women. *JAMA* 1996; 276:205–210.

65. Barengo NC, Hu G, Lakka TA, Pekkarinen H, Nissinen A, Tuomilehto J. Low physical activity as a predictor for total and cardiovascular disease mortality in middle-aged men and women in Finland. *Eur Heart J* 2004; 25:2204–2211.

66. Paffenbarger RS Jr, Hyde RT, Wing AL, Lee IM, Jung DL, Kampert JB. The association of changes in physical-activity level and other lifestyle characteristics with mortality among men. *N Engl J Med* 1993; 328:538–545.

67. Blair SN, Kohl HW 3rd, Barlow CE, Paffenbarger RS Jr, Gibbons LW, Macera CA. Changes in physical fitness and all-cause mortality. A prospective study of healthy and unhealthy men. *JAMA* 1995; 273:1093–1098.

68. Erikssen G, Liestol K, Bjornholt J, Thaulow E, Sandvik L, Erikssen J. Changes in physical fitness and changes in mortality. *Lancet* 1998; 352:759–762.

69. Wannamethee SG, Shaper AG, Walker M. Changes in physical activity, mortality, and incidence of coronary heart disease in older men. *Lancet* 1998; 351:1603–1608.
70. Paffenbarger RS Jr, Hyde RT, Wing AL, Steinmetz CH. A natural history of athleticism and cardiovascular health. *JAMA* 1984; 252:491–495.
71. Oguma Y, Shinoda-Tagawa T. Physical activity decreases cardiovascular disease risk in women: review and meta-analysis. *Am J Prev Med* 2004; 26:407–418.
72. Manson JE, Hu FB, Rich-Edwards JW *et al*. A prospective study of walking as compared with vigorous exercise in the prevention of coronary heart disease in women. *N Engl J Med* 1999; 341:650–658.
73. Lee IM, Rexrode KM, Cook NR, Manson JE, Buring JE. Physical activity and coronary heart disease in women: is 'no pain, no gain' passe? *JAMA* 2001; 285:1447–1454.
74. Manson JE, Greenland P, LaCroix AZ *et al*. Walking compared with vigorous exercise for the prevention of cardiovascular events in women. *N Engl J Med* 2002; 347:716–725.
75. Tanasescu M, Leitzmann MF, Rimm EB, Willett WC, Stampfer MJ, Hu FB. Exercise type and intensity in relation to coronary heart disease in men. *JAMA* 2002; 288:1994–2000.
76. Lee IM, Sesso HD, Paffenbarger RS Jr. Physical activity and coronary heart disease risk in men: does the duration of exercise episodes predict risk? *Circulation* 2000; 102:981–986.
77. Hu G, Tuomilehto J, Borodulin K, Jousilahti P. The joint associations of occupational, commuting, and leisure-time physical activity, and the Framingham risk score on the 10-year risk of coronary heart disease. *Eur Heart J* 2007; 28:492–498.
78. Wannamethee G, Shaper AG. Physical activity and stroke in British middle aged men. *BMJ* 1992; 304:597–601.
79. Abbott RD, Rodriguez BL, Burchfiel CM, Curb JD. Physical activity in older middle-aged men and reduced risk of stroke: the Honolulu Heart Program. *Am J Epidemiol* 1994; 139:881–893.
80. Kiely DK, Wolf PA, Cupples LA, Beiser AS, Kannel WB. Physical activity and stroke risk: the Framingham Study. *Am J Epidemiol* 1994; 140:608–620.
81. Gillum RF, Mussolino ME, Ingram DD. Physical activity and stroke incidence in women and men. The NHANES I Epidemiologic Follow-up Study. *Am J Epidemiol* 1996; 143:860–869.
82. Ellekjaer H, Holmen J, Ellekjaer E, Vatten L. Physical activity and stroke mortality in women. Ten-year follow-up of the Nord-Trondelag health survey, 1984–1986. *Stroke* 2000; 31:14–18.
83. Hu FB, Stampfer MJ, Colditz GA *et al*. Physical activity and risk of stroke in women. *JAMA* 2000; 283:2961–2967.
84. Kurl S, Laukkanen JA, Rauramaa R, Lakka TA, Sivenius J, Salonen JT. Cardiorespiratory fitness and the risk for stroke in men. *Arch Intern Med* 2003; 163:1682–1688.
85. Hu G, Sarti C, Jousilahti P, Silventoinen K, Barengo NC, Tuomilehto J. Leisure time, occupational, and commuting physical activity and the risk of stroke. *Stroke* 2005; 36:1994–1999.
86. Lee IM, Hennekens CH, Berger K, Buring JE, Manson JE. Exercise and risk of stroke in male physicians. *Stroke* 1999; 30:1–6.
87. Goldstein LB, Adams R, Becker K *et al*. Primary prevention of ischemic stroke: a statement for healthcare professionals from the Stroke Council of the American Heart Association. *Circulation* 2001; 103:163–182.
88. Sacco RL, Gan R, Boden-Albala B *et al*. Leisure-time physical activity and ischemic stroke risk: the Northern Manhattan Stroke Study. *Stroke* 1998; 29:380–387.
89. Hu FB, Stampfer MJ, Solomon C *et al*. Physical activity and risk for cardiovascular events in diabetic women. *Ann Intern Med* 2001; 134:96–105.
90. Batty GD, Shipley MJ, Marmot M, Smith GD. Physical activity and cause-specific mortality in men with Type 2 diabetes/impaired glucose tolerance: evidence from the Whitehall study. *Diabet Med* 2002; 19:580–588.
91. Gregg EW, Gerzoff RB, Caspersen CJ, Williamson DF, Narayan KM. Relationship of walking to mortality among US adults with diabetes. *Arch Intern Med* 2003; 163:1440–1447.
92. Tanasescu M, Leitzmann MF, Rimm EB, Hu FB. Physical activity in relation to cardiovascular disease and total mortality among men with type 2 diabetes. *Circulation* 2003; 107:2435–2439.
93. Hu G, Eriksson J, Barengo NC *et al*. Occupational, commuting, and leisure-time physical activity in relation to total and cardiovascular mortality among Finnish subjects with type 2 diabetes. *Circulation* 2004; 110:666–673.
94. Wei M, Gibbons LW, Kampert JB, Nichaman MZ, Blair SN. Low cardiorespiratory fitness and physical inactivity as predictors of mortality in men with type 2 diabetes. *Ann Intern Med* 2000; 132:605–611.

95. Oldridge NB, Guyatt GH, Fischer ME, Rimm AA. Cardiac rehabilitation after myocardial infarction. Combined experience of randomized clinical trials. *JAMA* 1988; 260:945–950.

96. O'Connor GT, Buring JE, Yusuf S *et al*. An overview of randomized trials of rehabilitation with exercise after myocardial infarction. *Circulation* 1989; 80:234–244.

97. Jolliffe JA, Rees K, Taylor RS, Thompson D, Oldridge N, Ebrahim S. Exercise-based rehabilitation for coronary heart disease. *Cochrane Database Syst Rev* 2001:CD001800.

98. Mittleman MA, Maclure M, Tofler GH, Sherwood JB, Goldberg RJ, Muller JE. Triggering of acute myocardial infarction by heavy physical exertion. Protection against triggering by regular exertion. Determinants of Myocardial Infarction Onset Study Investigators. *N Engl J Med* 1993; 329:1677–1683.

99. Albert CM, Mittleman MA, Chae CU, Lee IM, Hennekens CH, Manson JE. Triggering of sudden death from cardiac causes by vigorous exertion. *N Engl J Med* 2000; 343:1355–1361.

100. Reaven GM. Banting lecture 1988. Role of insulin resistance in human disease. *Diabetes* 1988; 37:1595–1607.

101. WHO Consultation. Definition, diagnosis and classification of diabetes mellitus and its complications. Part 1:diagnosis and classification of diabetes mellitus. World Health Organization, Geneva, 1999.

102. Pyörälä K. Relationship of glucose tolerance and plasma insulin to the incidence of coronary heart disease: results from two population studies in Finland. *Diabetes Care* 1979; 2:131–141.

103. Welborn TA, Wearne K. Coronary heart disease incidence and cardiovascular mortality in Busselton with reference to glucose and insulin concentrations. *Diabetes Care* 1979; 2:154–160.

104. Ducimetiere P, Eschwege E, Papoz L, Richard JL, Claude JR, Rosselin G. Relationship of plasma insulin levels to the incidence of myocardial infarction and coronary heart disease mortality in a middle-aged population. *Diabetologia* 1980; 19:205–210.

105. Pyörälä M, Miettinen H, Laakso M, Pyörälä K. Hyperinsulinemia predicts coronary heart disease risk in healthy middle-aged men : the 22-year follow-up results of the Helsinki Policemen Study. *Circulation* 1998; 98:398–404.

106. Folsom AR, Szklo M, Stevens J, Liao F, Smith R, Eckfeldt JH. A prospective study of coronary heart disease in relation to fasting insulin, glucose, and diabetes. The Atherosclerosis Risk in Communities (ARIC) Study. *Diabetes Care* 1997; 20:935–942.

107. Lempiäinen P, Mykkänen L, Pyörälä K, Laakso M, Kuusisto J. Insulin resistance syndrome predicts coronary heart disease events in elderly nondiabetic men. *Circulation* 1999; 100:123–128.

108. Lakka HM, Lakka TA, Tuomilehto J, Sivenius J, Salonen JT. Hyperinsulinemia and the risk of cardiovascular death and acute coronary and cerebrovascular events in men: the Kuopio Ischaemic Heart Disease Risk Factor Study. *Arch Intern Med* 2000; 160:1160–1168.

109. Hanley AJ, Williams K, Stern MP, Haffner SM. Homeostasis model assessment of insulin resistance in relation to the incidence of cardiovascular disease: the San Antonio Heart Study. *Diabetes Care* 2002; 25:1177–1184.

110. Hu G, Qiao Q, Tuomilehto J, Eliasson M, Feskens EJ, Pyörälä K. Plasma insulin and cardiovascular mortality in non-diabetic European men and women: a meta-analysis of data from eleven prospective studies. *Diabetologia* 2004; 47:1245–1256.

111. Collins VR, Dowse GK, Zimmet PZ *et al*. Serum insulin and ECG abnormalities suggesting coronary heart disease in the populations of Mauritius and Nauru: cross-sectional and longitudinal associations. *J Clin Epidemiol* 1993; 46:1373–1393.

112. Ferrara A, Barrett-Connor EL, Edelstein SL. Hyperinsulinemia does not increase the risk of fatal cardiovascular disease in elderly men or women without diabetes: the Rancho Bernardo Study, 1984–1991. *Am J Epidemiol* 1994; 140:857–869.

113. Lindberg O, Tilvis RS, Strandberg TE *et al*. Elevated fasting plasma insulin in a general aged population: an innocent companion of cardiovascular diseases. *J Am Geriatr Soc* 1997; 45:407–412.

114. Lindahl B, Dinesen B, Eliasson M *et al*. High proinsulin concentration precedes acute myocardial infarction in a nondiabetic population. *Metabolism* 1999; 48:1197–1202.

115. Wannamethee SG, Perry IJ, Shaper AG. Nonfasting serum glucose and insulin concentrations and the risk of stroke. *Stroke* 1999; 30:1780–1786.

116. Pyörälä M, Miettinen H, Laakso M, Pyorala K. Hyperinsulinemia and the risk of stroke in healthy middle-aged men: the 22-year follow-up results of the Helsinki Policemen Study. *Stroke* 1998; 29:1860–1866.

117. Folsom AR, Rasmussen ML, Chambless LE et al. Prospective associations of fasting insulin, body fat distribution, and diabetes with risk of ischemic stroke. The Atherosclerosis Risk in Communities (ARIC) Study Investigators. *Diabetes Care* 1999; 22:1077–1083.

118. DeFronzo R, Ferrannini E. Insulin resistance. A multifaceted syndrome responsible for NIDDM, obesity, hypertension, dyslipidemia, and atherosclerotic cardiovascular disease. *Diabetes Care* 1991; 14:173–194.

119. Kuusisto J, Mykkanen L, Pyörälä K, Laakso M. Hyperinsulinemic microalbuminuria. A new risk indicator for coronary heart disease. *Circulation* 1995; 91:831–837.

120. Imperatore G, Riccardi G, Iovine C, Rivellese AA, Vaccaro O. Plasma fibrinogen: a new factor of the metabolic syndrome. A population-based study. *Diabetes Care* 1998; 21:649–654.

121. Festa A, D'Agostino R Jr, Mykkanen L et al. Relative contribution of insulin and its precursors to fibrinogen and PAI-1 in a large population with different states of glucose tolerance. The Insulin Resistance Atherosclerosis Study (IRAS). *Arterioscler Thromb Vasc Biol* 1999; 19:562–568.

122. Meigs JB. Invited commentary: insulin resistance syndrome? Syndrome X? Multiple metabolic syndrome? A syndrome at all? Factor analysis reveals patterns in the fabric of correlated metabolic risk factors. *Am J Epidemiol* 2000; 152:908–911; discussion 912.

123. Lakka TA, Laaksonen DE, Lakka HM et al. Sedentary lifestyle, poor cardiorespiratory fitness, and the metabolic syndrome. *Med Sci Sports Exerc* 2003; 35:1279–1286.

124. Balkau B, Charles MA. Comment on the provisional report from the WHO consultation. European Group for the Study of Insulin Resistance (EGIR). *Diabet Med* 1999; 16:442–443.

125. National Institute of Health. Executive Summary of The Third Report of The National Cholesterol Education Program (NCEP) Expert Panel on Detection, Evaluation, And Treatment of High Blood Cholesterol In Adults (Adult Treatment Panel III). *JAMA* 2001; 285:2486–2497.

126. Grundy SM, Cleeman JI, Daniels SR et al. Diagnosis and management of the metabolic syndrome: an American Heart Association/National Heart, Lung, and Blood Institute Scientific Statement. *Circulation* 2005; 112:2735–2752.

127. Bloomgarden ZT. American Association of Clinical Endocrinologists (AACE) Consensus Conference on the Insulin Resistance Syndrome: 25–26 August 2002, Washington DC. *Diabetes Care* 2003; 26:933–939.

128. Einhorn D, Reaven GM, Cobin RH et al. American College of Endocrinology position statement on the insulin resistance syndrome. *Endocr Pract* 2003; 9:237–252.

129. Alberti KG, Zimmet P, Shaw J. The metabolic syndrome – a new worldwide definition. *Lancet* 2005; 366:1059–1062.

130. Ford ES, Giles WH, Dietz WH. Prevalence of the metabolic syndrome among US adults: findings from the third National Health and Nutrition Examination Survey. *JAMA* 2002; 287:356–359.

131. Hu G, Qiao Q, Tuomilehto J et al. Prevalence of the metabolic syndrome and its relation to all-cause and cardiovascular mortality in nondiabetic European men and women. *Arch Intern Med* 2004; 164:1066–1076.

132. Tan CE, Ma S, Wai D, Chew SK, Tai ES. Can we apply the National Cholesterol Education Program Adult Treatment Panel definition of the metabolic syndrome to Asians? *Diabetes Care* 2004; 27:1182–1186.

133. Kim MH, Kim MK, Choi BY, Shin YJ. Prevalence of the metabolic syndrome and its association with cardiovascular diseases in Korea. *J Korean Med Sci* 2004; 19:195–201.

134. Gu D, Reynolds K, Wu X et al. Prevalence of the metabolic syndrome and overweight among adults in China. *Lancet* 2005; 365:1398–1405.

135. Isomaa B, Almgren P, Tuomi T et al. Cardiovascular morbidity and mortality associated with the metabolic syndrome. *Diabetes Care* 2001; 24:683–689.

136. Lakka HM, Laaksonen DE, Lakka TA et al. The metabolic syndrome and total and cardiovascular disease mortality in middle-aged men. *JAMA* 2002; 288:2709–2716.

137. Ford ES. The metabolic syndrome and mortality from cardiovascular disease and all-causes: findings from the National Health and Nutrition Examination Survey II Mortality Study. *Atherosclerosis* 2004; 173:309–314.

138. Malik S, Wong ND, Franklin SS et al. Impact of the metabolic syndrome on mortality from coronary heart disease, cardiovascular disease, and all causes in United States adults. *Circulation* 2004; 110:1245–1250.

139. Hunt KJ, Resendez RG, Williams K, Haffner SM, Stern MP. National Cholesterol Education Program versus World Health Organization metabolic syndrome in relation to all-cause and cardiovascular mortality in the San Antonio Heart Study. *Circulation* 2004; 110:1251–1257.

140. Dekker JM, Girman C, Rhodes T *et al*. Metabolic syndrome and 10-year cardiovascular disease risk in the Hoorn Study. *Circulation* 2005; 112:666–673.

141. Eberly LE, Prineas R, Cohen JD *et al*. Metabolic syndrome: risk factor distribution and 18-year mortality in the multiple risk factor intervention trial. *Diabetes Care* 2006; 29:123–130.

142. Wilson PW, D'Agostino RB, Parise H, Sullivan L, Meigs JB. Metabolic syndrome as a precursor of cardiovascular disease and type 2 diabetes mellitus. *Circulation* 2005; 112:3066–3072.

143. Gami AS, Witt BJ, Howard DE *et al*. Metabolic syndrome and risk of incident cardiovascular events and death: a systematic review and meta-analysis of longitudinal studies. *J Am Coll Cardiol* 2007; 49:403–414.

144. McNeill AM, Rosamond WD, Girman CJ *et al*. The metabolic syndrome and 11-year risk of incident cardiovascular disease in the atherosclerosis risk in communities study. *Diabetes Care* 2005; 28:385–390.

145. Scuteri A, Najjar SS, Morrell CH, Lakatta EG. The metabolic syndrome in older individuals: prevalence and prediction of cardiovascular events: the Cardiovascular Health Study. *Diabetes Care* 2005; 28:882–887.

146. Wannamethee SG, Shaper AG, Lennon L, Morris RW. Metabolic syndrome vs Framingham Risk Score for prediction of coronary heart disease, stroke, and type 2 diabetes mellitus. *Arch Intern Med* 2005; 165:2644–2650.

147. Resnick HE, Jones K, Ruotolo G *et al*. Insulin resistance, the metabolic syndrome, and risk of incident cardiovascular disease in nondiabetic american indians: the strong heart study. *Diabetes Care* 2003; 26:861–867.

148. Ford ES. Risks for all-cause mortality, cardiovascular disease, and diabetes associated with the metabolic syndrome: a summary of the evidence. *Diabetes Care* 2005; 28:1769–1778.

149. Najarian RM, Sullivan LM, Kannel WB, Wilson PW, D'Agostino RB, Wolf PA. Metabolic syndrome compared with type 2 diabetes mellitus as a risk factor for stroke: the Framingham Offspring Study. *Arch Intern Med* 2006; 166:106–111.

150. Kurl S, Laukkanen J, Niskanen L *et al*. Metabolic syndrome and the risk of stroke in middle-aged men. *Stroke* 2006; 37:806–811.

151. World Health Organization. WHO Expert Committee on Diabetes Mellitus: second report. Geneva: World Health Organ Tech Rep Ser no 646, 1980.

152. Expert Committee on the Diagnosis and Classification of Diabetes Mellitus. Report of the Expert Committee on the Diagnosis and Classification of Diabetes Mellitus. *Diabetes Care* 1997; 20:1183–1197.

153. Genuth S, Alberti KG, Bennett P *et al*. Follow-up report on the diagnosis of diabetes mellitus. *Diabetes Care* 2003; 26:3160–3167.

154. Tominaga M, Eguchi H, Manaka H, Igarashi K, Kato T, Sekikawa A. Impaired glucose tolerance is a risk factor for cardiovascular disease, but not impaired fasting glucose. The Funagata Diabetes Study. *Diabetes Care* 1999; 22:920–924.

155. Qiao Q, Jousilahti P, Eriksson J, Tuomilehto J. Predictive properties of impaired glucose tolerance for cardiovascular risk are not explained by the development of overt diabetes during follow-up. *Diabetes Care* 2003; 26:2910–2914.

156. Kanaya AM, Herrington D, Vittinghoff E *et al*. Impaired fasting glucose and cardiovascular outcomes in postmenopausal women with coronary artery disease. *Ann Intern Med* 2005; 142:813–820.

157. Levitan EB, Song Y, Ford ES, Liu S. Is nondiabetic hyperglycemia a risk factor for cardiovascular disease? A meta-analysis of prospective studies. *Arch Intern Med* 2004; 164:2147–2155.

158. DECODE Study Group. Glucose tolerance and mortality: comparison of WHO and American Diabetes Association diagnostic criteria. The DECODE study group. European Diabetes Epidemiology Group. Diabetes Epidemiology: Collaborative analysis Of Diagnostic criteria in Europe. *Lancet* 1999; 354:617–621.

159. DECODE Study Group. Glucose tolerance and cardiovascular mortality: comparison of fasting and 2-hour diagnostic criteria. *Arch Intern Med* 2001; 161:397–405.

160. King H, Aubert RE, Herman WH. Global Burden of Diabetes, 1995–2025: prevalence, numerical estimates, and projections. *Diabetes Care* 1998; 21:1414–1431.

161. Zimmet P, Alberti KG, Shaw J. Global and societal implications of the diabetes epidemic. *Nature* 2001; 414:782–787.

162. Laakso M. Hyperglycemia and cardiovascular disease in type 2 diabetes. *Diabetes* 1999; 48:937–942.

163. Stamler J, Vaccaro O, Neaton JD, Wentworth D. Diabetes, other risk factors, and 12-yr cardiovascular mortality for men screened in the Multiple Risk Factor Intervention Trial. *Diabetes Care* 1993; 16:434–444.

164. Shaw JE, Hodge AM, de Courten M, Chitson P, Zimmet PZ. Isolated post-challenge hyperglycaemia confirmed as a risk factor for mortality. *Diabetologia* 1999; 42:1050–1054.

165. Barzilay JI, Spiekerman CF, Wahl PW *et al*. Cardiovascular disease in older adults with glucose disorders: comparison of American Diabetes Association criteria for diabetes mellitus with WHO criteria. *Lancet* 1999; 354:622–625.

166. Saydah SH, Loria CM, Eberhardt MS, Brancati FL. Subclinical states of glucose intolerance and risk of death in the U.S. *Diabetes Care* 2001; 24:447–453.

167. Haffner SM, Lehto S, Ronnemaa T, Pyörälä K, Laakso M. Mortality from coronary heart disease in subjects with type 2 diabetes and in nondiabetic subjects with and without prior myocardial infarction. *N Engl J Med* 1998; 339:229–234.

168. Hu FB, Stampfer MJ, Solomon CG *et al*. The impact of diabetes mellitus on mortality from all causes and coronary heart disease in women: 20 years of follow-up. *Arch Intern Med* 2001; 161:1717–1723.

169. Lotufo PA, Gaziano JM, Chae CU *et al*. Diabetes and all-cause and coronary heart disease mortality among US male physicians. *Arch Intern Med* 2001; 161:242–247.

170. Natarajan S, Liao Y, Cao G, Lipsitz SR, McGee DL. Sex differences in risk for coronary heart disease mortality associated with diabetes and established coronary heart disease. *Arch Intern Med* 2003; 163:1735–1740.

171. Becker A, Bos G, de Vegt F *et al*. Cardiovascular events in type 2 diabetes: comparison with nondiabetic individuals without and with prior cardiovascular disease. 10-year follow-up of the Hoorn Study. *Eur Heart J* 2003; 24:1406–1413.

172. Lee CD, Folsom AR, Pankow JS, Brancati FL. Cardiovascular events in diabetic and nondiabetic adults with or without history of myocardial infarction. *Circulation* 2004; 109:855–860.

173. Hu G, Jousilahti P, Qiao Q, Katoh S, Tuomilehto J. Sex differences in cardiovascular and total mortality among diabetic and non-diabetic individuals with or without history of myocardial infarction. *Diabetologia* 2005; 48:856–861.

174. Hu G, Jousilahti P, Qiao Q, Peltonen M, Katoh S, Tuomilehto J. The gender-specific impact of diabetes and myocardial infarction at baseline and during follow-up on mortality from all causes and coronary heart disease. *J Am Coll Cardiol* 2005; 45:1413–1418.

175. Lehto S, Ronnemaa T, Pyörälä K, Laakso M. Predictors of stroke in middle-aged patients with non-insulin-dependent diabetes. *Stroke* 1996; 27:63–68.

176. Tuomilehto J, Rastenyte D, Jousilahti P, Sarti C, Vartiainen E. Diabetes mellitus as a risk factor for death from stroke. Prospective study of the middle-aged Finnish population. *Stroke* 1996; 27:210–215.

177. Tanne D, Yaari S, Goldbourt U. Risk profile and prediction of long-term ischemic stroke mortality: a 21-year follow-up in the Israeli Ischemic Heart Disease (IIHD) Project. *Circulation* 1998; 98:1365–1371.

178. Iso H, Imano H, Kitamura A *et al*. Type 2 diabetes and risk of non-embolic ischaemic stroke in Japanese men and women. *Diabetologia* 2004; 47:2137–2144.

179. Lawes CM, Parag V, Bennett DA *et al*. Blood glucose and risk of cardiovascular disease in the Asia Pacific region. *Diabetes Care* 2004; 27:2836–2842.

180. Kissela BM, Khoury J, Kleindorfer D *et al*. Epidemiology of ischemic stroke in patients with diabetes: the greater Cincinnati/Northern Kentucky Stroke Study. *Diabetes Care* 2005; 28:355–359.

181. Haheim LL, Holme I, Hjermann I, Leren P. Risk factors of stroke incidence and mortality. A 12-year follow-up of the Oslo Study. *Stroke* 1993; 24:1484–1489.

182. Carrieri PB, Orefice G, Maiorino A, Provitera V, Balzano G, Lucariello A. Age-related risk factors for ischemic stroke in Italian men. *Neuroepidemiology* 1994; 13:28–33.

183. Simons LA, McCallum J, Friedlander Y, Simons J. Risk factors for ischemic stroke: Dubbo Study of the elderly. *Stroke* 1998; 29:1341–1346.

184. Bell DS. Stroke in the diabetic patient. *Diabetes Care* 1994; 17:213–219.

185. Tuomilehto J, Kuulasmaa K. WHO MONICA Project: assessing CHD mortality and morbidity. *Int J Epidemiol* 1989; 18:S38–S45.

186. Tunstall-Pedoe H, Kuulasmaa K, Amouyel P, Arveiler D, Rajakangas AM, Pajak A. Myocardial infarction and coronary deaths in the World Health Organization MONICA Project. Registration procedures, event rates, and case-fatality rates in 38 populations from 21 countries in four continents. *Circulation* 1994; 90:583–612.

187. Jousilahti P, Vartiainen E, Tuomilehto J, Puska P. Sex, age, cardiovascular risk factors, and coronary heart disease: a prospective follow-up study of 14 786 middle-aged men and women in Finland. *Circulation* 1999; 99:1165–1172.

188. Kannel WB, McGee DL. Diabetes and cardiovascular disease. The Framingham study. *JAMA* 1979; 241:2035–2038.
189. Barrett-Connor EL, Cohn BA, Wingard DL, Edelstein SL. Why is diabetes mellitus a stronger risk factor for fatal ischemic heart disease in women than in men? The Rancho Bernardo Study. *JAMA* 1991; 265:627–631.
190. Orchard TJ. The impact of gender and general risk factors on the occurrence of atherosclerotic vascular disease in non-insulin-dependent diabetes mellitus. *Ann Med* 1996; 28:323–333.
191. DECODE Study Group. Gender difference in all-cause and cardiovascular mortality related to hyperglycaemia and newly-diagnosed diabetes. *Diabetologia* 2003; 46:608–617.

7

Estimation of cardiovascular risk: close enough is not good enough

A. D. Sniderman, P. Couture

INTRODUCTION

Notwithstanding all we know as to its aetiology and notwithstanding all the treatments we have to prevent its complications, cardiovascular disease (CVD) is poised to become the most common cause of death worldwide [1]. If we know so much, why are we able to do so little? In large part the answer is that we apply our most potent therapies only after there is clinical evidence of vascular disease – too late to save the lives that have already been lost, too late to save the ventricle or the brain that has already been destroyed, too late to arrest arterial disease that is already too advanced: too little, too late, for too many.

This essay addresses a number of the assumptions that underlie the conventional approach to predicting vascular disease. We will argue that we have fallen into the trap of venerating the past rather than understanding it with the result that we overlook the methodological and conceptual limitations that restrict our ability to recognize high-risk subjects, limitations that are embedded in all the major conventional guidelines, limitations that must be recognized and corrected if primary prevention is to improve.

We will address three of these. The first is our failure to appreciate the error introduced into clinical decision-making by our use of an inaccurately calculated low-density lipoprotein (LDL) cholesterol as a surrogate for an accurately measured LDL cholesterol. The second is our failure to recognize the critical biological variance between the major proatherogenic lipoprotein-related risk factors – apolipoprotein B (apoB) and LDL cholesterol. The third is how arbitrarily restricted periods of observation artifactually reduce our appreciation of the role of factors such as apoB as causes of coronary disease, and following from this, whether we need to modify our interpretation of the statistical methods we use to assess the predictive power of the causes of vascular disease.

In this discussion, we will focus on the atherogenic plasma lipoproteins – the apoB lipoproteins – because they are the single most important and the single most treatable of the modifiable causes of premature vascular disease. We will also focus on prediction of the risk of vascular disease rather than therapy to reduce clinical events.

Allan D. Sniderman, MD, FRCP(C), Edwards Professor of Cardiology, McGill University, Mike Rosenbloom Laboratory for Cardiovascular Research, Royal Victoria Hospital, Montreal, Quebec, Canada

Patrick Couture, MD, FRCP(C), PhD, Associate Professor of Medicine, Lavel University, Québec City, Canada

WEAKNESS OF CALCULATED LDL CHOLESTEROL

Methodological: LDL cholesterol estimated by Friedewald versus LDL cholesterol measured by ultracentrifugation

LDL cholesterol remains the cornerstone of the lipid approach but LDL cholesterol, as esti-mated clinically, too often does not equal the mass of LDL cholesterol actually present in plasma. To accurately measure the amount of cholesterol in LDL, the triglyceride-rich lipoproteins, very low-density lipoprotein (VLDL) and chylomicrons, must first be removed by ultracentrifugation and the cholesterol in the infranate that remains quantitated before and after chemical precipitation of the apoB lipoproteins. This method is known as beta quantitation and is the gold standard to measure LDL cholesterol [2]. However, beta quan-titation is much too laborious and much too expensive for routine clinical use and therefore, in almost all clinical laboratories, LDL cholesterol is calculated from the Friedewald equa-tion [2]. This calculation assumes that chylomicrons are absent from plasma and that the ratio of triglyceride to cholesterol in VLDL is constant. Both assumptions are frequently vio-lated in clinical practice. To be sure, it is reasonably well-known that the calculation of LDL cholesterol breaks down so badly with triglycerides >400 mg/dl, that it can not be used. Less well-appreciated are the errors that occur at lower levels.

In principle, LDL cholesterol determined by the Friedewald calculation should equal LDL cholesterol measured by beta quantitation. In practice, they will differ somewhat. But how large can the difference be and how often does substantial difference occur? The answer is that it depends on how you look at it. In assessing error in laboratory tests, we generally focus on bias or accuracy – i.e., how close is the value achieved by the method we are using to the target value obtained using the reference method – and on precision or reproducibil-ity – i.e., what range of values are obtained with repetitive testing using the same method. We will show that this is not enough. We also need to look at the variance of the results obtained by the two methods.

In 9447 subjects, Tremblay *et al.* [3] found that the bias between the two methods was 4% or less across a wide range of values for LDL cholesterol. Moreover, the Friedewald result was reliable even at low levels of LDL cholesterol and with plasma triglycerides up to 9.0 mmol/l. This is the largest such study we are aware of and it demonstrates that across the full range of values encountered clinically, the means or averages by the two approaches differ little. So the issue should be settled.

Or is it: what about the variance between the two methods? In this case, variance is the range of values that are obtained by one method vs. the range of values obtained by the other. This can be displayed by dividing the group into deciles based on the LDL cholesterol calculated by each method. To fall within the same decile, i.e., within the same range of val-ues encompassed by 10% of the population, would not seem to represent a very severe test, particularly given the very small bias between the two methods in this study. The ideal results are shown in Table 7.1. The actual results are shown in Table 7.2. Agreement is not ideal. Indeed in the mid-range, it is far from ideal with the same ranking occurring only two-thirds of the time.

Let us relax our demand for agreement, double the interval, and use quintiles instead of deciles (Table 7.3). We are now only requiring that the two methods produce two values that lie within a range that covers 20% of the whole population. Agreement improves, but even now, even with what is a minimal requirement for agreement, within the mid-range, there is significant discordance for one patient in five.

Why is there such discordance? Chylomicron and VLDL remnants are almost certainly the major answer – remnants in which the triglyceride to cholesterol ratio differs from stand-ard VLDL, therefore violating both assumptions of the Friedewald equation: first that VLDL account for the vast majority of the plasma triglycerides and second that the ratio of plasma triglyceride to cholesterol within the triglyceride-rich lipoproteins is constant. The error is

Table 7.1   Theoretical agreement between calculated and measured LDL-c

						LDL-c (UC)					
		1	2	3	4	5	6	7	8	9	10
	1	100	0	0	0	0	0	0	0	0	0
	2	0	100	0	0	0	0	0	0	0	0
	3	0	0	100	0	0	0	0	0	0	0
	4	0	0	0	100	0	0	0	0	0	0
LDL-c (F)	5	0	0	0	0	100	0	0	0	0	0
	6	0	0	0	0	0	100	0	0	0	0
	7	0	0	0	0	0	0	100	0	0	0
	8	0	0	0	0	0	0	0	100	0	0
	9	0	0	0	0	0	0	0	0	100	0
	10	0	0	0	0	0	0	0	0	0	100

LDL-c = low-density lipoprotein cholesterol.

Table 7.2   Discordance between LDL-c (F) and LDL-c (UC) by deciles

						LDL-c (UC)					
		1	2	3	4	5	6	7	8	9	10
	1	85.50	14.40	0.10	0	0	0	0	0	0	0
	2	8.40	73.00	18.30	0.40	0	0	0	0	0	0
	3	2.30	8.70	68.00	20.10	0.90	0	0	0	0	0
	4	1.00	1.70	10.80	66.50	19.20	0.90	0	0	0	0
LDL-c (F)	5	0.86	0.74	1.40	11.70	66.10	18.80	0.40	0.10	0	0
	6	1.10	0.30	0.50	0.90	12.50	67.40	17.30	0	0	0
	7	0.60	0.50	0.50	0.40	0.10	11.70	71.30	14.00	0.10	0
	8	0	0.60	0.10	0	0.30	0.70	10.30	78.80	9.20	0
	9	0.30	0.10	0.30	0.10	0.30	0.30	0.50	7.00	87.00	4.30
	10	0	0	0.10	0	0	0.30	0.10	0.10	3.60	95.80

LDL-c = low-density lipoprotein cholesterol.

Table 7.3   Discordance between LDL-c (F) and LDL-c (UC) by quintiles

			LDL-c (UC)			
		1	2	3	4	5
	1	90.50	9.50	0	0	0
	2	7.00	82.40	10.60	0	0
LDL-c (F)	3	1.50	7.40	82.10	9.10	0
	4	0.90	0.50	6.90	87.00	4.80
	5	0.20	0.30	0.40	3.93	95.20

LDL-c = low-density lipoprotein cholesterol.
F = Friedwald Formula; UC = Ultracentrifugation.

officially acknowledged but not officially emphasized. To ensure that the estimate of LDL cholesterol is within a 10% error limit for any patient, the National Cholesterol Education Program (NCEP) has estimated that four samples on different days must be obtained and averaged [4]. Since the margin of error on an individual sample is at least 15 mg/dl, it is simply not possible, based on only one sample, to determine whether a patient is at any particular target. How often do physicians actually base their clinical decisions on multiple samples? How often do review articles or lectures mention that they are necessary?

The data in Tables 7.2 and 7.3 demonstrate that our clinical decisions are often no more than clinical guesses. Unfortunately these guesses are embedded in our clinical practice, sanctified by the summaries of guidelines. Dunbar and Rader [5] have written that the variance between calculated and measured LDL cholesterol is so common and so severe that, on this basis alone, the clinical value of the Friedewald calculation should be reassessed. We agree. What do diagnoses and targets mean if the estimate itself is so insecure? Unfortunately, direct measurements of LDL cholesterol do not solve the problem because they are not standardized and merely add further variance and substantial cost on top of what is already unacceptable variance [6].

As we shall see below, apoB has substantial biological advantage over LDL cholesterol in the estimation of vascular risk. But it also has methodological advantage. First, fasting samples are not required. ApoB48 particles, which carry triglyceride of intestinal origin, are recognized by the apoB antibody, but they are so few in number, even at the peak of the post-prandial period, that they do not significantly influence total plasma apoB [7]. Second, the measurement of apoB is standardized as is the measurement of apoA-I [8, 9] and therefore results from one method and one laboratory can be compared to the results obtained by another method in a different clinical laboratory. Third, the methods are automated and not expensive. Finally, as we have shown above, calculated LDL cholesterol is an estimate of the actual LDL cholesterol which is an estimate of LDL particle number. The Friedewald LDL cholesterol is therefore a surrogate of a surrogate. By contrast, apoB is an accurate measure of total number of lipoprotein particles, which can penetrate and injure the arterial wall. Thus apoB equals atherogenic particle number.

Biological variance between LDL cholesterol and apoB

A large body of published evidence indicates that apoB is a more accurate measure of the risk of vascular disease than any of the cholesterol indices (for review, please see [10–12]). Nevertheless, the absolute differences, whether expressed as odds ratios or receiver operator curves, between these markers have, to date, been relatively small, suggesting that the distinction may not be clinically significant. The narrowness of the difference is due, in large part, to the high correlation between them and that has been used to argue that they are equivalent. But correlation, as we have seen, is inadequate to judge whether two parameters are equivalent.

Similarly, comparing the mean value of two parameters is also inadequate to judge whether they are clinically equivalent because means ignore variance. With temperatures that drop to less than $-30°C$ in the winter and rise to more than $+30°C$ in the summer, it is the variance in temperature that influences how you dress in Montreal or Quebec City, not the mean. The same holds for LDL. Comparison of mean LDL cholesterol and apoB assumes that clinically significant variance in LDL composition across the range of values does not exist. This assumption is incorrect.

Figure 7.1 displays three LDL particles, each with different composition: one is cholesterol ester-enriched, one contains a normal amount of cholesterol ester, and one is cholesterol ester-depleted. When the majority of LDL particles are cholesterol-enriched, LDL cholesterol overestimates LDL particle number. Familial hypercholesterolaemia is the most extreme example of this finding, but in these patients LDL particle number is so high that the distinction between LDL cholesterol and LDL particle number is clinically irrelevant.

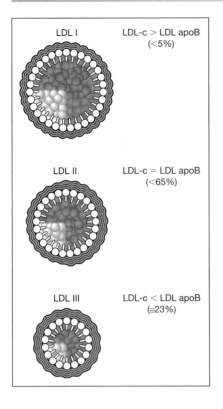

LDL I   LDL-c > LDL apoB
(<5%)

LDL II   LDL-c = LDL apoB
(<65%)

LDL III   LDL-c < LDL apoB
(≅23%)

Figure 7.1 The three principal subclasses of LDL: LDL I, LDL II, and LDL III, with subclasses in terms of the relative proportion of cholesterol to apoB and their frequency in the general population. LDL-c = low-density lipoprotein cholestorol; LDL apoB = low-density lipoprotein apolipoprotein B.

However, this discordance between LDL cholesterol and LDL particle number can be detected with less extreme values. Based on a small number of case–control studies, it has been suggested that cholesterol-enriched LDL particles might be particularly atherogenic. But the pattern is uncommon in patients with vascular disease. Moreover, the 13-year results of the prospective Quebec Cardiovascular Study have shown that when LDL cholesterol is disproportionately high compared to apoB, risk relates to apoB, not to LDL cholesterol, further strengthening the evidence that LDL particle number, not LDL composition, is the key variable that determines risk from LDL [13].

When the majority of LDL particles contain a normal amount of cholesterol ester, LDL cholesterol and LDL apoB will both closely approximate LDL particle number. This occurs in about two-thirds of individuals and accounts in large part for the very strong correspondence in the overall risk estimates of LDL cholesterol and apoB. For this group, LDL cholesterol and apoB will perform equally well. However, for individuals within this group, as we have shown, the variance in the laboratory estimation of calculated LDL cholesterol will play havoc with clinical decision-making.

Let us focus on the group in whom small dense cholesterol-depleted LDL particles predominate. Within this group, LDL cholesterol significantly underestimates LDL particle number. Since LDL particles make up just over 90% of total apoB particles, LDL particle number effectively determines plasma apoB [7]. It is within this group that apoB substantially outperforms LDL cholesterol. This superiority will obtain both for the diagnostic accuracy of the risk of vascular disease as well as the evaluation of the adequacy of LDL-lowering therapy [10–12, 14, 15]. To be sure, even within the group, there will be a trend towards higher LDL cholesterol levels with higher values of apoB. However, it is the absolute difference between them that matters for the individual and that is unpredictable from the group results [14, 15]. The variance between LDL cholesterol and apoB is greatest in this group and that is why apoB is essential to measure and to treat.

This group is sizeable by any reasonable standards as it includes about 25% of the overall population. This atherogenic phenotype is, however, much more common in those with abdominal obesity, insulin resistance, type 2 diabetes or vascular disease, and is the rule rather than the exception in patients with hypertriglyceridaemia [8].

ROC curves and cardiovascular risk assessment

A receiver operating characteristic (ROC) curve quantifies the diagnostic accuracy of a test for a particular disease [16]. This has become the standard method to compare the value of different diagnostic tests, a position in favour of which Pepe *et al.* [17] have argued strongly and coherently. But all tests are context-dependent and the issue we will explore is how well the standard interpretation of a ROC curve fits the context of cardiovascular risk prediction. The c-index summarizes the diagnostic accuracy of a ROC curve [18]. For orientation, a value of 0.500 means the test result is no more predictive than chance alone, a value of 1.00 is perfect, values between 0.700 and 0.800 are acceptable and those between 0.800 and 0.900 are excellent [19].

How do the classical cardiovascular risk factors fare using this approach? One way to tell is to estimate how much each raise the c-index and how high is the final total? Except for age, the answers are disappointing to say the least. Take the results of Cook *et al.* [20], which detail the impact of the conventional cardiovascular risk factors in women [20]. Age alone produces a c-index of 0.731. Adding LDL cholesterol increases it to only 0.746. Age plus systolic blood pressure plus smoking produces a c-index of 0.791. Add LDL cholesterol and the sum changes only trivially to 0.796. If this is the test, except for age, we would have to reject the classical risk factors for CVD. That would be difficult given all we know, particularly the evidence that treatment reduces risk.

Nevertheless, we have to address why the results of ROC analyses are so unsatisfactory when it comes to CVD. We believe the weakness lies in how we calculate the false-positive fraction (FPF) and the significance we attach to the FPF. Most epidemiological studies do not take time into account. Moreover, the clinical significance of a suboptimal FPF depends on the balance between the ultimate risk and benefit of therapy. We will deal with each in turn.

Time and ROC curves

Take any suitably large and representative group of subjects with an average age of 50 who will be followed for 10 years for cardiovascular events. At the beginning, there are no cases, only controls. Over the time of follow-up, only a small minority will suffer clinical events. The calculation of the impact of any factor on clinical risk depends, in the first instance, on the accuracy with which cases and controls are separated. In our hypothetical study, if the criteria to recognize clinical events are valid and faithfully applied, all those designated as cases will, in fact, have suffered clinical events. These can be classified securely. But what about the rest: all those who did not suffer a clinical event and who will be labelled controls?

The incidence of CVD rises dramatically with age. In developed countries, in men, clinical events occur at a discernible rate in the fifth decade, but only become common during the sixth, rising ever more dramatically thereafter. In women, the same schedule applies, but delayed roughly by a decade [21]. As is the case in most of the large epidemiological studies, most of the subjects in our study were below the age at which vascular events are commonplace and the restricted period of observation has consequence.

If we follow the subjects in our study for another decade, all cases will, of course, remain cases, whether they suffer another clinical event or not. However, many of the controls will suffer clinical events. They then become cases and, given the increase in age for the study population, the number of cases amongst the controls in this extended period is almost certain to be much larger than the number of cases in the initial period of observation.

By definition, the FPF in the original calculation of the ROC curve for any particular risk factor such as apoB would be based on the results and would include all the controls with an elevated apoB who did not suffer a clinical event. By lengthening the period of observation, the fragility of the FPF we originally calculated becomes evident. Indeed, if we extend the period of observation over their lifetime, approximately 45% of males and 35% of females will die of CVD. Thus, what we mean by control depends on the time of observation since 40% of controls will eventually become cases. The bottom line is that in any standard epidemiological study of the determinants of CVD, the inaccuracy in controls will lead to substantial underestimation of the importance of the risk factor.

If examined from a broader perspective, the error is even larger. LDL causes atherosclerosis and atherosclerosis results in clinical events. Of all the atherosclerotic lesions that exist within any particular individual, only a trivial number ever produce a clinical cardiovascular event. Based on the reduction in clinical events that follows statin therapy, LDL obviously plays an important role in the pathological processes that lead to plaque rupture. But other factors must also come into play and therefore it seems highly likely that the relation of LDL to arteriosclerosis will be more direct than the relation of LDL to clinical events. In any case, the total number with significant intramural atherosclerosis will certainly be larger than the total number with clinical events.

Risk, benefit and ROC curves

The clinical choices we make should be conditioned not only by the likelihood of disease but by the safety and efficacy of therapy. If the aim of a test is to detect a cancer which has a low incidence and whose diagnosis or treatment involves substantial risk, not only must the true-positive fraction (TPF-positive by test/positive for disease) be very high but the false-positive fraction (FPF-positive by test/negative for disease) must be very low.

Change the example to CVD. Let us assume we are older than 50 and that our level of apoB is sufficiently high that we have a TPF of 0.800 – i.e., our level of apoB would be found in 80% of those who suffer a cardiovascular event. Let us assume also that our FPF is only 0.500 – i.e., only 50% with a level of apoB this high will suffer a cardiovascular event over the time of observation. Whatever the calculated c-index may be, given the effectiveness and safety of statin therapy, virtually all would want to consider statin therapy. We are not confronting the possibility of a rare cancer that demands therapy that carries substantial risk. We are considering the commonest cause of human death in the world in which potent pharmacological therapy is associated with extremely low levels of serious risk. With CVD, the risk is from the disease not the therapy.

HOW CAN WE IMPROVE PREVENTION OF CARDIOVASCULAR DISEASE?

Stop relying on LDL cholesterol: start using apoB

LDL cholesterol remains the fundamental index of the proatherogenic risk of the plasma lipoproteins. Other than habit and convenience, there is little to support this choice. Not only is LDL cholesterol frequently a poor index of LDL particle number, as we have demonstrated, calculated LDL cholesterol is frequently a poor index of LDL cholesterol. As the evidence from clinical trials that LDL lowering saves lives and reduces events has become stronger and stronger, so the therapeutic targets for LDL cholesterol have become lower and lower [22]. The methodological problem is noted by clinical biochemists [23] but not by clinical guidelines.

Against the disadvantages of calculated LDL cholesterol, consider the advantages of apoB. ApoB is a measurement not a calculation. Moreover, what it measures – total atherogenic particle number – is what matters, biologically and clinically. Fasting samples are not required and the measurement is automated, standardized and not expensive. One number – apoB – is superior to three: total cholesterol, LDL cholesterol and non-HDL cholesterol.

What is the disadvantage of apoB? Education of healthcare givers and patients would be required. It has been argued that this would cause confusion and make the price too high [24]. But what patient would choose a poorer clinical outcome because they were more attached to one word than another? Our modern medical world is defined by change, change which allows us to measure more accurately and intervene more precisely, change which moves us closer to better care and better outcomes.

Stop relying entirely on short-term estimates of risk with arbitrary cutpoints

All of the major models such as Framingham calculate risk only over the short term. Obviously the short term matters but it is not the only time-frame that matters. We need to take our whole lifetime into account not just a decade of it [25]. The possibilities for safe evacuation are limited when the tsunami is spotted just off shore. Similarly, prevention will not be most successful if it starts just when the highest risk of death and clinical events starts.

The standard calculations to estimate risk can create an arbitrary boundary between coherent action and medical neglect, a boundary defined more by budgetary than by clinical concerns. Not only are the boundaries in guidelines arbitrary but the methods to calculate them do not work well in discriminating individuals who will suffer clinical events from those who will not. This conclusion should be indisputable given the ROC analyses of the risk of CVD.

SUMMARY: IS CLOSE ENOUGH GOOD ENOUGH?

The question is not whether apoB is a better marker of vascular risk than LDL cholesterol. It is. The question is not whether apoB is a better marker of the adequacy of LDL-lowering therapy than LDL cholesterol. It is. The question is whether it is worth the time and trouble to move from cholesterol to apoB. The answer might well depend on who is asked: those who have been the strongest supporters of cholesterol, those who have achieved so much, those who are used to seeing themselves as the leading edge of care – for many of them, close enough appears to be good enough. On the other hand, those who would benefit: those with small dense LDL, the group whose risk would be more precisely recognized and those whose therapy could be more precisely gauged and adjusted would almost certainly say that close enough is not good enough.

ApoB is not a cost, or laboratory, or convenience issue. The measurement of apolipoproteins is not expensive, is standardized, and can be done on non-fasting samples. Indeed, a system based on apoB and apoA-I would be simpler to establish and administer in most developing countries than one based on fasting samples and measuring triglycerides, total cholesterol, HDL cholesterol and calculating LDL cholesterol.

Given that abdominal obesity, insulin resistance and diabetes are on the rise worldwide, it is a certainty that the group with small dense LDL – the group in which LDL cholesterol importantly underestimates LDL particle number – will increase substantially as well. In this very large group, the evidence demonstrates that LDL cholesterol is not close enough and not good enough. ApoB is a more accurate clinical marker when accuracy means that more lives can be saved and more infarcts can be prevented.

REFERENCES

1. Levenson JW, Skerrett PJ, Gaziano JM. Reducing the global burden of cardiovascular disease: the role of risk factors. *Prev Cardiol* 2002; 5:188–199.
2. Friedewald WT, Levy RI, Fredrickson DS. Estimation of the concentration of low-density lipoprotein cholesterol in plasma, without use of the preparative ultracentrifuge. *Clin Chem* 1972; 18:499–502.
3. Tremblay AJ, Morissette H, Gagne JM, Bergeron J, Gagre C, Couture P. Validation of the Friedewald formula for the determination of low-density lipoprotein cholesterol compared with beta-quantitation in a large population. *Clin Biochem* 2004; 37:785–790.

4. Bachorik PS, Ross JW. National Cholesterol Education Program recommendations for measurement of low-density lipoprotein cholesterol: executive summary. The National Cholesterol Education Program Working Group on Lipoprotein Measurement. *Clin Chem* 1995; 41:1414–1420.

5. Dunbar RL, Rader DJ. Measurement of atherogenic lipoproteins. In: Morrow DA (ed.). *Cardiovascular Risk Assessment in Contemporary Cardiology: Cardiovascular Biomarkers: Pathophysiology and Disease Management.* Humana Press, Totowa, NJ, 2006.

6. Marcovina S, Packard CJ. Measurement and meaning of apolipoprotein AI and apolipoprotein B levels. *J Intern Med* 2006; 259:437–446.

7. Sniderman AD, Scantlebury T, Cianflone K. Hypertriglyceridemic hyperapoB: the unappreciated atherogenic dyslipoproteinemia in type 2 diabetes mellitus. *Ann Intern Med* 2001; 135:447–459.

8. Marcovina SM, Albers JJ, Henderson LO, Hannon WH. International Federation of Clinical Chemistry standardization project for measurements of apolipoproteins A-I and B. III. Comparability of apolipoprotein A-I values by use of international reference material. *Clin Chem* 1993; 39:773–781.

9. Marcovina SM, Albers JJ, Kennedy H, Mei JV, Henderson LO, Hannon WH. International Federation of Clinical Chemistry standardization project for measurements of apolipoproteins A-I and B. IV. Comparability of apolipoprotein B values by use of International Reference Material. *Clin Chem* 1994; 40:586–592.

10. Barter PJ, Ballantyne CM, Carmena R *et al*. ApoB versus cholesterol to estimate cardiovascular risk and to guide therapy: report of the thirty person/ten country panel. *J Intern Med* 2006; 259:247–258.

11. Chan DC, Watts GF. Apolipoproteins as markers and managers of coronary risk Q. *J Med* 2006; 99:277–287.

12. Walldius G, Jungner I. The apoB/apoA-1 ratio: a strong, new risk factor for cardiovascular disease and a target for lipid-lowering therapy – a review of the evidence. *J Intern Med* 2006; 259:493–519.

13. St-Pierre AC, Cantin B, Dagenais GR, Despres JP, Lamarche B. Apolipoprotein-B, low density lipoprotein cholesterol, and the long-term risk of coronary heart disease in men. *Am J Cardiol* 2006; 97:997–1001.

14. Sniderman AD, Furberg CD, Keech A *et al*. Apolipoproteins versus lipids as indices of coronary risk and as targets for statin therapy treatment. *Lancet* 2003; 361:777–780.

15. Stein EA, Sniderman A, Laskarzewski P. Assessment of reaching goal in patients with combined hyperlipidemia: low-density lipoprotein cholesterol, non-high-density lipoprotein cholesterol, or apolipoprotein B. *Am J Cardiol* 2005; 96:36–43.

16. Hanley JA, McNeil BJ. The meaning and use of the area under a receiver operating characteristic (ROC) curve. *Radiology* 1982; 143:29–36.

17. Pepe MS, Janes H, Longton G, Leisenring W, Newcom P. Limitations of the odds ratio in gauging the performance of a diagnostic, prognostic, or screening marker. *Am J Epidemiol* 2004; 159:882–890.

18. Harrell FEJ. Regression modelling strategies. Springer, New York, 2001.

19. Hosmer DW, Lemeshow S. *Applied Logistic Regression*, 2nd edition. J Wiley, New York, 2000.

20. Cook NR, Buring JE, Ridker PM. The effect of including C-reactive protein in cardiovascular risk prediction models for women. *Ann Intern Med* 2006; 145:21–29.

21. Booth GL, Kapral MK, Fung K, Tu JV. Relation between age and cardiovascular disease in men and women with diabetes compared with non-diabetic people: a population-based retrospective cohort study. *Lancet* 2006; 368:29–36.

22. Grundy SM, Cleeman JI, Merz CN *et al*. Implications of recent clinical trials for the National Cholesterol Education Program Adult Treatment Panel III guidelines. *Circulation* 2004; 110:227–239.

23. Contois J. Why do lipid results differ between laboratories? *The Fats of Life.* 2006; 2–3.

24. Denke MA. Weighing in before the fight: low-density lipoprotein cholesterol and non-high-density lipoprotein cholesterol versus apolipoprotein B as the best predictor for coronary heart disease and the best measure of therapy. *Circulation* 2005; 112:3368–3370.

25. Lloyd-Jones DM, Leip EP, Larson MG *et al*. Prediction of lifetime risk for cardiovascular disease by risk factor burden at 50 years of age. *Circulation* 2006; 113:791–798.

8

New biomarkers of cardiovascular disease

E. Ingelsson, R. S. Vasan

INTRODUCTION

Cardiovascular disease (CVD) is the leading cause of morbidity and mortality in the United States [1] and globally [2]. CVD is a life course disease, beginning with the development of risk factors in young people, which then contribute to the evolution of subclinical atherosclerosis [3, 4] that in turn culminates in clinical CVD events [5, 6]. Primary and secondary prevention of CVD are considered, therefore, to be public health priorities [7].

Clinical evaluation still is, and probably will remain, the cornerstone of all patient management. However, such assessment has been demonstrated to have its limitations [8–11]. Therefore, clinicians use additional tools to complement clinical evaluation with the objective of better characterizing the heterogeneity in disease risk among patients who have similar clinical profiles, with the expectation of identifying patients at greater risk for CVD [12, 13]. Biomarkers (biological markers) are useful adjuncts to clinical evaluation that can aid the identification of high-risk individuals, facilitate the screening for and diagnosis of CVD quickly and more correctly, and assist treatment and prognostication of patients with established disease. In this chapter, we discuss practical considerations in the clinical use of CVD biomarkers and provide an overview of the newer biomarkers.

CVD BIOMARKERS – CHARACTERISTICS AND PRACTICAL CONSIDERATIONS

CVD BIOMARKERS – A DEFINITION

Biomarkers are: *'measurable and quantifiable biological parameters (e.g. specific enzyme concentration, specific hormone concentration, specific gene phenotype distribution in a population, presence of biological substances) which serve as indices for health- and physiology-related assessments, such as disease risk, psychiatric disorders, environmental exposure and its effects, disease diagnosis, metabolic processes, substance abuse, pregnancy, cell line development, epidemiologic studies, etc.'* [14]. Thus, a CVD biomarker can be measured in biological samples (e.g. blood, urine or tissue), recorded on a person (e.g. blood pressure [BP] or an electrocardiogram), or it can be an imaging test (echocardiogram, magnetic resonance imaging, or computerized tomographic scan). Further, CVD biomarkers can be divided broadly into serological (e.g. C-reactive protein or troponin I), structural (e.g. carotid intimal-medial thickness) or functional (e.g. BP) markers. An alternative way to categorize biomarkers is based on their potential clinical

Erik Ingelsson, MD, PhD, Post-Doctoral Fellow, The Framingham Study, Boston University School of Medicine, Framingham, Massachusetts, USA and Department of Public Health and Caring Sciences, Uppsala University, Uppsala, Sweden

Ramachandran S. Vasan, MBBS, MD, DM, FACC, Professor of Medicine, Departments of Preventive Medicine and Cardiology, Boston University School of Medicine and Senior Investigator, The Framingham Heart Study, Framingham, Massachusetts, USA

use: *antecedent biomarkers* help identify risk of developing CVD, *screening biomarkers* assist screening for subclinical disease, *diagnostic biomarkers* are used to test for presence of overt disease in symptomatic patients, and *prognostic biomarkers* aid the prediction of recurrences and sequelae of CVD, and may contribute to the monitoring of effectiveness of therapeutic agents [15].

CHARACTERISTICS OF AN IDEAL CVD BIOMARKER

The purpose of a CVD biomarker is to help the clinician to optimally manage the patient with or at risk for CVD. For example, in a person with recurrent chest pain, a biomarker could aid identification of patients with possible angina pectoris (e.g. an exercise stress test), or help characterize the extent and severity of disease (e.g. coronary angiogram). Of note, a new CVD biomarker will be of clinical value only if it is accurate, acceptable (to the patient), easy to interpret by clinicians and reproducibly measured. Further, it should have both high sensitivity and specificity for the specific CVD outcome it is used to identify, explain a considerable proportion of the outcome, and knowledge of biomarker levels should change management strategies [16]. Understandably, the optimal properties of a specific CVD biomarker may vary with its potential use [17]. For instance, a screening CVD biomarker will be obtained on asymptomatic people, and therefore should have features of both high sensitivity, specificity, and predictive values combined with reasonably low cost. For diagnostic biomarkers of acute coronary ischaemia or cardiac injury, desirable features include high sensitivity, rapid and sustained elevation, tissue specificity indicating myocardial origin, release proportional to tissue injury, and assay features that are compatible with point-of-care testing [18].

DEFINING REFERENCE VALUES FOR NEW CVD BIOMARKERS

It is important to define 'normal' and 'abnormal' biomarker values before a putative CVD biomarker can be used in clinical settings [17]. This means that studies must characterize adequately the variations in levels with age, sex, ethnicity, presence of known risk factors, and prevalent disease [19]. There are three main approaches for defining abnormal biomarker levels that are complementary.

(1) *Reference limits* are generated using cross-sectional studies of healthy reference samples, and choosing a statistically-derived cutpoint (typically the 95th or 97.5th percentile) to define the lower threshold of the abnormal range of values [20–22]. The reference limits can be changed up or down to strike an optimal balance between false-negative and false-positive results, i.e. by considering the consequences of missing CVD, and the potential benefits of treating people with abnormal values, factoring in the costs associated with follow-up of abnormal results.

(2) *Discrimination limits* are generated by evaluating the overlap of biomarker values in patients with vs. those without CVD in cross-sectional studies [23]. Discrimination limits mark clinical decision thresholds; they can vary depending on the relative importance of missing CVD vs. that of misclassifying non-diseased individuals. For example, a blood brain natriuretic peptide (BNP) value above 200 pg/ml has been suggested as a threshold identifying presence of heart failure with reasonable certainty [24].

(3) *'Undesirable' biomarker levels* are defined by relating the range of values in community-dwelling people to the incidence of CVD events, and assessing if there is a threshold beyond which CVD risk escalates. For most CVD risk factors, a majority of individuals in a population could be classified as having 'undesirable' levels, since there is a continuous gradient of risk across the range of risk factors. For instance, a desirable systolic BP may be as low as ≤115 mmHg, because incidence of vascular disease increases linearly above this level [25]. However, 'treatment' levels (especially for pharmacological

treatment) of risk factors often differ from 'undesirable levels'. Treatment levels are defined based on scientific evidence that treatment for values above a limit does more benefit than harm, typically in randomized controlled trials.

EVALUATION OF NEW CVD BIOMARKERS

The evaluation of a new CVD biomarker requires an independent comparison of the performance of the biomarker with a reference standard [26]. Such appraisal includes initial assessment of biomarker performance in a *derivation set*, followed by an investigation in a *validation set* [27]. The accuracy of a biomarker is evaluated in terms of sensitivity (identification of true positives) and specificity (identification of true negatives) at different cutpoints. Since many CVD biomarkers are continuously distributed variables, it is critical to evaluate performance over a range of biomarker values, typically using receiver operating characteristic curves, or *ROC curves* [28–30]. The ROC curves exemplify the trade-off between sensitivity and specificity when different biomarker levels are used clinically to identify disease. Which cutpoint should be chosen is dependent on the planned use of the biomarker. For instance, a biomarker used to screen for an uncommon asymptomatic condition (e.g. asymptomatic left ventricular systolic dysfunction) should have high specificity because a *'rule in'* strategy is more important in this context (the *SpIN* rule [31]); the costs of mislabelling healthy individuals may outweigh those of missing a rare disease. On the other hand, a biomarker that is used to diagnose a potentially life-threatening condition in a symptomatic sick patient (e.g. acute MI) should have a high sensitivity because a *'rule out'* strategy is vital in this setting (the *SnOUT* rule [31]); costs of missing a potentially life-threatening illness overshadow the costs of any additional testing or a false-positive diagnosis.

For a new CVD biomarker to be clinically useful, it must be demonstrated that it adds risk information over and beyond that readily available from measurement of established CVD risk factors. Thus, investigators must demonstrate that higher (or in some cases lower) levels of the new biomarker are associated with elevated CVD risk, after accounting for standard risk factors. It is important to emphasize that a high relative risk of CVD associated with a new biomarker does not necessarily translate into better CVD risk prediction. Very strong associations of markers with CVD are required for a given biomarker to have good discrimination properties [32]. The reason for this is that even when a biomarker threshold is associated with very high odds of CVD, it will often identify only a small proportion of people with CVD if false-positive results are to be kept low [32]. Stated simply, CVD risk factors may not be good screening tools [33]. Also, the critical question we must answer is whether a new CVD biomarker improves the predictive accuracy of the best available model (representing the standard of care for that disease) that incorporates several known CVD risk factors [34]. Thus, to really establish a biomarker as being additive to the existing prediction models for CVD, studies incorporating multimarker scores are highly warranted. The most established multimarker scores are the Framingham Risk Score [35] and the recent European variant, SCORE [36], and a novel biomarker should generally have an additional predictive value when added to these scores to be really useful in the clinical setting, at least if it is intended for use for screening for CVD risk.

OVERVIEW OF NEWER CVD BIOMARKERS

The following sections will provide an overview of the newer CVD biomarkers, categorized empirically as markers of arterial vulnerability (i.e. markers of the vascular wall function and the arthrosclerosis process), blood vulnerability (i.e. indicators of the coagulation process that occurs in the blood), and myocardial vulnerability (i.e. indicating myocardial pathology). Further, each of these sections is also divided into serological, structural and functional markers.

MARKERS OF ARTERIAL VULNERABILITY

As arterial pathology, such as atherosclerosis, is a fundamental substrate for the development of CVD, many currently available CVD biomarkers measure different aspects/phases of atherogenesis and clinical CVD events. The markers include circulating (serological) markers (e.g. lipids or inflammation markers), structural markers (e.g. coronary calcium) and functional markers (e.g. BP). A list of biomarkers of arterial vulnerability is shown in Table 8.1.

Serological markers of arterial vulnerability

Lipids

The blood lipid profile, including cholesterol fractions, was one of the first biomarkers to be established as a risk factor for CVD. Even though it is not a new biomarker, we have included it in this chapter, since it is widely accepted and included in most CVD guidelines and risk evaluation tools [37]. A closely related marker is the low-density lipoprotein (LDL) particle concentration, which has also been associated with CVD [38, 39], even though it does not seem to add predictive value to that of the ordinary lipid profile [38]. Over recent years, there has been much interest in the association between apolipoproteins and CVD. Indeed, there is strong evidence that apolipoprotein B (apoB) [40–45] and also lipoprotein (a) (Lp(a)) [46], are associated with CVD incidence. Also, there are some studies indicating that apoB may have a better predictive value compared to the usual lipid fractions [40, 42, 45], but this has been questioned in several other studies [41, 43, 47]. One proposed reason for the inconsistent results in these studies is that the study samples evaluated have varied with regard to CVD risk. Thus, apoB might not perform better than lipid fractions for identifying CVD risk in low-risk populations, whereas it may outperform these fractions in high-risk populations [48]. Some of the major arguments for using apoB instead of non-high-density lipoprotein (non-HDL) cholesterol (which seemingly is the best CVD predictor of the different lipid fraction measurements) are: apoB represents the total number of atherogenic particles, leading to a better measurement of atherosclerotic risk; measurement is standardized, automated, inexpensive, and does not require fasting samples; it is better predictive of risk in people on lipid-lowering treatment [48, 49]. The main arguments against the routine clinical use of apoB (in preference to established lipid markers) are: apoB assays are not as widely available relative to standard lipid fractions; there is more information about the distribution of cholesterol fractions in populations and therapeutic cutpoints for apoB may not be defined as readily; and extensive educational campaigns have taken place for health professionals and the public regarding the importance of measuring serum cholesterol, and replacing cholesterol measurement in clinical practice may create confusion [50].

Another new lipid biomarker that seems to track with CVD incidence is lipoprotein-associated phospholipase A2 (Lp-PLA2), measured either as mass [51–56] or as activity [57]. Although Lp-PLA2 significantly increased the C statistic when added to a risk factor model including established risk factors in a study, this increase was very modest [58]. One more recently proposed lipid biomarker is cholesteryl ester transfer protein (CETP), which was associated with an increased risk of future coronary artery disease in relatively healthy individuals, but only in those with increased triglycerides [59].

Inflammatory markers

Atherosclerosis is currently viewed as an inflammatory disorder [60]. Therefore, inflammatory markers have been the focus of intense research in recent years as potential biomarkers of CVD risk. The most studied inflammatory biomarker is high-sensitive C-reactive protein (hs-CRP), which is measured in a standardized fashion with a convenient and reproducible

Table 8.1 Biomarkers for identifying arterial vulnerability

Biomarker	Methodology standardized	Methodology available/convenient	Linked to disease prospectively	Additive to FHS risk score	Tracks with disease treatment
Serological biomarkers of arterial vulnerability					
Lipids					
Abnormal lipid profile	+++[243–246]	+++	+++[37]	Part of score	+++[37]
LDL particle number	±[247]	−	+[38, 39]	−[38]	?
ApoB	+[248]	+	+++[40–45]	+[40, 42, 45]/−[41, 43, 47]	+[49, 249, 250]
Lp(a)	±	+	+++(reviewed in [46])	−	?
CETP	±[251]	±	+[59]	?	?
Lp-PLA2	−[252]	−	+[51–58]	?	?[253, 254]
Inflammation					
hs-CRP	+++[61]	+++	+++(reviewed in [62])	+[64]/?[65]	+/?(reviewed in [63])
sICAM-1	±[255]	±	+++(reviewed in [79])	?	?
IL-6	−[256]	−	++[67–73]	?	?
IL-18	−	−	++[74, 75]	?	?
SAA	−[257]	−	−[77, 78]/+[76]	?	?
MPO	?[258]	−	−[80–82]	?	−
sCD40L	−[255]	?	+[83–86]	?	?[259, 260]
MCP-1	−	−	+[87, 88]	?	?
PAPP-A	−	−	+[89, 90]	?	?
PlGF	−	−	+[91, 92]	?	?
Oxidative stress					
Oxidized LDL	−	+	+[95]	?[95]	?
GPX1 activity	−	−	+[96, 97]	?[97]	?
Nitrotyrosine	−	−	+[98]	+/?	+[98]
Homocysteine	+++	+++	+++(reviewed in [99, 100])/−[101, 102]	?	?

Table 8.1 (continued)

Biomarker	Methodology standardized	Methodology available/ convenient	Linked to disease prospectively	Additive to FHS risk score	Tracks with disease treatment
Neurohormonal					
Natriuretic peptides	+[118]	++	+++[104-114]	+[119]	+[115-117]
Aldosterone	+[261]	-	+[120, 121]	?	+[262]
Renin	+[261]	-	-[122]/+[123-125]	?	?
Extracellular matrix					
MMP-9	-	-	+[130]	?	?
TIMP-1	+	-	+[131]	?	?
Others					
Cystatin-C	+	-	+[126-129]	?	?
ADMA	+[263-265]	-	++[132-139]	?	?[135]
Structural biomarkers of arterial vulnerability					
Carotid ultrasonography	++[140]	+/?	++[141-148]	+/?[142-144]	++[266-268]
Coronary artery calcium	+++	+	+[151-155]	+/?[153]	?
Functional markers of arterial vulnerability					
Blood pressure	+++[158]	++	+++(reviewed in [25])	Part of score	+++[25]
Ambulatory blood pressure	++[158]	+	++[159-161]	?	+
Endothelial dysfunction	+[162,163]	+	+[164-179]	?	+[269]
Arterial stiffness	++[270-273]	++	+[180-187]	?	+[274]
Ankle-brachial index	+++[188, 189]	+++	++(reviewed in [190])	+/?[275]	?
Urine albumin excretion	++[276]	++	++[192, 194-199]	+/?	++[192]

- = no data; ? = unknown or questionable/equivocal data; + = some evidence; ++ = good evidence; +++ = strong evidence.
ADMA = asymmetrical dimethyl arginine; ApoB = apolipoprotein B; CETP = cholesterol ester transfer protein; GPX1 = glutathione peroxidase 1; IL = interleukin; IMT = intimal-medial thickness; LDL = low-density lipoprotein cholesterol; Lp(a) = lipoprotein a; Lp-PLA2 = lipoprotein-associated phospholipase A2; MPO = myeloperoxidase; SAA = serum amyloid A; sCD40L = soluble CD40 ligand; MCP-1 = monocyte chemoattractant protein-1; PAPP-A = pregnancy-associated plasma protein A; PlGF = placental growth factor; sICAM = soluble intercellular adhesion molecule.

Schema of criteria for risk factors adapted from reference with permission [277].

assay [61]. Hs-CRP has repeatedly been demonstrated to be associated with incident CVD [62] and some studies indicate that it tracks with disease treatment [63]. A recent report from the Women's Health Study highlighted that it may have an additive value when added to risk prediction instruments, such as the Framingham Risk Score [64]. Among women initially classified as having a 10-year CVD risk between 5% and 20%, the additional use of hs-CRP resulted in the reclassification of approximately 20% of the women into 'more accurate' risk categories. However, the evidence for an additive predictive value of hs-CRP to multivariable risk models is still sparse and confined to people with intermediate risk of CVD, in whom it has been advocated as a 'tiebreaker' test [65]. In the latest scientific statement from the American Heart Association and the Centers for Disease Control and Prevention on this subject, experts concluded that hs-CRP seemed to add predictive value above that of currently established risk factors, but that the evidence was not entirely consistent across published studies and, in particular, additional prospective studies are needed to more precisely define risk at various strata, and to assure consistency of performance within age, sex, and ethnicity groups. Therefore, the experts recommended against screening of the entire adult population for hs-CRP as a public health measure, but stated that it was reasonable to measure hs-CRP as an adjunct to the major risk factors to further assess absolute risk for primary prevention of coronary disease in selected cases [66].

Interleukins (ILs) have also been investigated in several studies as potential biomarkers for CVD, and both IL-6 [67–73] and IL-18 [74, 75] have consistently been demonstrated to be associated with CVD incidence. Serum amyloid A (SAA) protein has been shown to provide similar CVD risk information as hs-CRP in some [76, 77] but not in other studies [78]. Different soluble cell adhesion molecules have also been evaluated as potential biomarkers for CVD; there are data indicating that soluble intercellular adhesion molecule-1 (ICAM-1) is associated with CVD incidence [79]. Also, other indicators of inflammation, such as myeloperoxidase (MPO) [80–82], soluble CD40 ligand [83–86], monocyte chemoattractant protein-1 (MCP-1) [87, 88], pregnancy-associated plasma protein A (PAPP-A) [89, 90], and placental growth factor (PlGF) [91, 92] have been associated with CVD incidence in different reports and constitute putative new candidates for further assessment and validation.

Oxidative stress
Oxidative stress is a state of excess formation of reactive oxygen species, or free radicals (independent molecules with at least one unpaired electron). Intracellular generation of free radicals is a crucial activator of the final common pathway for the prothrombotic and proinflammatory maladaptive cellular behaviour that is associated with vascular injury [93, 94]. Several indicators of oxidative stress have been proposed as biomarkers for CVD. Those with some supportive scientific evidence at the time include oxidized LDL [95], glutathione peroxidase activity [96, 97], and nitrotyrosine [98]. A biomarker that has been much in focus in recent years, and that could be included among markers of oxidative stress, is homocysteine. Homocysteine is measured by a standardized and convenient method, and it has repeatedly been demonstrated to track with CVD development in observational studies [99, 100]. However, the results of two landmark studies, Heart Outcomes Prevention Evaluation-2 (HOPE 2) [101] and Norwegian Vitamin (NORVIT) [102] did not support the 'homocysteine hypothesis of atherogenesis'. Both these studies were large, randomized, double-blind secondary prevention trials, comparing treatment with vitamin B12 and/or folic acid for lowering plasma homocysteine with administration of a placebo. The treatment resulted in lower plasma homocysteine levels, but there was no reduction of morbidity or mortality, raising doubts about the value of plasma homocysteine as a CVD biomarker. There are, however, several possible explanations for the discrepancy between the results of observational and interventional studies: treatment doses in the latter may have been too low leading to very small decrements in plasma homocysteine levels; intervention studies may have been

underpowered to detect very modest benefits from homocysteine lowering; possible deleterious effects of vitamin B12 or folic acid mediated *via* mechanisms independent of CVD risk; hyperhomocysteinaemia may simply be a 'marker' of increased risk of CVD, without 'causing' it [103].

Neurohormones

As disturbances in the neurohormonal axis are considered to have a fundamental role in the development and progression of CVD, considerable interest has focused on the hormones of the renin–angiotensin–aldosterone (RAAS) system as potential biomarkers of CVD. Among the most promising neurohormonal biomarkers are the natriuretic peptides; there is strong evidence for association of these markers with disease risk [104–114]. Further, plasma BNP has been demonstrated to track with treatment [115–117], and can be measured in a standardized fashion and with a convenient assay [118]. Also, a recent study has demonstrated that n-terminal pro-BNP significantly increased the C statistic when added to a CVD risk prediction model that included traditional risk factors [119]. Although pro-BNP is an emerging and promising biomarker, these initial results should be confirmed in additional large-scale studies of community-based samples before considering this biomarker for routine clinical use. Data relating other neurohormonal biomarkers to CVD risk are more limited, and less unequivocal. Serum aldosterone has been demonstrated to track prospectively with hypertension incidence [120] and with in-stent restenosis [121] in separate reports. Even though plasma renin activity was not associated with ischaemic heart disease in an earlier study [122], several more recent studies have linked higher renin levels with vascular risk [123–125].

Other CVD biomarkers

Cystatin C, a serum measure of renal function, has been demonstrated to be associated with CVD risk in several reports [126–129], and it may be a better predictor of the risk of death and CVD events in elderly persons compared to serum creatinine or estimated glomerular filtration rate [129]. Matrix metalloproteinases (MMPs) are proteolytic enzymes, which breakdown the extracellular matrix, and influence cardiac remodelling. They are inhibited by tissue inhibitors of metalloproteinases (TIMPs). Recent studies have highlighted MMP-9 [130], and TIMP-1 [131] as potential biomarkers for incident CVD. Asymmetrical dimethyl-arginine (ADMA) is an endogenous nitric oxide synthase inhibitor, and a putative biomarker of endothelial dysfunction. It has been associated with CVD risk in multiple reports [132–139]. Endothelial function can also be measured using functional markers of arterial vulnerability, as described below.

Structural markers of arterial vulnerability

Carotid ultrasonography is a widely used and established method for measuring atherosclerotic burden. The most commonly assessed ultrasonographic carotid measurement is the intimal–medial thickness (IMT) because it is measured in a standardized, convenient, and reproducible way [140], and has been shown to be strongly associated with an increased risk of myocardial infarction and stroke [141–144]. Also, other carotid characteristics measured with ultrasonography, such as focal wall thickening (i.e. carotid plaques or stenosis) [145, 146], plaque echogenicity (i.e. how much ultrasound is reflected) [147] and plaque heterogeneity [148], have been demonstrated to predict CVD incidence. Newer techniques to detect vulnerable plaques are also undergoing evaluation, including techniques such as optical coherence tomography [149], and thermography [150]. However, it still remains to be established if these newer plaque imaging methods can be used as CVD biomarkers prospectively.

Another structural marker of arterial vulnerability is coronary artery calcium, which is measured using computed tomography (CT) in a standardized and convenient way, although the method confers a high level of radiation exposure. Coronary artery calcium score (determined with CT) is predictive of future CVD [151–155]. Additionally, there are some data to support the notion that a high coronary artery calcium score may add risk information to risk evaluation tools, such as the Framingham Risk Score, especially in people in the intermediate-risk category in whom clinical decision-making is most uncertain [153]. In 2000, the American College of Cardiology/American Heart Association issued a joint statement [156] that noted a lack of supportive evidence for the use of coronary artery calcium score as a screening procedure for coronary heart disease except in selected clinically referred individuals with intermediate clinical risk, due to the low specificity (high percentage of false-positive results) of the method, which could result in additional expensive and unnecessary testing to rule out a diagnosis. These recommendations are still considered to be valid [157].

Functional markers of arterial vulnerability

BP is definitely not a new biomarker, but it is usually considered to be among the most important of all CVD biomarkers, so it is included in this section for the sake of completeness [25, 158]. Further, recent investigations have highlighted the importance of ambulatory BP patterns in the development of CVD [159–161]. Studies have demonstrated that a non-dipping night/day BP pattern (i.e. BP that does not decrease during nighttime) is a strong predictor of CVD [160, 161]. Further, 24-hour BP monitoring is easily accessible, reproducible and non-invasive. However, before using 24-hour monitoring of BP in clinical practice, additional investigations are warranted, including studies performing cost–benefit analyses and clinical interventions using 24-hour BP as the target.

In addition to measuring circulating ADMA noted above, endothelial dysfunction can be assessed *via* functional measurements, such as ultrasound assessment of endothelial-dependent flow-mediated vasodilatation (FMD) of the brachial artery [162] or tonometric assessment of finger arterial pulse wave amplitude (PWA) [163]. There is some evidence for associations between these markers of endothelial function and CVD risk [164–179]. Although endothelial function testing remains a research tool at the present time, this technology may contribute to CVD risk assessment strategies in the future. Further, arterial stiffness quantified non-invasively using tonometry of the carotid or radial artery, has also been demonstrated to predict incident CVD in several studies [180–187].

Another functional marker of arterial vulnerability that has been in use for many years is the ankle-brachial index, measured using a standardized and easily performed methodology [188, 189]. The evidence for ankle-brachial index as a CVD biomarker is robust; the specificity of a low ankle-brachial index for predicting future CVD outcomes is high, but its sensitivity is low [190]. Interestingly, a recent study established that the association between high ankle-brachial index and mortality was similar to that for a low index and mortality, highlighting a U-shaped association [191]. This observation merits further investigation.

Finally, urine albumin excretion may be considered a functional marker of arterial vulnerability, since it mirrors target organ damage caused by hypertension. Urine albumin excretion has been demonstrated to predict future CVD events in multiple reports [192–198], and even in healthy individuals with levels well below the current threshold defining microalbuminuria [199]. Urine albumin excretion as a predictor of CVD and general mortality was first established in subjects with diabetes [195–198], and patients with hypertensive nephrosclerosis [192], but has since been confirmed in non-diabetics and non-hypertensive subjects as well [194, 195, 199]. Whether it constitutes a clinically useful addition to multivariable risk prediction models remains to be established.

MARKERS OF BLOOD VULNERABILITY

Whereas markers of arterial vulnerability are indicators of vascular wall function and the atherosclerotic process, markers of blood vulnerability are indicators of the actual coagulation process that occurs within the blood vessels. A list of biomarkers of blood vulnerability is provided in Table 8.2.

Table 8.2   Biomarkers for identifying blood vulnerability

Biomarker	Methodology standardized	Methodology available/ convenient	Linked to disease prospectively	Additive to FHS risk score	Tracks with disease treatment
Serological markers of blood vulnerability					
Hypercoagulability					
Fibrinogen	++[278]	++	+++(reviewed in [201])	?	?
D-dimer	+	+	++(reviewed in [202])	?	?
von Willebrand Factor	++	++	+(reviewed in [203])	?	?
Decreased fibrinolysis					
TPA/PAI-1	±[279]	+	++ (reviewed in [204])	?	?

− = no data; ? = unknown or questionable/equivocal data; + = some evidence; ++ = good evidence; +++ = strong evidence.

PAI-1 = plasminogen activator inhibitor; TPA = tissue plasminogen activator.

Schema of criteria for risk factors adapted from reference with permission [277].

Serological markers of blood vulnerability

Hypercoagulation

Fibrinogen, the major coagulation protein in blood and the precursor of fibrin, is an important determinant of blood viscosity and platelet aggregation [200]. There is strong evidence for an association between an elevated fibrinogen level and future CVD events [201], but whether this adds information above that contained in traditional risk score instruments is still to be examined. Also, there is evidence linking D-dimer [202], and von Willebrand factor [203] to increased incidence of coronary heart disease.

Decreased fibrinolysis

Tissue plasminogen activator (TPA) activates clot dissolution by cleaving cross-linked fibrin to D-dimer and other degradation products. TPA and its major plasma inhibitor, plasminogen activator inhibitor-1 (PAI-1), have been associated with incident CVD [204], but additional studies are needed to determine to what extent this association is independent of established CVD risk factors.

In a recent report from the Caerphilly Study [205], 11 haemostatic biomarkers were evaluated to determine which had prognostic value for CVD incidence after accounting for traditional CVD risk factors. The results showed that fibrinogen, D-dimer, PAI-1 activity, and factor VIIc each had incremental predictive value in a multivariable model that included traditional CVD risk factors and haemostatic factors conjointly.

MARKERS OF MYOCARDIAL VULNERABILITY

Markers of myocardial vulnerability indicate myocardial pathology, such as myocardial damage, remodelling and dysfunction. A list of biomarkers of myocardial vulnerability can be found in Table 8.3.

Table 8.3 Biomarkers for identifying myocardial vulnerability

Biomarker	Methodology standardized	Methodology available/ convenient	Linked to disease prospectively	Additive to FHS risk score	Tracks with disease treatment
Serological markers of myocardial vulnerability					
Troponins	++[280, 281]	++	++(reviewed in [206, 207])	?	?
Ischaemia-modified albumin	+	−	+[208, 209]	?	?
H-FABP	+[282]	−	+[210]	?	?
Structural markers of myocardial vulnerability					
LVH	++[212–214]	++	++[215–221, 226, 227]	?	++[222–225]
Functional markers of myocardial vulnerability					
LV dysfunction	++[213]	++	++[226–228]	?	++[229, 230]
Exercise stress test/stress echo	++	++	++[231–233]	++[283, 284]	++

− = no data; ? = unknown or questionable/equivocal data; + = some evidence; ++ = good evidence; +++ = strong evidence.

H-FABP = heart-type fatty acid binding protein; LVH = left ventricular hypertrophy; LV = left ventricle.

Schema of criteria for risk factors adapted from reference with permission [277].

Serological markers of myocardial vulnerability

Cardiac troponins have largely replaced creatine kinase-MB as the preferred biomarkers for establishing a diagnosis of myocardial infarction [206]. Troponins are well-established markers of myocardial damage, and have a prognostic value in acute coronary syndromes [207]. A novel biomarker that has been studied in the same setting as troponins is ischaemia-modified albumin, a marker with a high sensitivity for myocardial ischaemia, making it a promising *'rule-out'* marker in the emergency room [208, 209]. Another promising biomarker in patients with acute coronary syndrome is heart-type fatty acid binding protein (H-FABP), which has been demonstrated to provide complementary predictive information above and beyond that offered by troponin I and BNP [210]. Plasma myoglobin has been shown to rise quickly after onset of myocardial ischaemia, but its value for risk stratification has been inconsistent, and its use is limited by poor specificity in the presence of concomitant renal insufficiency or muscle trauma [211].

Structural markers of myocardial vulnerability

An echocardiographic examination, assessing left ventricular hypertrophy and other structural elements of the heart, is a very common examination for establishing current and future CVD. The methodology is fairly standardized, available and convenient [212–214], and different structural measures have been associated with CVD risk in many studies [215–221]. Further, the regression of left ventricular hypertrophy assessed with echocardiography tracks with treatment with antihypertensives [222–225]. In recent years, computed axial tomography (CAT) and magnetic resonance imaging (MRI) have been used to assess the myocardial structure in studies, but these methods are still confined to research, and have not been examined in relation to incident CVD in the community.

Functional markers of myocardial vulnerability

Echocardiographic examinations are also useful for examining myocardial function, i.e. both systolic and diastolic ventricular function. In addition, echocardiographic markers have been prospectively associated with incident CVD in several studies [226–228], and track with treatment [229, 230]. Exercise stress tests are also routinely used as functional markers of myocardial vulnerability. This methodology is widely used, standardized, and convenient. Further, it has consistently been associated with the risk of future CVD events [231–233]. MRI and positron emission tomography (PET) can also be used to assess myocardial function, but this is a newer research area; these modalities have not been evaluated in studies of predictors of incident CVD in the community.

GENETIC MARKERS OF CVD

An emerging and very interesting group of biomarkers are the genetic markers. Although research in this area has been ongoing for some years now, there still are no established genetic markers for CVD risk prediction. A major problem in this research is that there seem to be many reports of false-positive associations with disease (or phenotypes). The failure of replication could result from numerous factors, such as true genetic heterogeneity across samples, publication bias, confounding by population structure, misclassification of outcomes, allelic heterogeneity, small sample sizes and failure to account for multiple testing (including the possibility that findings are due to chance) [234, 235]. A more detailed discussion of the factors contributing to the lack of replication and the future potential genetic biomarkers is beyond the scope of this chapter, but for those interested, there is a recent review on the topic by Gibbons *et al.* [236].

Genetic markers can also be useful in observational epidemiology by utilizing the concept of Mendelian randomization, which is the term for the random assortment of alleles at the time of gamete formation. This means that the genetic variants are distributed in the population independently of behavioural and environmental factors that usually confound associations between the suggestive risk factors and disease. By using these concepts one can avoid the usual problems in observational epidemiology, such as reverse causation, associative selection bias, and regression dilution bias [237]. An example of how this concept has been used is for examining the association between fibrinogen and CVD. Blood concentrations of fibrinogen have been associated with coronary heart disease risk in several epidemiological studies as discussed above, but it is uncertain whether this association is causal or reflects residual confounding by other risk factors. This has been examined by relating fibrinogen genotypes and CVD risk, however with inconsistent results [238, 239]. This method of linking genotypes to outcomes is an efficient way of strengthening the potential association of biomarkers with outcomes.

ILLUSTRATING THE USE OF NEW CVD BIOMARKERS

The potential use of newer CVD biomarkers is readily illustrated by the clinical setting of an acute coronary syndrome. Acute coronary syndromes are heralded by dynamic obstruction superimposed on progressive mechanical arterial stenosis, associated plaque inflammation, instability and rupture, followed by thrombosis. This cascade of events leads to myocardial ischaemia and necrosis, followed in due course by ventricular remodelling. Consequently, diverse sets of biomarkers are activated during the different phases of the process and these biomarkers may be detected in the peripheral circulation [12, 13, 240] as illustrated in Figure 8.1. Atherosclerotic arterial lesions that are prone to rupture are rich in macrophages (which release lytic enzymes like metalloproteinases), have a reduced smooth muscle layer, a low-grade stenosis, and a thin fibrous cap. Plaque rupture is associated with release of several soluble biomarkers, such as the CD40 ligand, PlGF, PAPP-A and adhesion molecules [240].

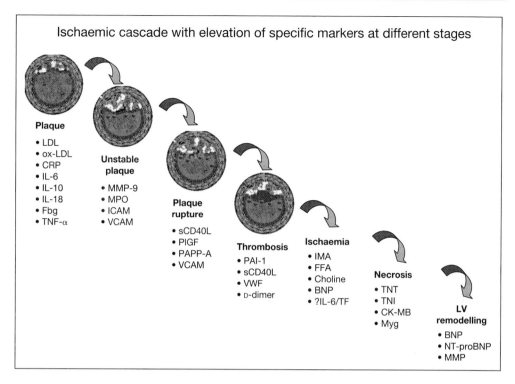

Figure 8.1   Biomarkers of acute coronary syndromes. The arrows indicate the sequence of events during an acute coronary syndrome. Biomarkers that may be elevated at each phase of the disease are displayed. BNP = B-type natriuretic peptide; sCD40L = soluble CD40 ligand; CK-MB = creatine kinase–MB isoform; CRP = C-reactive protein; Fbg = fibrinogen; FFA = free fatty acid; ICAM = intercellular adhesion molecule; IL = interleukin; IMA = ischaemia-modified albumin; LDL = low-density lipoprotein; MMP = matrix metalloproteinases; MPO = myeloperoxidase; Myg = myoglobin; NT-proBNP = N-terminal proBNP; ox-LDL = oxidized LDL; PAI-1 = plasminogen activator inhibitor; PAPP-A = pregnancy-associated plasma protein-A; PlGF = placental growth factor; TF = tissue factor; TNF = tumour necrosis factor; TNI = troponin I; TNT = troponin T; VCAM = vascular cell adhesion molecule; VWF = von Willebrand Factor.

Adapted with permission from references [12, 13, 240].

Superimposed thrombosis may be indicated by elevation of circulating D-dimer, PAI-1 and von Willebrand factor levels [240]. Before the beginning of symptomatic ischaemia, ischaemia-modified albumin is released for a few hours. The development of myocardial necrosis results in release of myocyte components in a time-dependent manner, i.e. elevation of troponins, myoglobin and creatine kinase (MB). It has been suggested that elevation of blood troponin levels in a patient with non-ST segment elevation MI is a marker of myocyte necrosis, but is also an indicator of intracoronary thrombus formation and the distal microembolization of platelet microaggregates [241]. So, troponin release in acute coronary syndromes has been related to an increased likelihood of response to antiplatelet and antithrombin therapy [241]. An elevation of plasma natriuretic peptide levels indicates the haemodynamic consequences of ischaemia and/or infarction. Ultimately, the choice of the biomarkers assayed in patients with suspected acute coronary syndromes depends on several factors [242], such as where the test is being performed (emergency room vs. clinician's office), the duration of ischaemic symptoms, the discrimination limits used for the selected biomarkers, and it varies based on whether the test is being done for diagnosis or for prognostication.

SUMMARY

Biomarkers, defined as measured changes in the components of body fluids or tissues, are emerging as powerful tools for understanding manifestations across the entire CVD spectrum. CVD biomarkers are used for screening, diagnosis, prognostication, prediction of disease recurrence and therapeutic monitoring. Recent biotechnological advances have provided numerous putative markers that may be informative in the various stages of CVD. A prerequisite for clinical use of biomarkers is clarification of the specific indications, standardization of analytical methods, assessment of performance characteristics, demonstration of incremental predictive value for given clinical indications (above standard risk factors), and the demonstration of cost-effectiveness, especially when considering biomarkers in screening programmes. There is rapid scientific progress in the area of biomarker discovery, combining the traditional approaches to biomarker discovery (such as serological, structural, or functional markers) with newer approaches, including functional genomics, proteomics, and metabolomics. These advances will likely identify an increasing array of CVD biomarkers. In the future, it is conceivable that many CVD markers will constitute comprehensive multimarker panels, providing opportunities for individual risk profiling and for individualizing the diagnosis and treatment of CVD.

ACKNOWLEDGEMENTS

This work was supported through the Foundation of Thuréus and the Foundation of Gustaf Adolf Johansson (Dr Ingelsson), and National Institute of Health/National Heart, Lung & Blood Institute Contract N01-HC-25195, 1R01HL67288, and 2K24HL04334 (Dr Vasan).

REFERENCES

1. American Heart Association. *Heart Disease and Stroke Statistics – 2005 Update*. American Heart Association, Dallas, Texas, 2005.
2. World Health Association. *The World Health Report 2002: Risks to Health 2002*. World Health Organization, Geneva, 2002.
3. Berenson GS, Srinivasan SR, Bao W *et al*. Association between multiple cardiovascular risk factors and atherosclerosis in children and young adults. *N Engl J Med* 1998; 338:1650–1656.
4. Raitakari OT, Juonala M, Kahonen M *et al*. Cardiovascular risk factors in childhood and carotid artery intima-media thickness in adulthood: the Cardiovascular Risk in Young Finns Study. *JAMA* 2003; 290:2277–2283.
5. Kuller LH, Shemanski L, Psaty BM *et al*. Subclinical disease as an independent risk factor for cardiovascular disease. *Circulation* 1995; 92:720–726.
6. Psaty BM, Furberg CD, Kuller LH *et al*. Traditional risk factors and subclinical disease measures as predictors of first myocardial infarction in older adults: The Cardiovascular Health Study. *Arch Intern Med* 1999; 159:1339–1347.
7. Pearson TA, Blair SN, Daniels SR *et al*. AHA guidelines for primary prevention of cardiovascular disease and stroke: 2002 update: Consensus panel guide to comprehensive risk reduction for adult patients without coronary or other atherosclerotic vascular diseases. *Circulation* 2002; 106:388–391.
8. Kita Chun A, McGee SR. Bedside diagnosis of coronary artery disease: a systematic review. *Am J Med* 2004; 117:334–343.
9. Panju AA, Hemmelgarn BR, Guyatt GH, Simel DL. Is this patient having a myocardial infarction? *JAMA* 1998; 280:1256–1263.
10. Pope JH, Aufderheide TP, Ruthazer R *et al*. Missed diagnoses of acute cardiac ischemia in the emergency department. *N Engl J Med* 2000; 342:1163–1170.
11. Swap CJ, Nagurney JT. Value and limitations of chest pain history in the evaluation of patients with suspected acute coronary syndromes. *JAMA* 2005; 294:2623–2629.
12. Naghavi M, Libby P, Falk E *et al*. From vulnerable plaque to vulnerable patient: a call for new definitions and risk assessment strategies: Part I. *Circulation* 2003; 108:1664–1672.

13. Naghavi M, Libby P, Falk E *et al.* From vulnerable plaque to vulnerable patient: a call for new definitions and risk assessment strategies: Part II. *Circulation* 2003; 108:1772–1778.

14. National Library of Medicine. http://www.ncbi.nlm.nih.gov/entrez/query.fcgi?db=MeSH. 2006. 10-7-2006.

15. Atkinson AJ, Colburn WA, De Gruttola VG *et al.* Biomarkers and surrogate endpoints: Preferred definitions and conceptual framework. *Clin Pharmacol Ther* 2001; 69:89–95.

16. Manolio T. Novel risk markers and clinical practice. *N Engl J Med* 2003; 349:1587–1589.

17. LaBaer J. So, you want to look for biomarkers (Introduction to the special biomarkers issue). *J Proteome Res* 2005; 4:1053–1059.

18. Morrow DA, de Lemos JA, Sabatine MS, Antman EM. The search for a biomarker of cardiac ischemia. *Clin Chem* 2003; 49:537–539.

19. Fortmann SP, Ford E, Criqui MH *et al.* CDC/AHA workshop on markers of inflammation and cardiovascular disease: application to clinical and public health practice: report from the Population Science Discussion Group. *Circulation* 2004; 110:e554–e559.

20. Solberg HE. Approved recommendations (1986) on the theory of reference values, I: the concept of reference values. *J Clin Chem Clin Biochem* 1987; 25:337–342.

21. Solberg HE. Approved recommendations (1987) on the theory of reference values, II: selection of individuals for the production of reference values. *J Clin Chem Clin Biochem* 1987; 25:639–644.

22. Solberg HE. Approved recommendations (1987) on the theory of reference values, V: statistical treatment of collected reference values. Determination of reference limits. *J Clin Chem Clin Biochem* 1987; 25:645–656.

23. Sunderman FW Jr. Current concepts of 'normal values,' 'reference values,' and 'discrimination values,' in clinical chemistry. *Clin Chem* 1975; 21:1873–1877.

24. Shapiro BP, Chen HH, Burnett JC Jr, Redfield MM. Use of plasma brain natriuretic peptide concentration to aid in the diagnosis of heart failure. *Mayo Clin Proc* 2003; 78:481–486.

25. Prospective Studies Collaboration. Age-specific relevance of usual blood pressure to vascular mortality: a meta-analysis of individual data for one million adults in 61 prospective studies. *Lancet* 2002; 360:1903–1913.

26. Bossuyt PM, Reitsma JB, Bruns DE *et al.* Towards complete and accurate reporting of studies of diagnostic accuracy: The STARD Initiative. *Clin Chem* 2003; 49:1–6.

27. Wade A. Derivation versus validation. *Arch Dis Child* 2000; 83:459–460.

28. Hanley JA, McNeil BJ. The meaning and use of the area under a Receiver Operating Characteristic (ROC) curve. *Radiology* 1982; 143:29–36.

29. Swets JA. Measuring the accuracy of diagnostic systems. *Science* 1988; 240:1285–1293.

30. Baker SG. The central role of Receiver Operating Characteristic (ROC) curves in evaluating tests for the early detection of cancer. *J Natl Cancer Inst* 2003; 95:511–515.

31. Sackett DL, Haynes RB, Guyatt GH, Tugwell P. The interpretation of diagnostic data. Clinical epidemiology, a basic science for clinical medicine. Little Brown, Boston, 1991, pp 69–152.

32. Pepe MS, Janes H, Longton G, Leisenring W, Newcomb P. Limitations of the odds ratio in gauging the performance of a diagnostic, prognostic, or screening marker. *Am J Epidemiol* 2004; 159:882–890.

33. Wald NJ, Hackshaw AK, Frost CD. When can a risk factor be used as a worthwhile screening test? *BMJ* 1999; 319:1562–1565.

34. Kattan MW. Evaluating a new marker's predictive contribution. *Clin Cancer Res* 2004; 10:822–824.

35. Wilson PWF, D'Agostino RB, Levy D, Belanger AM, Silbershatz H, Kannel WB. Prediction of coronary heart disease using risk factor categories. *Circulation* 1998; 97:1837–1847.

36. Conroy RM, Pyörälä K, Fitzgerald AP *et al.* Estimation of ten-year risk of fatal cardiovascular disease in Europe: the SCORE project. *Eur Heart J* 2003; 24:987–1003.

37. Expert Panel on Detection, Evaluation and Treatment of High Blood Cholesterol in Adults. Executive Summary of the Third Report of the National Cholesterol Education Program (NCEP) Expert Panel on Detection, Evaluation, and Treatment of High Blood Cholesterol in Adults (Adult Treatment Panel III). *JAMA* 2001; 285:2486–2497.

38. Blake GJ, Otvos JD, Rifai N, Ridker PM. Low-density lipoprotein particle concentration and size as determined by nuclear magnetic resonance spectroscopy as predictors of cardiovascular disease in women. *Circulation* 2002; 106:1930–1937.

39. Kuller L, Arnold A, Tracy R *et al.* Nuclear magnetic resonance spectroscopy of lipoproteins and risk of coronary heart disease in the cardiovascular health study. *Arterioscler Thromb Vasc Biol* 2002; 22:1175–1180.

40. Pischon T, Girman CJ, Sacks FM, Rifai N, Stampfer MJ, Rimm EB. Non-high-density lipoprotein cholesterol and apolipoprotein B in the prediction of coronary heart disease in men. *Circulation* 2005; 112:3375–3383.

41. Shai I, Rimm EB, Hankinson SE *et al*. Multivariate assessment of lipid parameters as predictors of coronary heart disease among postmenopausal women: potential implications for clinical guidelines. *Circulation* 2004; 110:2824–2830.

42. Walldius G, Jungner I, Holme I, Aastveit AH, Kolar W, Steiner E. High apolipoprotein B, low apolipoprotein A-I, and improvement in the prediction of fatal myocardial infarction (AMORIS study): a prospective study. *Lancet* 2001; 358:2026–2033.

43. Sharrett AR, Ballantyne CM, Coady SA *et al*. Coronary heart disease prediction from lipoprotein cholesterol levels, triglycerides, lipoprotein(a), apolipoproteins A-I and B, and HDL density subfractions: The Atherosclerosis Risk in Communities (ARIC) Study. *Circulation* 2001; 104:1108–1113.

44. Talmud PJ, Hawe E, Miller GJ, Humphries SE. Nonfasting apolipoprotein B and triglyceride levels as a useful predictor of coronary heart disease risk in middle-aged UK men. *Arterioscler Thromb Vasc Biol* 2002; 22:1918–1923.

45. Lamarche B, Moorjani S, Lupien PJ *et al*. Apolipoprotein A-I and B Levels and the Risk of Ischemic Heart Disease During a Five-Year Follow-up of Men in the Quebec Cardiovascular Study. *Circulation* 1996; 94:273–278.

46. Danesh J, Collins R, Peto R. Lipoprotein(a) and coronary heart disease: Meta-analysis of prospective studies. *Circulation* 2000; 102:1082–1085.

47. Ridker PM, Rifai N, Cook NR, Bradwin G, Buring JE. Non-HDL cholesterol, apolipoproteins A-I and B100, standard lipid measures, lipid ratios, and CRP as risk factors for cardiovascular disease in women. *JAMA* 2005; 294:326–333.

48. Sniderman AD. Apolipoprotein B versus non-high-density lipoprotein cholesterol: and the winner is. *Circulation* 2005; 112:3366–3367.

49. Gotto AM Jr, Whitney E, Stein EA *et al*. Relation between baseline and on-treatment lipid parameters and first acute major coronary events in the Air Force/Texas Coronary Atherosclerosis Prevention Study (AFCAPS/TexCAPS). *Circulation* 2000; 101:477–484.

50. Denke MA. Weighing in before the fight: low-density lipoprotein cholesterol and non-high-density lipoprotein cholesterol versus apolipoprotein B as the best predictor for coronary heart disease and the best measure of therapy. *Circulation* 2005; 112:3368–3370.

51. Ballantyne CM, Hoogeveen RC, Bang H *et al*. Lipoprotein-associated phospholipase A2, high-sensitivity C-reactive protein, and risk for incident coronary heart disease in middle-aged men and women in the Atherosclerosis Risk in Communities (ARIC) Study. *Circulation* 2004; 109:837–842.

52. Ballantyne CM, Hoogeveen RC, Bang H *et al*. Lipoprotein-associated phospholipase A2, high-sensitivity C-reactive protein, and risk for incident ischemic stroke in middle-aged men and women in the Atherosclerosis Risk in Communities (ARIC) Study. *Arch Intern Med* 2005; 165:2479–2484.

53. Blake GJ, Dada N, Fox JC, Manson JE, Ridker PM. A prospective evaluation of lipoprotein-associated phospholipase A2 levels and the risk of future cardiovascular events in women. *J Am Coll Cardiol* 2001; 38:1302–1306.

54. Brilakis ES, McConnell JP, Lennon RJ, Elesber AA, Meyer JG, Berger PB. Association of lipoprotein-associated phospholipase A2 levels with coronary artery disease risk factors, angiographic coronary artery disease, and major adverse events at follow-up. *Eur Heart J* 2005; 26:137–144.

55. Koenig W, Khuseyinova N, Lowel H, Trischler G, Meisinger C. Lipoprotein-associated phospholipase A2 adds to risk prediction of incident coronary events by C-reactive protein in apparently healthy middle-aged men from the general population: results from the 14-Year Follow-up of a Large Cohort from Southern Germany. *Circulation* 2004; 110:1903–1908.

56. Boekholdt SM, Keller TT, Wareham NJ *et al*. Serum levels of type II secretory phospholipase A2 and the risk of future coronary artery disease in apparently healthy men and women: the EPIC-Norfolk Prospective Population Study. *Arterioscler Thromb Vasc Biol* 2005; 25:839–846.

57. Oei HH, van der Meer IM, Hofman A *et al*. Lipoprotein-associated phospholipase A2 activity is associated with risk of coronary heart disease and ischemic stroke: The Rotterdam Study. *Circulation* 2005; 111:570–575.

58. Folsom AR, Chambless LE, Ballantyne CM *et al*. An assessment of incremental coronary risk prediction using C-reactive protein and other novel risk markers: the Atherosclerosis Risk in Communities Study. *Arch Intern Med* 2006; 166:1368–1373.

59. Boekholdt SM, Kuivenhoven JA, Wareham NJ *et al*. Plasma levels of cholesteryl ester transfer protein and the risk of future coronary artery disease in apparently healthy men and women. The Prospective

EPIC (European Prospective Investigation into Cancer and nutrition)-Norfolk Population Study. *Circulation* 2004; 110:1418–1423.

60. Libby P, Theroux P. Pathophysiology of coronary artery disease. *Circulation* 2005; 111:3481–3488.

61. Ledue TB, Rifai N. Preanalytic and analytic sources of variations in C-reactive protein measurement: implications for cardiovascular disease risk assessment. *Clin Chem* 2003; 49:1258–1271.

62. Danesh J, Wheeler JG, Hirschfield GM *et al.* C-reactive protein and other circulating markers of inflammation in the prediction of coronary heart disease. *N Engl J Med* 2004; 350:1387–1397.

63. Smith SC Jr, Anderson JL, Cannon RO III *et al.* CDC/AHA workshop on markers of inflammation and cardiovascular disease: application to clinical and public health practice: Report From the Clinical Practice Discussion Group. *Circulation* 2004; 110:e550–e553.

64. Cook NR, Buring JE, Ridker PM. The effect of including C-reactive protein in cardiovascular risk prediction models for women. *Ann Intern Med* 2006; 145:21–29.

65. Lloyd-Jones DM, Liu K, Tian L, Greenland P. Narrative review: Assessment of C-reactive protein in risk prediction for cardiovascular disease. *Ann Intern Med* 2006; 145:35–42.

66. Pearson TA, Mensah GA, Alexander RW *et al.* Markers of inflammation and cardiovascular disease: application to clinical and public health practice: a statement for healthcare professionals from the centers for disease control and prevention and the American Heart Association. *Circulation* 2003; 107:499–511.

67. Cesari M, Penninx BWJH, Newman AB *et al.* Inflammatory markers and onset of cardiovascular events: Results From the Health ABC Study. *Circulation* 2003; 108:2317–2322.

68. Lindmark E, Diderholm E, Wallentin L, Siegbahn A. Relationship between interleukin 6 and mortality in patients with unstable coronary artery disease: Effects of an early invasive or noninvasive strategy. *JAMA* 2001; 286:2107–2113.

69. Luc G, Bard JM, Juhan-Vague I *et al.* C-reactive protein, interleukin-6, and fibrinogen as predictors of coronary heart disease: The PRIME Study. *Arterioscler Thromb Vasc Biol* 2003; 23:1255–1261.

70. Pai JK, Pischon T, Manson JE *et al.* Inflammatory markers and the risk of coronary heart disease in men and women. *N Engl J Med* 2004; 351:2599–2610.

71. Pradhan AD, Manson JE, Rossouw JE *et al.* Inflammatory biomarkers, hormone replacement therapy, and incident coronary heart disease: Prospective Analysis from the Women's Health Initiative Observational Study. *JAMA* 2002; 288:980–987.

72. Ridker PM, Rifai N, Stampfer MJ, Hennekens CH. Plasma concentration of interleukin-6 and the risk of future myocardial infarction among apparently healthy men. *Circulation* 2000; 101:1767–1772.

73. Volpato S, Guralnik JM, Ferrucci L *et al.* Cardiovascular disease, interleukin-6, and risk of mortality in older women: The Women's Health and Aging Study. *Circulation* 2001; 103:947–953.

74. Blankenberg S, Tiret L, Bickel C *et al.* Interleukin-18 is a strong predictor of cardiovascular death in stable and unstable angina. *Circulation* 2002; 106:24–30.

75. Blankenberg S, Luc G, Ducimetiere P *et al.* Interleukin-18 and the risk of coronary heart disease in European men: The Prospective Epidemiological Study of Myocardial Infarction (PRIME). *Circulation* 2003; 108:2453–2459.

76. Johnson BD, Kip KE, Marroquin OC *et al.* Serum amyloid A as a predictor of coronary artery disease and cardiovascular outcome in women: The National Heart, Lung, and Blood Institute-Sponsored Women's Ischemia Syndrome Evaluation (WISE). *Circulation* 2004; 109:726–732.

77. Biasucci LM, Liuzzo G, Grillo RL *et al.* Elevated levels of C-reactive protein at discharge in patients with unstable angina predict recurrent instability. *Circulation* 1999; 99:855–860.

78. Haverkate E, Thompson SG, Pyke SD, Gallimore JR, Group MBP. Production of C-reactive protein and risk of coronary events in stable and unstable angina. *Lancet* 1997; 349:462–466.

79. Malik I, Danesh J, Whincup P *et al.* Soluble adhesion molecules and prediction of coronary heart disease: a prospective study and meta-analysis. *Lancet* 2001; 358:971–976.

80. Baldus S, Heeschen C, Meinertz T *et al.* Myeloperoxidase serum levels predict risk in patients with acute coronary syndromes. *Circulation* 2003; 108:1440–1445.

81. Brennan ML, Penn MS, van Lente F *et al.* Prognostic value of myeloperoxidase in patients with chest pain. *N Engl J Med* 2003; 349:1595–1604.

82. Zhang R, Brennan ML, Fu X *et al.* Association between myeloperoxidase levels and risk of coronary artery disease. *JAMA* 2001; 286:2136–2142.

83. Heeschen C, Dimmeler S, Hamm CW *et al.* Soluble CD40 ligand in acute coronary syndromes. *N Engl J Med* 2003; 348:1104–1111.

84. Schonbeck U, Varo N, Libby P, Buring J, Ridker PM. Soluble CD40L and cardiovascular risk in women. *Circulation* 2001; 104:2266–2268.

85. Varo N, Libby P, Morrow DA *et al*. Soluble CD40L: risk prediction after acute coronary syndromes. *Circulation* 2003; 108:1049–1052.

86. Yan JC, Zhu J, Gao L *et al*. The effect of elevated serum soluble CD40 ligand on the prognostic value in patients with acute coronary syndromes. *Clinica Chimica Acta* 2004; 343:155–159.

87. Hoogeveen RC, Morrison A, Boerwinkle E *et al*. Plasma MCP-1 level and risk for peripheral arterial disease and incident coronary heart disease: Atherosclerosis Risk in Communities Study. *Atherosclerosis* 2005; 183:301–307.

88. Piemonti L, Calori G, Mercalli A *et al*. Fasting plasma leptin, tumor necrosis factor-alpha receptor 2, and monocyte chemoattracting protein 1 concentration in a population of glucose-tolerant and glucose-intolerant women: impact on cardiovascular mortality. *Diabetes Care* 2003; 26:2883–2889.

89. Bayes-Genis A, Conover CA, Overgaard MT *et al*. Pregnancy-associated plasma protein A as a marker of acute coronary syndromes. *N Engl J Med* 2001; 345:1022–1029.

90. Lund J, Qin QP, Ilva T *et al*. Circulating pregnancy-associated plasma protein A predicts outcome in patients with acute coronary syndrome but no troponin I elevation. *Circulation* 2003; 108:1924–1926.

91. Heeschen C, Dimmeler S, Fichtlscherer S, Zeiher AM, Hamm CW, Simoons ML. Pregnancy-associated plasma protein-A levels in patients with acute coronary syndromes: comparison with markers of systemic inflammation, platelet activation, and myocardial necrosis. *J Am Coll Cardiol* 2005; 45:229–237.

92. Heeschen C, Dimmeler S, Fichtlscherer S *et al*. Prognostic value of placental growth factor in patients with acute chest pain. *JAMA* 2004; 291:435–441.

93. Griendling KK, FitzGerald GA. Oxidative stress and cardiovascular injury: Part II: animal and human studies. *Circulation* 2003; 108:2034–2040.

94. Griendling KK, FitzGerald GA. Oxidative stress and cardiovascular injury: Part I: basic mechanisms and in vivo monitoring of ROS. *Circulation* 2003; 108:1912–1916.

95. Meisinger C, Baumert J, Khuseyinova N, Loewel H, Koenig W. Plasma oxidized low-density lipoprotein, a strong predictor for acute coronary heart disease events in apparently healthy, middle-aged men from the general population. *Circulation* 2005; 112:651–657.

96. Blankenberg S, Rupprecht HJ, Bickel C *et al*. Glutathione peroxidase 1 activity and cardiovascular events in patients with coronary artery disease. *N Engl J Med* 2003; 349:1605–1613.

97. Schnabel R, Lackner KJ, Rupprecht HJ *et al*. Glutathione peroxidase-1 and homocysteine for cardiovascular risk prediction: Results from the AtheroGene Study. *J Am Coll Cardiol* 2005; 45:1631–1637.

98. Shishehbor MH, Aviles RJ, Brennan ML *et al*. Association of nitrotyrosine levels with cardiovascular disease and modulation by statin therapy. *JAMA* 2003; 289:1675–1680.

99. Homocysteine Studies Collaboration. Homocysteine and risk of ischemic heart disease and stroke: a meta-analysis. *JAMA* 2002; 288:2015–2022.

100. Wald DS, Law M, Morris JK. Homocysteine and cardiovascular disease: evidence on causality from a meta-analysis. *BMJ* 2002; 325:1202–1206.

101. Lonn E, Yusuf S, Arnold MJ *et al*. Homocysteine lowering with folic acid and B vitamins in vascular disease. *N Engl J Med* 2006; 354:1567–1577.

102. Bonaa KH, Njolstad I, Ueland PM *et al*. Homocysteine lowering and cardiovascular events after acute myocardial infarction. *N Engl J Med* 2006; 354:1578–1588.

103. Rosenberg IH, Mulrow CD. Trials that matter: should we routinely measure homocysteine levels and 'treat' mild hyperhomocysteinemia? *Ann Intern Med* 2006; 145:226–227.

104. de Lemos JA, Morrow DA, Bentley JH *et al*. The prognostic value of B-type natriuretic peptide in patients with acute coronary syndromes. *N Engl J Med* 2001; 345:1014–1021.

105. Galvani M, Ottani F, Oltrona L *et al*. N-terminal pro-brain natriuretic peptide on admission has prognostic value across the whole spectrum of acute coronary syndromes. *Circulation* 2004; 110:128–134.

106. Heeschen C, Hamm CW, Mitrovic V, Lantelme NH, White HD, for the Platelet Receptor Inhibition in Ischemic Syndrome Management (PRISM) Investigators. N-terminal pro-B-type natriuretic peptide levels for dynamic risk stratification of patients with acute coronary syndromes. *Circulation* 2004; 110:3206–3212.

107. Kistorp C, Raymond I, Pedersen F, Gustafsson F, Faber J, Hildebrandt P. N-terminal pro-brain natriuretic peptide, C-reactive protein, and urinary albumin levels as predictors of mortality and cardiovascular events in older adults. *JAMA* 2005; 293:1609–1616.

108. Kragelund C, Grønning B, Hildebrandt P, Køber L, Steffensen R. N-terminal pro-B-type natriuretic peptide and long-term mortality in stable coronary heart disease. *N Engl J Med* 2005; 352:666–675.

109. Morrow DA, Sabatine MS, McCabe CH et al. Evaluation of B-type natriuretic peptide for risk assessment in unstable angina/non-ST-elevation myocardial infarction: B-type natriuretic peptide and prognosis in TACTICS-TIMI 18. *J Am Coll Cardiol* 2003; 41:1264–1272.

110. Morrow DA, de Lemos JA, Blazing MA et al. Prognostic value of serial B-type natriuretic peptide testing during follow-up of patients with unstable coronary artery disease. *JAMA* 2005; 294:2866–2871.

111. Omland T, Richards AM, Wergeland R, Vik-Mo H. B-type natriuretic peptide and long-term survival in patients with stable coronary artery disease. *Am J Cardiol* 2005; 95:24–28.

112. Sabatine MS, Morrow DA, de Lemos JA et al. Multimarker approach to risk stratification in non-ST elevation acute coronary syndromes: simultaneous assessment of troponin I, C-reactive protein, and B-type natriuretic peptide. *Circulation* 2002; 105:1760–1763.

113. Suzuki S, Yoshimura M, Nakayama M et al. Plasma level of B-type natriuretic peptide as a prognostic marker after acute myocardial infarction: a long-term follow-up analysis. *Circulation* 2004; 110:1387–1391.

114. Wang TJ, Larson MG, Levy D et al. Plasma natriuretic peptide levels and the risk of cardiovascular events and death. *N Engl J Med* 2004; 350:655–663.

115. Gackowski A, Isnard R, Golmard JL et al. Comparison of echocardiography and plasma B-type natriuretic peptide for monitoring the response to treatment in acute heart failure. *Eur Heart J* 2004; 25:1788–1796.

116. Logeart D, Thabut G, Jourdain P et al. Predischarge B-type natriuretic peptide assay for identifying patients at high risk of re-admission after decompensated heart failure. *J Am Coll Cardiol* 2004; 43:635–641.

117. Troughton RW, Frampton CM, Yandle TG, Espine EA, Nicholls MG, Richards AM. Treatment of heart failure guided by plasma aminoterminal brain natriuretic peptide (N-BNP) concentrations. *Lancet* 2000; 355:1126–1130.

118. Apple FS, Panteghini M, Ravkilde J et al. Quality specifications for B-type natriuretic peptide assays. *Clin Chem* 2005; 51:486–493.

119. Blankenberg S, McQueen MJ, Smieja M et al. Comparative impact of multiple biomarkers and N-terminal pro-brain natriuretic peptide in the context of conventional risk factors for the prediction of recurrent cardiovascular events in the Heart Outcomes Prevention Evaluation (HOPE) Study. *Circulation* 2006; 114:201–208.

120. Vasan RS, Evans JC, Larson MG et al. Serum aldosterone and the incidence of hypertension in nonhypertensive persons. *N Engl J Med* 2004; 351:33–41.

121. Amano T, Matsubara T, Izawa H et al. Impact of plasma aldosterone levels for prediction of in-stent restenosis. *Am J Cardiol* 2006; 97:785–788.

122. Meade TW, Cooper JA, Peart WS. Plasma renin activity and ischemic heart disease. *N Engl J Med* 1993; 329:616–619.

123. Alderman MH, Ooi WL, Cohen H, Madhavan S, Sealey JE, Laragh JH. Plasma renin activity: a risk factor for myocardial infarction in hypertensive patients. *Am J Hypertens* 1997; 10:1–8.

124. Blumenfeld JD, Sealey JE, Alderman MH et al. Plasma renin activity in the emergency department and its independent association with acute myocardial infarction. *Am J Hypertens* 2000; 13:855–863.

125. Campbell DJ, Woodward M, Chalmers JP et al. Prediction of myocardial infarction by N-terminal-pro-B-type natriuretic peptide, C-reactive protein, and renin in subjects with cerebrovascular disease. *Circulation* 2005; 112:110–116.

126. Koenig W, Twardella D, Brenner H, Rothenbacher D. Plasma concentrations of cystatin C in patients with coronary heart disease and risk for secondary cardiovascular events: more than simply a marker of glomerular filtration rate. *Clin Chem* 2005; 51:321–327.

127. Luc G, Bard JM, Lesueur C et al. Plasma cystatin-C and development of coronary heart disease: The PRIME Study. *Atherosclerosis* 2006; 185:375–380.

128. O'Hare AM, Newman AB, Katz R et al. Cystatin C and incident peripheral arterial disease events in the elderly: results from the Cardiovascular Health Study. *Arch Intern Med* 2005; 165:2666–2670.

129. Shlipak MG, Sarnak MJ, Katz R et al. Cystatin C and the risk of death and cardiovascular events among elderly persons. *N Engl J Med* 2005; 352:2049–2060.

130. Blankenberg S, Rupprecht HJ, Poirier O et al. Plasma concentrations and genetic variation of matrix metalloproteinase 9 and prognosis of patients with cardiovascular disease. *Circulation* 2003; 107:1579–1585.

131. Lubos E, Schnabel R, Rupprecht HJ et al. Prognostic value of tissue inhibitor of metalloproteinase-1 for cardiovascular death among patients with cardiovascular disease: results from the AtheroGene study. *Eur Heart J* 2006; 27:150–156.

132. Krempl TK, Maas R, Sydow K, Meinertz T, Böger RH, Kähler J. Elevation of asymmetric dimethylarginine in patients with unstable angina and recurrent cardiovascular events. *Eur Heart J* 2005; 26:1846–1851.

133. Valkonen VP, Paiva H, Salonen JT *et al*. Risk of acute coronary events and serum concentration of asymmetrical dimethylarginine. *Lancet* 2001; 358:2127–2128.
134. Zoccali C, Bode-Boger S, Mallamaci F *et al*. Plasma concentration of asymmetrical dimethylarginine and mortality in patients with end-stage renal disease: a prospective study. *Lancet* 2001; 358:2113–2117.
135. Bae SW, Stuhlinger MC, Yoo HS *et al*. Plasma asymmetric dimethylarginine concentrations in newly diagnosed patients with acute myocardial infarction or unstable angina pectoris during two weeks of medical treatment. *Am J Cardiol* 2005; 95:729–733.
136. Boger RH, Zoccali C. ADMA: a novel risk factor that explains excess cardiovascular event rate in patients with end-stage renal disease. *Atheroscler Suppl* 2003; 4:23–28.
137. Mallamaci F, Tripepi G, Cutrupi S, Malatino LS, Zoccali C. Prognostic value of combined use of biomarkers of inflammation, endothelial dysfunction, and myocardiopathy in patients with ESRD. *Kidney Int* 2005; 67:2330–2337.
138. Ravani P, Tripepi G, Malberti F, Testa S, Mallamaci F, Zoccali C. Asymmetrical dimethylarginine predicts progression to dialysis and death in patients with chronic kidney disease: a competing risks modeling approach. *J Am Soc Nephrol* 2005; 16:2449–2455.
139. Tarnow L, Hovind P, Teerlink T, Stehouwer CD, Parving HH. Elevated plasma asymmetric dimethylarginine as a marker of cardiovascular morbidity in early diabetic nephropathy in type 1 diabetes. *Diabetes Care* 2004; 27:765–769.
140. Riley WA, Barnes RW, Applegate WB *et al*. Reproducibility of noninvasive ultrasonic measurement of carotid atherosclerosis. The Asymptomatic Carotid Artery Plaque Study. *Stroke* 1992; 23:1062–1068.
141. Bots ML, Hoes AW, Koudstaal PJ, Hofman A, Grobbee DE. Common carotid intima-media thickness and risk of stroke and myocardial infarction: The Rotterdam Study. *Circulation* 1997; 96:1432–1437.
142. Chambless LE, Heiss G, Folsom AR *et al*. Association of coronary heart disease incidence with carotid arterial wall thickness and major risk factors: the Atherosclerosis Risk in Communities (ARIC) Study, 1987–1993. *Am J Epidemiol* 1997; 146:483–494.
143. Hodis HN, Mack WJ, LaBree L *et al*. The role of carotid arterial intima-media thickness in predicting clinical coronary events. *Ann Intern Med* 1998; 128:262–269.
144. O'Leary DH, Polak JF, Kronmal RA *et al*. Carotid-artery intima and media thickness as a risk factor for myocardial infarction and stroke in older adults. *N Engl J Med* 1999; 340:14–22.
145. Joakimsen O, Bonaa KH, Mathiesen EB, Stensland-Bugge E, Arnesen E. Prediction of mortality by ultrasound screening of a general population for carotid stenosis: the Tromso Study. *Stroke* 2000; 31:1871–1876.
146. Lernfelt B, Forsberg M, Blomstrand C, Mellstrom D, Volkmann R. Cerebral atherosclerosis as predictor of stroke and mortality in representative elderly population. *Stroke* 2002; 33:224–229.
147. Mathiesen EB, Bonaa KH, Joakimsen O. Echolucent plaques are associated with high risk of ischemic cerebrovascular events in carotid stenosis: the Tromso Study. *Circulation* 2001; 103:2171–2175.
148. Aburahma AF, Thiele SP, Wulu JT Jr. Prospective controlled study of the natural history of asymptomatic 60% to 69% carotid stenosis according to ultrasonic plaque morphology. *J Vasc Surg* 2002; 36:437–442.
149. Jang IK, Tearney GJ, MacNeill B *et al*. In vivo characterization of coronary atherosclerotic plaque by use of optical coherence tomography. *Circulation* 2005; 111:1551–1555.
150. Madjid M, Naghavi M, Malik BA, Litovsky S, Willerson JT, Casscells W. Thermal detection of vulnerable plaque. *Am J Cardiol* 2002; 90:36L–39L.
151. Arad Y, Spadaro LA, Goodman K *et al*. Predictive value of electron beam computed tomography of the coronary arteries: 19-month follow-up of 1173 asymptomatic subjects. *Circulation* 1996; 93:1951–1953.
152. Arad Y, Goodman KJ, Roth M, Newstein D, Guerci AD. Coronary calcification, coronary disease risk factors, C-reactive protein, and atherosclerotic cardiovascular disease events: The St. Francis Heart Study. *J Am Coll Cardiol* 2005; 46:158–165.
153. Greenland P, LaBree L, Azen SP, Doherty TM, Detrano RC. Coronary artery calcium score combined with Framingham score for risk prediction in asymptomatic individuals. *JAMA* 2004; 291:210–215.
154. Kondos GT, Hoff JA, Sevrukov A *et al*. Electron-beam tomography coronary artery calcium and cardiac events: a 37-month follow-up of 5635 initially asymptomatic low- to intermediate-risk adults. *Circulation* 2003; 107:2571–2576.
155. Vliegenthart R, Oudkerk M, Hofman A *et al*. Coronary calcification improves cardiovascular risk prediction in the elderly. *Circulation* 2005; 112:572–577.
156. O'Rourke RA, Brundage BH, Froelicher VF *et al*. American College of Cardiology/American Heart Association Expert Consensus document on electron-beam computed tomography for the diagnosis and prognosis of coronary artery disease. *Circulation* 2000; 102:126–140.

157. Gibbons RJ, Eckel RH, Jacobs AK. The utilization of cardiac imaging. *Circulation* 2006; 113:1715–1716.

158. Pickering TG, Hall JE, Appel LJ *et al*. Recommendations for blood pressure measurement in humans and experimental animals: Part 1: Blood Pressure Measurement in Humans: a statement for professionals from the subcommittee of Professional and Public Education of the American Heart Association Council on High Blood Pressure Research. *Circulation* 2005; 111:697–716.

159. Clement DL, de Buyzere ML, de Bacquer DA *et al*. Prognostic value of ambulatory blood-pressure recordings in patients with treated hypertension. *N Engl J Med* 2003; 348:2407–2415.

160. Ingelsson E, Björklund-Bodegård K, Lind L, Ärnlöv J, Sundström J. Diurnal blood pressure pattern and risk of congestive heart failure. *JAMA* 2006; 295:2859–2866.

161. Staessen JA, Thijs L, Fagard R *et al*. Predicting cardiovascular risk using conventional vs ambulatory blood pressure in older patients with systolic hypertension. Systolic Hypertension in Europe Trial Investigators. *JAMA* 1999; 282:539–546.

162. Corretti MC, Anderson TJ, Benjamin EJ *et al*. Guidelines for the ultrasound assessment of endothelial-dependent flow-mediated vasodilation of the brachial artery: a report of the International Brachial Artery Reactivity Task Force. *J Am Coll Cardiol* 2002; 39:257–265.

163. Kuvin JT, Patel AR, Sliney KA *et al*. Assessment of peripheral vascular endothelial function with finger arterial pulse wave amplitude. *Am Heart J* 2003; 146:168–174.

164. Bonetti PO, Lerman LO, Lerman A. Endothelial dysfunction: a marker of atherosclerotic risk. *Arterioscler Thromb Vasc Biol* 2003; 23:168–175.

165. Brevetti G, Silvestro A, Schiano V, Chiariello M. Endothelial dysfunction and cardiovascular risk prediction in peripheral arterial disease: additive value of flow-mediated dilation to ankle-brachial pressure index. *Circulation* 2003; 108:2093–2098.

166. Chan SY, Mancini GB, Kuramoto L, Schulzer M, Frohlich J, Ignaszewski A. The prognostic importance of endothelial dysfunction and carotid atheroma burden in patients with coronary artery disease. *J Am Coll Cardiol* 2003; 42:1037–1043.

167. Fichtlscherer S, Breuer S, Zeiher AM. Prognostic value of systemic endothelial dysfunction in patients with acute coronary syndromes: further evidence for the existence of the 'vulnerable' patient. *Circulation* 2004; 110:1926–1932.

168. Gokce N, Keaney JF Jr, Hunter LM, Watkins MT, Menzoian JO, Vita JA. Risk stratification for postoperative cardiovascular events via noninvasive assessment of endothelial function: a prospective study. *Circulation* 2002; 105:1567–1572.

169. Gokce N, Keaney JF Jr, Hunter LM *et al*. Predictive value of noninvasively determined endothelial dysfunction for long-term cardiovascular events in patients with peripheral vascular disease. *J Am Coll Cardiol* 2003; 41:1769–1775.

170. Halcox JP, Schenke WH, Zalos G *et al*. Prognostic value of coronary vascular endothelial dysfunction. *Circulation* 2002; 106:653–658.

171. Heitzer T, Schlinzig T, Krohn K, Meinertz T, Munzel T. Endothelial dysfunction, oxidative stress, and risk of cardiovascular events in patients with coronary artery disease. *Circulation* 2001; 104:2673–2678.

172. Neunteufl T, Heher S, Katzenschlager R *et al*. Late prognostic value of flow-mediated dilation in the brachial artery of patients with chest pain. *Am J Cardiol* 2000; 86:207–210.

173. Perticone F, Ceravolo R, Pujia A *et al*. Prognostic significance of endothelial dysfunction in hypertensive patients. *Circulation* 2001; 104:191–196.

174. Schachinger V, Britten MB, Zeiher AM. Prognostic impact of coronary vasodilator dysfunction on adverse long-term outcome of coronary heart disease. *Circulation* 2000; 101:1899–1906.

175. Schindler TH, Hornig B, Buser PT *et al*. Prognostic value of abnormal vasoreactivity of epicardial coronary arteries to sympathetic stimulation in patients with normal coronary angiograms. *Arterioscler Thromb Vasc Biol* 2003; 23:495–501.

176. Suwaidi JA, Hamasaki S, Higano ST, Nishimura RA, Holmes DR Jr, Lerman A. Long-term follow-up of patients with mild coronary artery disease and endothelial dysfunction. *Circulation* 2000; 101:948–954.

177. Targonski PV, Bonetti PO, Pumper GM, Higano ST, Holmes DR Jr, Lerman A. Coronary endothelial dysfunction is associated with an increased risk of cerebrovascular events. *Circulation* 2003; 107:2805–2809.

178. Verma S, Buchanan MR, Anderson TJ. Endothelial function testing as a biomarker of vascular disease. *Circulation* 2003; 108:2054–2059.

179. von Mering GO, Arant CB, Wessel TR *et al*. Abnormal coronary vasomotion as a prognostic indicator of cardiovascular events in women: results from the national heart, lung, and blood institute-sponsored Women's Ischemia Syndrome Evaluation (WISE). *Circulation* 2004; 109:722–725.

180. Blacher J, Asmar R, Djane S, London GM, Safar ME. Aortic pulse wave velocity as a marker of cardiovascular risk in hypertensive patients. *Hypertension* 1999; 33:1111–1117.
181. Boutouyrie P, Tropeano AI, Asmar R *et al*. Aortic stiffness is an independent predictor of primary coronary events in hypertensive patients: a Longitudinal Study. *Hypertension* 2002; 39:10–15.
182. London GM, Blacher J, Pannier B, Guerin AP, Marchais SJ, Safar ME. Arterial wave reflections and survival in end-stage renal failure. *Hypertension* 2001; 38:434–438.
183. Safar ME, Blacher J, Pannier B *et al*. Central pulse pressure and mortality in end-stage renal disease. *Hypertension* 2002; 39:735–738.
184. Stork S, van den Beld AW, von Schacky C *et al*. Carotid artery plaque burden, stiffness, and mortality risk in elderly men: A Prospective, Population-Based Cohort Study. *Circulation* 2004; 110:344–348.
185. Weber T, Auer J, O'Rourke MF *et al*. Arterial stiffness, wave reflections, and the risk of coronary artery disease. *Circulation* 2004; 109:184–189.
186. Weber T, Auer J, O'Rourke MF *et al*. Increased arterial wave reflections predict severe cardiovascular events in patients undergoing percutaneous coronary interventions. *Eur Heart J* 2005; 26:2657–2663.
187. Grey E, Bratteli C, Glasser SP *et al*. Reduced small artery but not large artery elasticity is an independent risk marker for cardiovascular events. *Am J Hypertens* 2003; 16:265–269.
188. Kaiser V, Kester ADM, Stoffers HEJH, Kitslaar PJEH, Knottnerus JA. The influence of experience on the reproducibility of the ankle-brachial systolic pressure ratio in peripheral arterial occlusive disease. *Eur J Vasc Endovasc Surg* 1999; 18:25–29.
189. Matzke S, Franckena M, Alback A, Railo M, Lepantalo M. Ankle brachial index measurements in critical leg ischaemia – the influence of experience on reproducibility. *Scand J Surg* 2003; 92:144–147.
190. Doobay AV, Anand SS. Sensitivity and specificity of the ankle-brachial index to predict future cardiovascular outcomes: a systematic review. *Arterioscler Thromb Vasc Biol* 2005; 25:1463–1469.
191. Resnick HE, Lindsay RS, McDermott MM *et al*. Relationship of high and low ankle brachial index to all-cause and cardiovascular disease mortality: the Strong Heart Study. *Circulation* 2004; 109:733–739.
192. Agodoa LY, Appel L, Bakris GL *et al*. Effect of Ramipril vs Amlodipine on renal outcomes in hypertensive nephrosclerosis: a Randomized Controlled Trial. *JAMA* 2001; 285:2719–2728.
193. Ballard DJ, Humphrey LL, Melton LJ *et al*. Epidemiology of persistent proteinuria in type II diabetes mellitus. Population-based study in Rochester, Minnesota. *Diabetes* 1988; 37:405–412.
194. Borch-Johnsen K, Feldt-Rasmussen B, Strandgaard S, Schroll M, Jensen JS. Urinary albumin excretion: an independent predictor of ischemic heart disease. *Arterioscler Thromb Vasc Biol* 1999; 19:1992–1997.
195. Miettinen H, Haffner SM, Lehto S, Ronnemaa T, Pyörälä K, Laakso M. Proteinuria predicts stroke and other atherosclerotic vascular disease events in nondiabetic and non-insulin-dependent diabetic subjects. *Stroke* 1996; 27:2033–2039.
196. Mogensen CE. Microalbuminuria predicts clinical proteinuria and early mortality in maturity-onset diabetes. *N Engl J Med* 1984; 310:356–360.
197. Neil A, Hawkins M, Potok M, Thorogood M, Cohen D, Mann J. A prospective population-based study of microalbuminuria as a predictor of mortality in NIDDM. *Diabetes Care* 1993; 16:996–1003.
198. Nelson RG, Pettitt DJ, Carraher MJ, Baird HR, Knowler WC. Effect of proteinuria on mortality in NIDDM. *Diabetes* 1988; 37:1499–1504.
199. Ärnlöv J, Evans JC, Meigs JB *et al*. Low-grade albuminuria and incidence of cardiovascular disease events in nonhypertensive and nondiabetic individuals: the Framingham Heart Study. *Circulation* 2005; 112:969–975.
200. Smith EB. Fibrinogen, fibrin and the arterial wall. *Eur Heart J* 1995; 16(suppl A):11–14.
201. Fibrinogen Studies Collaboration. Plasma fibrinogen level and the risk of major cardiovascular diseases and nonvascular mortality: an individual participant meta-analysis. *JAMA* 2005; 294:1799–1809.
202. Danesh J, Whincup P, Walker M *et al*. Fibrin D-dimer and coronary heart disease: Prospective study and meta-analysis. *Circulation* 2001; 103:2323–2327.
203. Whincup PH, Danesh J, Walker M *et al*. von Willebrand factor and coronary heart disease. Prospective study and meta-analysis. *Eur Heart J* 2002; 23:1764–1770.
204. Lowe GDO, Danesh J, Lewington S *et al*. Tissue plasminogen activator antigen and coronary heart disease: Prospective study and meta-analysis. *Eur Heart J* 2004; 25:252–259.
205. Smith *et al*. Which hemostatic markers add to the predictive value of conventional risk factors for coronary heart disease and ischaemic stroke? The Caerphilly Study. *Circulation* 2005; 112:3080–3087.
206. Scirica BM, Morrow DA. Troponins in acute coronary syndromes. *Prog Cardiovasc Dis* 2004; 47:177–188.

207. Heidenreich PA, Alloggiamento T, Melsop K, McDonald KM, Go AS, Hlatky MA. The prognostic value of troponin in patients with non-ST elevation acute coronary syndromes: A meta-analysis. *J Am Coll Cardiol* 2001; 38:478–485.

208. Peacock F, Morris DL, Anwaruddin S *et al*. Meta-analysis of ischemia-modified albumin to rule out acute coronary syndromes in the emergency department. *Am Heart J* 2006; 152:253–262.

209. Sinha MK, Gaze DC, Tippins JR, Collinson PO, Kaski JC. Ischemia modified albumin is a sensitive marker of myocardial ischemia after percutaneous coronary intervention. *Circulation* 2003; 107:2403–2405.

210. O'Donoghue M, de Lemos JA, Morrow DA *et al*. Prognostic utility of heart-type fatty acid binding protein in patients with acute coronary syndromes. *Circulation* 2006; 114:550–557.

211. McCord J, Nowak RM, Hudson MP *et al*. The prognostic significance of serial myoglobin, troponin I, and creatine kinase-MB measurements in patients evaluated in the emergency department for acute coronary syndrome. *Ann Emerg Med* 2003; 42:343–350.

212. Devereux RB, Alonso DR, Lutas EM *et al*. Echocardiographic assessment of left ventricular hypertrophy: comparison to necropsy findings. *Am J Cardiol* 1986; 57:450–458.

213. Palmieri V, Dahlof B, DeQuattro V *et al*. Reliability of echocardiographic assessment of left ventricular structure and function: the PRESERVE Study. *J Am Coll Cardiol* 1999; 34:1625–1632.

214. Wachtell K, Bella JN, Liebson PR *et al*. Impact of different partition values on prevalences of left ventricular hypertrophy and concentric geometry in a large hypertensive population: The LIFE Study. *Hypertension* 2000; 35:6–12.

215. Aronow BJ, Toyokawa T, Canning A *et al*. Divergent transcriptional responses to independent genetic causes of cardiac hypertrophy. *Physiol Genomics* 2001; 6:19–28.

216. Bikkina M, Levy D, Evans JC *et al*. Left ventricular mass and risk of stroke in an elderly cohort. The Framingham Heart Study. *JAMA* 1994; 272:33–36.

217. Kannel WB, Abbott RD. A prognostic comparison of asymptomatic left ventricular hypertrophy and unrecognized myocardial infarction: the Framingham Study. *Am Heart J* 1986; 111:391–397.

218. Koren MJ, Devereux RB, Casale PN, Savage DD, Laragh JH. Relation of left ventricular mass and geometry to morbidity and mortality in uncomplicated essential hypertension. *Ann Intern Med* 1991; 114:345–352.

219. Levy D, Garrison RJ, Savage DD, Kannel WB, Castelli WP. Prognostic implications of echocardiographically determined left ventricular mass in the Framingham Heart Study. *N Engl J Med* 1990; 322:1561–1566.

220. Schillaci G, Verdecchia P, Porcellati C, Cuccurullo O, Cosco C, Perticone F. Continuous relation between left ventricular mass and cardiovascular risk in essential hypertension. *Hypertension* 2000; 35:580–586.

221. Vakili BA, Okin PM, Devereux RB. Prognostic implications of left ventricular hypertrophy. *Am Heart J* 2001; 141:334–341.

222. Verdecchia P, Schillaci G, Borgioni C *et al*. Prognostic significance of serial changes in left ventricular mass in essential hypertension. *Circulation* 1998; 97:48–54.

223. Devereux RB, Wachtell K, Gerdts E *et al*. Prognostic significance of left ventricular mass change during treatment of hypertension. *JAMA* 2004; 292:2350–2356.

224. Mathew J, Sleight P, Lonn E *et al*. Reduction of cardiovascular risk by regression of electrocardiographic markers of left ventricular hypertrophy by the angiotensin-converting enzyme inhibitor ramipril. *Circulation* 2001; 104:1615–1621.

225. Okin PM, Devereux RB, Jern S *et al*. Regression of electrocardiographic left ventricular hypertrophy during antihypertensive treatment and the prediction of major cardiovascular events. *JAMA* 2004; 292:2343–2349.

226. Liao Y, Cooper RS, McGee DL, Mensah GA, Ghali JK. The relative effects of left ventricular hypertrophy, coronary artery disease, and ventricular dysfunction on survival among black adults. *JAMA* 1995; 273:1592–1597.

227. Quinones MA, Greenberg BH, Kopelen HA *et al*. Echocardiographic predictors of clinical outcome in patients with left ventricular dysfunction enrolled in the SOLVD registry and trials: significance of left ventricular hypertrophy. Studies of Left Ventricular Dysfunction. *J Am Coll Cardiol* 2000; 35:1237–1244.

228. Wang TJ, Evans JC, Benjamin EJ, Levy D, LeRoy EC, Vasan RS. Natural history of asymptomatic left ventricular systolic dysfunction in the community. *Circulation* 2003; 108:977–982.

229. Randomised, placebo-controlled trial of carvedilol in patients with congestive heart failure due to ischaemic heart disease. Australia/New Zealand Heart Failure Research Collaborative Group. *Lancet* 1997; 349:375–380.

230. Wachtell K, Bella JN, Rokkedal J et al. Change in diastolic left ventricular filling after one year of antihypertensive treatment: the Losartan Intervention For Endpoint Reduction in Hypertension (LIFE) Study. *Circulation* 2002; 105:1071–1076.

231. Ekelund LG, Suchindran CM, McMahon RP et al. Coronary heart disease morbidity and mortality in hypercholesterolemic men predicted from an exercise test: the Lipid Research Clinics Coronary Primary Prevention Trial. *J Am Coll Cardiol* 1989; 14:556–563.

232. Gibbons LW, Mitchell TL, Wei M, Blair SN, Cooper KH. Maximal exercise test as a predictor of risk for mortality from coronary heart disease in asymptomatic men. *Am J Cardiol* 2000; 86:53–58.

233. Rautaharju PM, Prineas RJ, Eifler WJ et al. Prognostic value of exercise electrocardiogram in men at high risk of future coronary heart disease: Multiple Risk Factor Intervention Trial experience. *J Am Coll Cardiol* 1986; 8:1–10.

234. Colhoun HM, McKeigue PM, Smith GD. Problems of reporting genetic associations with complex outcomes. *Lancet* 2003; 361:865–872.

235. Wacholder S, Chanock S, Garcia-Closas M, El Ghormli L, Rothman N. Assessing the probability that a positive report is false: an approach for Molecular Epidemiology Studies. *J Natl Cancer Inst* 2004; 96:434–442.

236. Gibbons GH, Liew CC, Goodarzi MO et al. Genetic markers: progress and potential for cardiovascular disease. *Circulation* 2004; 109(suppl 1):IV-47–58.

237. Davey SG, Ebrahim S. 'Mendelian randomization': can genetic epidemiology contribute to understanding environmental determinants of disease? *Int J Epidemiol* 2003; 32:1–22.

238. Keavney B, Danesh J, Parish S et al. Fibrinogen and coronary heart disease: test of causality by 'Mendelian randomization'. *Int J Epidemiol* 2006; 35:935–943.

239. Mannila MN, Eriksson P, Lundman P et al. Contribution of haplotypes across the fibrinogen gene cluster to variation in risk of myocardial infarction. *Thromb Haemost* 2005; 93:570–577.

240. Apple FS, Wu AHB, Mair J et al. Future biomarkers for detection of ischemia and risk stratification in acute coronary syndrome. *Clin Chem* 2005; 51:810–824.

241. Morrow DA, Braunwald E. Future of biomarkers in acute coronary syndromes: moving toward a multimarker strategy. *Circulation* 2003; 108:250–252.

242. Ravkilde J. Risk stratification of acute coronary syndrome patients. A multi-marker approach. *Scand J Clin Lab Invest Suppl* 2005; 240:25–29.

243. Current status of blood cholesterol measurement in clinical laboratories in the United States: a report from the Laboratory Standardization Panel of the National Cholesterol Education Program. *Clin Chem* 1988; 34:193–201.

244. Bachorik PS, Ross JW. National Cholesterol Education Program recommendations for measurement of low-density lipoprotein cholesterol: executive summary. The National Cholesterol Education Program Working Group on Lipoprotein Measurement. *Clin Chem* 1995; 41:1414–1420.

245. Stein EA, Myers GL. National Cholesterol Education Program recommendations for triglyceride measurement: executive summary. The National Cholesterol Education Program Working Group on Lipoprotein Measurement. *Clin Chem* 1995; 41:1421–1426.

246. Warnick GR, Wood PD. National Cholesterol Education Program recommendations for measurement of high-density lipoprotein cholesterol: executive summary. The National Cholesterol Education Program Working Group on Lipoprotein Measurement. *Clin Chem* 1995; 41:1427–1433.

247. Otvos JD, Jeyarajah EJ, Bennett DW, Krauss RM. Development of a proton nuclear magnetic resonance spectroscopic method for determining plasma lipoprotein concentrations and subspecies distributions from a single, rapid measurement. *Clin Chem* 1992; 38:1632–1638.

248. Marcovina SM, Albers JJ, Kennedy H, Mei JV, Henderson LO, Hannon WH. International Federation of Clinical Chemistry standardization project for measurements of apolipoproteins A-I and B. IV. Comparability of apolipoprotein B values by use of International Reference Material. *Clin Chem* 1994; 40:586–592.

249. Ballantyne CM, Andrews TC, Hsia JA, Kramer JH, Shear C. Correlation of non-high-density lipoprotein cholesterol with apolipoprotein B: effect of 5 hydroxymethylglutaryl coenzyme A reductase inhibitors on non-high-density lipoprotein cholesterol levels. *Am J Cardiol* 2001; 88:265–269.

250. Simes RJ, Marschner IC, Hunt D et al. Relationship between lipid levels and clinical outcomes in the Long-term Intervention with Pravastatin in Ischemic Disease (LIPID) trial: to what extent is the reduction in coronary events with pravastatin explained by on-study lipid levels? *Circulation* 2002; 105:1162–1169.

251. Mezdour H, Kora I, Parra HJ, Tartar A, Marcel YL, Fruchart JC. Two-site enzyme immunoassay of cholesteryl ester transfer protein with monoclonal and oligoclonal antibodies. *Clin Chem* 1994; 40:593–597.

252. Hoogeveen RC, Ballantyne CM. PLAC test for identification of individuals at increased risk for coronary heart disease. *Expert Rev Mol Diagn* 2005; 5:9–14.

253. Tsimihodimos V, Karabina SA, Tambaki AP *et al.* Atorvastatin preferentially reduces LDL-associated platelet-activating factor acetylhydrolase activity in dyslipidemias of type IIA and type IIB. *Arterioscler Thromb Vasc Biol* 2002; 22:306–311.

254. Schaefer EJ, McNamara JR, Asztalos BF *et al.* Effects of atorvastatin versus other statins on fasting and postprandial C-reactive protein and lipoprotein-associated phospholipase A2 in patients with coronary heart disease versus control subjects. *Am J Cardiol* 2005; 95:1025–1032.

255. Roberts WL. CDC/AHA workshop on markers of inflammation and cardiovascular disease: application to clinical and public health practice: laboratory tests available to assess inflammation – performance and standardization: a Background Paper. *Circulation* 2004; 110:e572–e576.

256. Gaines Das RE, Poole S. The international standard for interleukin-6. Evaluation in an International Collaborative Study. *J Immunol Methods* 1993; 160:147–153.

257. Poole S, Walker D, Gaines Das RE, Gallimore JR, Pepys MB. The first international standard for serum amyloid A protein (SAA). Evaluation in an International Collaborative Study. *J Immunol Methods* 1998; 214:1–10.

258. Halldorsdottir AM, Stoker J, Porche-Sorbet R, Eby CS. Soluble CD40 ligand measurement inaccuracies attributable to specimen type, processing time, and ELISA method. *Clin Chem* 2005; 51:1054–1057.

259. Kinlay S, Schwartz GG, Olsson AG *et al.* Effect of atorvastatin on risk of recurrent cardiovascular events after an acute coronary syndrome associated with high soluble CD40 ligand in the Myocardial Ischemia Reduction with Aggressive Cholesterol Lowering (MIRACL) Study. *Circulation* 2004; 110:386–391.

260. Sanguigni V, Pignatelli P, Lenti L *et al.* Short-term treatment with atorvastatin reduces platelet CD40 ligand and thrombin generation in hypercholesterolemic patients. *Circulation* 2005; 111:412–419.

261. Sealey JE, Gordon RD, Mantero F. Plasma renin and aldosterone measurements in low renin hypertensive states. *Trends Endocrinol Metab* 2005; 16:86–91.

262. Cohn JN, Anand IS, Latini R, Masson S, Chiang YT, Glazer R. Sustained reduction of aldosterone in response to the angiotensin receptor blocker valsartan in patients with chronic heart failure: results from the Valsartan Heart Failure Trial. *Circulation* 2003; 108:1306–1309.

263. Teerlink T. Measurement of asymmetric dimethylarginine in plasma: methodological considerations and clinical relevance. *Clin Chem Lab Med* 2005; 43:1130–1138.

264. Schwedhelm E, Tan-Andresen J, Maas R, Riederer U, Schulze F, Boger RH. Liquid chromatography-tandem mass spectrometry method for the analysis of asymmetric dimethylarginine in human plasma. *Clin Chem* 2005; 51:1268–1271.

265. Vishwanathan K, Tackett RL, Stewart JT, Bartlett MG. Determination of arginine and methylated arginines in human plasma by liquid chromatography-tandem mass spectrometry. *J Chrom Biomed Sci Appl* 2000; 748:157–166.

266. Lonn E. Use of carotid ultrasound to stratify risk. *Can J Cardiol* 2001; 17(suppl A):22A–25A.

267. Mancini GB. Carotid intima-media thickness as a measure of vascular target organ damage. *Curr Hypertens Rep* 2000; 2:71–77.

268. Mukherjee D, Yadav JS. Carotid artery intimal-medial thickness: indicator of atherosclerotic burden and response to risk factor modification. *Am Heart J* 2002; 144:753–759.

269. Modena MG, Bonetti L, Coppi F, Bursi F, Rossi R. Prognostic role of reversible endothelial dysfunction in hypertensive postmenopausal women. *J Am Coll Cardiol* 2002; 40:505–510.

270. Brinton BS, Cotter MD, Kailasam MBBS, Brown MD, Chio P. Development and validation of a noninvasive method to determine arterial pressure and vascular compliance. *Am J Cardiol* 1997; 80:323–330.

271. Karamanoglu M, Gallagher DE, Avolio AP, O'Rourke MF. Pressure wave propagation in a multibranched model of the human upper limb. *Am J Physiol Heart Circ Physiol* 1995; 269:H1363–H1369.

272. McVeigh GE, Bratteli CW, Morgan DJ *et al.* Age-related abnormalities in arterial compliance identified by pressure pulse contour analysis: aging and arterial compliance. *Hypertension* 1999; 33:1392–1398.

273. Mitchell GF, Lacourciere Y, Ouellet JP *et al.* Determinants of elevated pulse pressure in middle-aged and older subjects with uncomplicated systolic hypertension: the role of proximal aortic diameter and the aortic pressure-flow relationship. *Circulation* 2003; 108:1592–1598.

274. Schiffrin EL, Park JB, Intengan HD, Touyz RM. Correction of arterial structure and endothelial dysfunction in human essential hypertension by the angiotensin receptor antagonist losartan. *Circulation* 2000; 101:1653–1659.

275. Criqui MH, Langer RD, Fronek A *et al*. Mortality over a period of 10 years in patients with peripheral arterial disease. *N Engl J Med* 1992; 326:381–386.

276. National Kidney Foundation. K/DOQI clinical practice guidelines for chronic kidney disease: evaluation, classification, and stratification. *Am J Kidney Dis* 2002; 39(suppl 1):S1–S266.

277. Vasan RS. Biomarkers of cardiovascular disease: molecular basis and practical considerations. *Circulation* 2006; 113:2335–2362.

278. Whitton CM, Sands D, Hubbard AR, Gaffney PJ. A Collaborative Study to establish the 2nd International Standard for Fibrinogen, Plasma. *Thromb Haemost* 2000; 84:258–262.

279. Longstaff C, Whitton CM. A proposed reference method for plasminogen activators that enables calculation of enzyme activities in SI units. *J Thromb Haemost* 2004; 2:1416–1421.

280. Apple FS, Parvin CA, Buechler KF, Christenson RH, Wu AHB, Jaffe AS. Validation of the 99th percentile cutoff independent of assay imprecision (CV) for cardiac troponin monitoring for ruling out myocardial infarction. *Clin Chem* 2005; 51:2198–2200.

281. Panteghini M. Standardization of cardiac troponin I measurements: the way forward? *Clin Chem* 2005; 51:1594–1597.

282. Chan CP, Sum KW, Cheung KY *et al*. Development of a quantitative lateral-flow assay for rapid detection of fatty acid-binding protein. *J Immunol Methods* 2003; 279:91–100.

283. Balady GJ, Larson MG, Vasan RS, Leip EP, O'Donnell CJ, Levy D. Usefulness of exercise testing in the prediction of coronary disease risk among asymptomatic persons as a function of the Framingham risk score. *Circulation* 2004; 110:1920–1925.

284. Mora S, Redberg RF, Sharrett AR, Blumenthal RS. Enhanced risk assessment in asymptomatic individuals with exercise testing and Framingham risk scores. *Circulation* 2005; 112:1566–1572.

9

Risk in those with established disease

L. Wilhelmsen, H. Wedel

INTRODUCTION

It is established that patients who have suffered cardiovascular disease (CVD) such as a myocardial infarction (MI), angina pectoris (AP) or a stroke have often had risk factors such as elevated blood pressure, smoking, diabetes mellitus and, for MI at least, elevated blood cholesterol levels, just to mention some of the most important. When these persons suffer an event and become patients, this event carries with it another set of important predictors for future outcome. The above-mentioned cardiovascular diseases are generally regarded as different manifestations of an underlying atherothrombotic process and the general understanding is that risk factors enhance this process. There are similarities between the manifestations, but recently certain differences have also been pointed out [1]. The underlying athero-thrombotic lesion is a chronic, continuing process and the predisposing risk factors are thought of as continuing to act as promoters of the process. If so, the risk factors should continue to be of importance after established disease as well. However, the new predictors that occur as a consequence of the disease event may take over as more important for the immediate prognosis and it may be difficult to see the association with the original 'pre-disease' risk factors. Long-term follow-up is often needed to establish the prognostic factors of importance. One example is that female sex has been regarded as protective against MI and sudden coronary death, but when a woman has suffered an MI this protection seems to be lost; her prognosis is no better than that of a man. Treatment of patients with established cardiovascular diseases aims to lower the risk factor burden, though it may be difficult to assess the importance of such factors during follow-up. Older studies may therefore be better aimed at analysing such associations. Furthermore, diagnostics have changed; events that were earlier diagnosed as MI are nowadays often named acute coronary syndromes, because diagnostic criteria for MI may not have been fulfilled due to early interventions. Thus, prognosis in a person who has had a clinical atherothrombotic event will depend upon a complex interplay between preceding risk factors, variations over time in the natural history of the disease, the impact of the event itself and the effect of subsequent interventions. Advances in diagnostic tests with consequent changes in diagnostic criteria add to the difficulties in isolating key prognostic markers. Nevertheless, a plethora of randomized controlled trials have isolated major interventions that determine prognosis.

In the following, we analyse factors of importance for follow-up after an MI, AP, coronary surgery and a stroke, which are attached manifestations for which relatively good predictions are available.

Lars Wilhelmsen, MD, PhD, Professor, Cardiovascular Institute, Göteborg University Göteborg, Sweden

Hans Wedel, PhD, Professor of Epidemiology and Biostatistics, Nordic School of Public Health, Göteborg, Sweden

RISK FACTORS FOR RECURRENCE OR DEATH AFTER A MYOCARDIAL INFARCTION

Immediate prognosis after MI is determined by age and the size of the infarct and consequent complications. This effect wanes over several years and the impact of conventional risk factors becomes more apparent. Women appear to have a worse prognosis than men, at least in part because of a higher prevalance of diabetes and other complicating factors [2, 3]. The impact of factors associated with the index MI will be considered first.

FACTORS ASSOCIATED WITH THE INDEX INFARCTION THAT DETERMINE SUBSEQUENT PROGNOSIS

It has been known for a long time that the *size of the index MI*, the *number of previous MIs*, as well as the presence of *ventricular arrhythmias*, are serious prognostic factors after an MI [4]. Refined methods to measure the extent of myocardial damage have proved that this is also an important predictor. The number and severity of coronary occlusions are important and this has led to the increased use of acute percutaneous revascularization procedures. Thus, Cantor *et al.* [5] recently reported from a series of 8286 patients with acute coronary syndromes on in-hospital cardiac catheterization (performed in 44% of patients) with following interventions if necessary. They found significantly lower mortality associated with interventions in high-risk patients, but no effect in low-risk patients.

Pre-discharge exercise testing of MI patients was performed in a Danish study [6] of patients with ST-elevation who were randomized to primary angioplasty or fibrinolysis. Exercise testing was performed in 1164 out of 1462 patients discharged alive. Multivariable predictors of death or re-infarction were: age, gender, diabetes, previous stroke, anterior MI, randomization to fibrinolysis and exercise capacity.

Several prospective studies indicate the adverse outcome among patients with signs of more extensive coronary artery disease. Thus, patients with AP both before and after their MI [7, 8] have a worse outcome than those without such symptoms, and the extent of vascular lesions at coronary angiography is prognostically important. It is logical, therefore, to improve the blood flow in an attempt to improve outcome.

Hellermann *et al.* [9] analysed the outcome in 1915 MI patients without a prior history of heart failure. Four to five years after the MI, 41% had suffered heart failure and only 45% of the heart failure patients were alive.

Magnetic resonance imaging was used by Hombach *et al.* [10] in 110 MI patients. During follow-up there were only 16 events and among them 7 deaths, but multivariable analysis revealed high left ventricular end-diastolic volume, low ejection fraction, and persistent microvascular obstruction to be significant predictors for outcome.

There are few if any therapeutic possibilities to heal the damaged myocardium with resulting cardiac failure. However, improved cardiac function and amelioration of heart failure has been followed by improved prognosis [11, 12].

Drug trials of arrhythmia suppression have not demonstrated any therapeutic benefit [13].

It has been questioned whether risk factors determined in the pre-vascularization era are still of importance in patients who have undergone such procedures. A recent study [14] conducted with MI patients, 70% of whom underwent coronary revascularization, showed that Holter monitoring conveyed significant information on prognosis in multivariable analysis. Age, diabetes and ejection fraction, as well as reduced post-ectopic turbulence and non-sustained ventricular tachycardia, were predictive, but these associations were only seen in patients with ejection fraction >35%.

It can be argued that the underlying atherothrombotic vascular process will continue after the intervention, and that action to reduce risk factors therefore ought to be useful.

IMPORTANCE OF PRIMARY RISK FACTORS AFTER A MYOCARDIAL INFARCTION

Blood lipids

Elevated total or low-density cholesterol are well-known to increase the risk of an MI in many populations and this factor has also been prognostically negative after an MI [15–17]. In the latter study, there was a relatively higher number of patients who had suffered their MI more than 5 years ago compared to several other studies, which might have influenced the risk associations. Interestingly, it was found that total serum cholesterol was a significant predictor in multivariable analysis and was better than low-density lipoprotein (LDL) cholesterol, and that high-density lipoprotein (HDL) cholesterol (of borderline significance in bi-variable analysis) did not improve prediction in men in the placebo group of the study. Serum triglycerides were significant predictors of outcome in bi-variable analysis, but not in multivariable analysis. The beta-coefficient for serum cholesterol was 0.168, corresponding to an approximately 17% increase in risk for 1 mmol/l increase in serum cholesterol, which is similar to the beta-coefficients reported in other prospective studies of post-MI studies [15, 16], but smaller than those reported in prospective studies in clinical healthy populations [18]. The post-MI trials showed an important reduction of mortality and recurrences with treatment with a lipid-lowering statin [19], which strengthens the importance of serum cholesterol as a significant factor in the process leading up to an MI and the progress after an MI.

Elevated blood pressure

All studies that have analysed the prognostic importance of elevated blood pressure – hypertension – have found it to be independently associated with increased risk of recurrence and death [7, 16, 20, 21]. In the previously discussed Scandinavian Simvastatin Survival Study (4S) trial [17] it was a significant predictor of outcome in both the placebo and the simvastatin groups. It is important to notice that it is a history of hypertension known before the index MI that influences prognosis rather than the blood pressure level measured immediately after the MI. Blood pressure falls with an MI and the amount of decline in blood pressure is related to infarct size and prognosis [22]. Furthermore, even treated blood pressure elevation has been related to deteriorated prognosis [7]. So far no specific blood pressure-lowering drug has been superior to others, but drugs that have been valuable after MI for other reasons than their blood pressure-lowering effect, such as beta-blockers and angiotensin-converting enzyme (ACE) inhibitors, are generally recommended.

C-reactive protein

C-reactive protein (CRP) has attracted great interest during recent years as an independent risk factor for a first MI, and recently it was also shown to be related to outcome after acute coronary syndromes in 3745 patients [23]. The findings were independent of the LDL cholesterol levels, and the authors conclude that CRP levels ought to be monitored after MI.

Similar results were reported from the Fragmin and fast Revascularisation during Instability in Coronary artery disease (FRISC) study [24], in which 2 457 patients with unstable coronary artery disease were randomized to an invasive or a non-invasive strategy. In the group who were not subjected to an invasive strategy it was found that age >70 years, male sex, diabetes, previous MI, ST-depression and increased concentrations of troponins and markers of inflammation (interleukin 6 or CRP) independently increased the risk for death or MI during one year's follow-up. So far no study has shown any effect of improvement of normalization of CRP levels.

Endothelial dysfunction

Another recently discussed factor of importance for a first MI as well as recurrence is endothelial dysfunction [25]. These authors found in 198 patients with acute coronary syndromes that disturbed endothelial function was a significant predictor of cardiovascular events during 47.7 ± 15.1 months among the 31 patients who had recurrent events. Furthermore, recovery of endothelial function was associated with longer event-free survival.

Diabetes mellitus

In the studies referred to above [16, 17] diabetes has often been significantly involved in the multivariable analyses.

The previously mentioned study [16] showed that diabetes mellitus, as well as increased blood glucose levels, carries independent negative prognostic information after an MI, and that was true also in the group treated with simvastatin, but only in the placebo group of the 4S trial [17].

The importance of diabetes is shown in several older studies [26, 27]. The negative effect of diabetes is seen both during the acute, hospital phase and during long-term follow-up.

Franklin et al. [28] analysed a patient register with 5403 MI patients with ST-elevation MI and 4725 with non-ST-elevation, and found that about 25% of patients had diabetes, and that they were more often older women with a greater prevalence of comorbidities. The diabetic patients in general had higher hospital mortality.

These results are very similar to those reported by Casella et al. [29] from Italy, as well as in the Atherosclerosis Risk in Communities (ARIC) study [30] with 3242 hospitalized MI patients with diabetes and 9826 non-diabetic patients.

It has also been recently reported from Sweden that glucose intolerance detected during hospitalization for an MI among 168 patients not known to have diabetes is associated with increased risk during 34 months' follow-up [31].

In a Danish study [32] 494 MI patients were followed for 6–8 years and it was found that high plasma insulin levels increased risk for all-cause mortality in multivariable analysis.

In this context it is of interest too that the metabolic syndrome has also been associated with increased risk of heart failure after MI [33], as well as death and cardiovascular events [34].

Prognosis after an MI is definitely worse when diabetes control is not good, but so far there is no proof that better antidiabetic treatment may improve prognosis [35, 36].

Homocysteine

Homocysteine has been an independent risk factor for various cardiovascular events, and was shown to be significantly related to outcome after an MI and angiographically documented coronary artery disease in a Norwegian study [37]. Trials to analyse whether lowering of the levels also improves prognosis are being carried out.

Tobacco smoking

Tobacco smoking is a well-known risk factor for MI. When analysing the importance of smoking after an MI it is important to keep in mind the process whereby patients have suffered their MI. Non-smokers who suffer an MI have as a group had higher levels of other risk factors than smokers. This selection is important because any comparison of the effect of smoking habits has to be between those who continue and those who stop smoking after an MI. The effect of stopping smoking was not related to the amount smoked before the MI [38]. Different studies, most of them performed long ago, have found a significantly better prognosis among both male and female post-MI patients who stopped smoking compared to continuing smokers [38–46]. The mortality reduction varied between 38% and 70%, and the reduction in rate of non-fatal recurrences has been of at least the same magnitude. In a later multivariable analysis, Greenwood et al. [47] found that stopping smoking was significantly related to prognosis regarding mortality in addition to diabetes, AP and treatment with anti-arrhythmics. Those findings are similar to the result of the previously mentioned multivariable analysis [17]. The mechanism through which smoking increases risk of MI has not been elucidated completely. There were, however, some interesting observations by Grines *et al.* [48] in a study of outcome after thrombolytic therapy for MI. Smokers had less extensive coronary disease with larger diameter of the normal reference segment of the - coronary arteries, and lesser prevalence of three-vessel disease, and the authors conclude that smokers seem to have a relatively hypercoagulable state and that the mechanism of the MI could be a spasm or thrombosis of a less critically atherosclerotic lesion than for non-smokers. This is also compatible with the relatively rapid effect of stopping smoking on risk both of a first MI and a recurrence.

Psychosocial factors

Most studies on psychosocial factors have been rather short – often with only 1–1½ years' follow-up. A relatively recent review by Hemingway and Marmot [49] considered all factors that had been related to risk of a first MI as well as prognosis after an MI. Prognosis was related to depression, anxiety and lack of social support, but not to type A personality pattern.

In a 10-year follow-up study of 230 men and 45 women with MI [50], it was studied whether prognosis was related to psychological stress, lack of social support, anxiety and a tendency to be depressed, as well as marital status, education, extra work, mental strain at work, mental strain in the marriage, dissatisfaction with family life, problems with children, dissatisfaction with financial situation, life events, irritability, type A behaviour and also sleep problems. All-cause mortality was significantly related to left ventricular failure, ventricular dysrhythmias, and high depression scores with borderline significance for low social support, but not to any of the other variables mentioned above. Prognosis regarding non-fatal MI recurrences was not related to any of these psychosocial variables.

van Melle *et al.* [51] reported from a study of 1989 MI patients that there was a significant relation between depression and left ventricular function, but they did not report on short- or long-term prognosis of their patients, and consequently not on the independent prognosis of these two variables.

Mookadam and Arthur [52] reported in a review that low social support network could be a common determinant of 1-year mortality after MI, and was equivalent to several of the classical risk factors.

Taylor *et al.* [53] studied 2481 depressed and/or socially isolated MI patients during a mean of 29 months in relation to use of antidepressants. The risk of death or recurrent MI was significantly lower among patients taking selective serotonin reuptake inhibitors compared to those not taking such drugs. It should be emphasized that this was not a randomized trial.

Genetic determinants

Few studies on the effect of genetic determinants on prognosis after MI have been performed, but Liu *et al.* [54] reported that stromelysin-1 promoter 5A/6A polymorphism is an independent prognostic factor and interacts with smoking cessation after MI in 162 patients aged 27–45 years followed for 4.43 years.

MULTIVARIATE ANALYSES OF FACTORS COLLECTED BEFORE MYOCARDIAL INFARCTION

In a still not published study of risk factors for the prognosis after a non-fatal MI performed in the Primary Prevention Study in Göteborg, data were available for all factors included in a multivariable analysis from 1154 surviving MI patients. Baseline age, presence of diabetes mellitus, high systolic blood pressure and smoking were all significant, but not family history, low physical activity, psychological stress, social class, body mass index or serum cholesterol.

RISK FACTORS FOR MYOCARDIAL INFARCTION OR DEATH AFTER DIAGNOSIS OF ANGINA PECTORIS

Compared to the extensive studies of prognostic factors after an MI there are relatively few reports of prognostic factors after AP. Beginning with the Framingham and other prospective population studies, the prognosis relating to some clinical data was published [55–57]. High blood pressure, cardiac enlargement, pathological electrocardiograph (ECG) findings, as well as a complicating MI, increased the risk of a fatal outcome. The introduction of coronary angiography and ventriculography made it possible to relate prognosis to number of diseased vessels and left ventricular function. Thus, it has been shown that the number of coronary vessels involved, with three-vessel disease and left main disease, carries the worst prognosis during 15 years' follow-up [58]. Severity of AP symptoms predicted prognosis during the first 2 years, but not thereafter, in the Veterans Administration Study [59].

Prognosis in relation to baseline factors was studied in a random population sample of men aged 47–55 years at baseline in Göteborg, Sweden [60, 61]. It was found that during 16 years' follow-up, survival was 72% among men without coronary disease at baseline, 53% among men with AP uncomplicated with MI, and 34% among men with MI at baseline. Elevated serum cholesterol (relative risk [RR] per mmol/l 1.34 [1.13–1.23]), systolic blood pressure (RR per 10 mmHg 1.13 [1.02–1.25]), tobacco smoking (RR 1.74 [1.09–2.78]), as well as diabetes (RR 2.63 [1.45–4.77]), were all independently related to deteriorated prognosis.

Thus, these findings show a very similar risk factor pattern as seen for an MI.

In a recent report, a risk score for predicting death, MI and stroke in patients with AP has been constructed [62]. Among 7311 patients it was found that during 4.9 years the following factors independently predicted adverse prognosis in order of decreasing contribution: age, left ventricular ejection fraction, smoking, white blood cell count, diabetes, casual blood glucose concentration, creatinine concentration, previous stroke, at least one angina attack per week, coronary angiographic findings, lipid-lowering treatment, QT interval, systolic blood pressure ≥155 mmHg, number of drugs used for angina, previous MI, and sex.

PROGNOSTIC FACTORS AFTER CORONARY SURGERY

Coronary artery by-pass surgery (CABG) or percutaneous coronary interventions (PCI) have a beneficial impact on the prognosis of these patients [63], but relatively few reports have analysed the combined effect of common cardiovascular risk factors as well as myocardial and coronary artery anatomy on prognosis. In the Post-Coronary Artery Bypass Graft study [64], it was found that maximum stenosis of the graft at coronary angiography immediately after the operation, small minimum graft diameter, male sex, prior MI, high triglyceride levels, low HDL cholesterol level, high LDL cholesterol level, high blood pressure and tobacco smoking were predictors of atherosclerosis progression. Similar factors with the addition of diabetes mellitus have also been associated with long-term prognosis after surgery [65–67]. In accordance with the studies after an MI it was found that smoking patients who stopped after the operation had a significantly better prognosis than those who continued [68, 69].

RISK FACTORS AMONG MEN WITH 'NON-SPECIFIC' CHEST PAIN

In the previously discussed population study [60], all men with chest pain at the second screening examination 4 years after the baseline examination were further examined by a single experienced physician and the examination was supplemented with exercise testing and coronary angiography (in a few men) if deemed necessary [70]. Four groups were formed: (1) no chest pain; (2) chest pain according to the general questionnaire, but not typical AP according to the detailed examination: 'non-specific chest pain'; (3) typical AP; (4) men who had suffered an MI. There were 441 men in group 2 and it was found that their cardiovascular mortality was twice that of men without any chest pain and only marginally less than in men with typical AP. Serum cholesterol, systolic blood pressure, diabetes and smoking were significant predictors of outcome in multivariable analysis, both with respect to fatal coronary disease and total mortality during the 16-year follow-up period. Thus, 'non-specific' chest pain ought to be taken seriously among people (at least men), especially with elevated coronary risk factors.

RISK FACTORS FOR RECURRENCE OR DEATH AFTER A STROKE

There is a remarkable difference in the number of risk factors known for coronary disease and the limited number found for stroke, and there is also rather little known about prognostic factors after a stroke or transitory ischaemic attacks (TIA). As previously stated, there are differences in incidence, case fatality and risk factors between stroke and coronary disease [1], but the prognosis of stroke is influenced by presence of signs of atherothrombosis and coronary disease. In conformity with the discussion on prognosis after MI, we will first analyse the importance of factors associated with the underlying atherothrombotic disease and the index stroke.

FACTORS ASSOCIATED WITH THE INDEX STROKE AND SIGNS OF ATHEROTHROMBOSIS

A German register study of 13 400 ischaemic stroke patients [71] found that in both men and women, older age, the severity of the index stroke and atrial fibrillation were associated with higher in-hospital mortality. In addition, in men, previous stroke and diabetes mellitus were important.

Hankey [72] reported from Australia that 1–5 years after a stroke, increasing age, a history of previous CVD and cardiovascular risk factors are predictors of adverse prognosis.

Similarly, in a Japanese study, Yokota et al. [73] found that a history of TIA, atrial fibrillation, ischaemic heart disease and disability at discharge were independent predictors for recurrence and death 3 years after a first-ever stroke.

In a smaller Spanish study, of 240 patients with ischaemic stroke, Varona et al. [74] during a mean follow-up of 12.3 years found that age over 35 years, male gender, presence of cardiovascular risk factors and atherosclerosis of large arteries were predictors of negative outcome.

Hypertension
Hypertension is the strongest risk factor for a first stroke.

In a study of 30 days' prognosis, Okumura et al. [75] found that in 1004 cases of brain infarction there was a U-shaped relationship between blood pressure and prognosis with a nadir at systolic blood pressure of 150–169 mmHg and at diastolic of 100–110 mmHg. In subjects with previous hypertension, the relationship between prognosis and systolic blood pressure shifted to higher pressures by about 10 mmHg. In 1097 cases with haemorrhage the relationship between blood pressure and mortality showed a J-shape in systolic pressure, and a U-shape in diastolic pressure.

We have earlier in this summary presented data from follow-up of a random population study of men who suffered MI during follow-up. In the same study, 575 men with complete data survived a stroke for 28 days, and their fate during up to 28 years from the basal examination at age 47–55 years was investigated. Only age and high systolic blood pressure (treated or untreated) were prognostic factors during follow-up. It is of interest that neither diabetes nor smoking habits were predictive as was seen among MI patients. However, in comparison with other studies regarding prognosis in stroke, in which diabetes has been found to be strongly predictive of outcome, diabetes status was not re-assessed during follow-up in this study.

Diabetes mellitus

The effect of diabetes was studied in 6105 patients with stroke or TIA among whom 761 had diabetes [76]. They found that diabetes increased the risk of recurrent stroke by 35%, and found that blood pressure reduction with the antihypertensive agent perindopril reduced recurrence as much in diabetes patients as in those without diabetes.

A Finnish register study [77] found that diabetes, which was present in 25% of patients, was a significant ($P = 0.020$) predictor of death during 4 weeks after onset of ischaemic stroke in 4390 patients.

A 10-year follow-up of patients after minor stroke or TIA in 2447 patients was reported by van Wijk et al. [78] who documented that risk factors for worse prognosis were a history of claudication, previous vascular surgery and pathological Q-waves on the baseline electrocardiogram, as well as diabetes (RR 2.10 [1.79–2.48]).

Serum cholesterol

There is an interesting difference between prospective epidemiological studies, which in general showed no association between stroke incidence and total cholesterol levels [79], whereas statin therapy reduced stroke incidence by about 17% for all stroke types taken together. There was no effect on haemorrhagic strokes [19].

Tobacco smoking

The risk of a first stroke is significantly higher among tobacco smokers as well as among subjects with high blood fibrinogen levels. Continued smoking has been associated with adverse prognosis after a stroke [72], and it is generally agreed that stroke patients should stop smoking.

Inflammatory markers

Grau et al. [80] investigated whether inflammatory makers, which predict a first stroke event, are also involved in a recurrent event, in the Clopidogoel versus Aspirin in Patients at risk of Ischaemic Events (CAPRIE) trial with 18 556 patients. They found that, compared with the quartile with the lowest leukocyte count at baseline, patients in the top quartile had higher risk for ischaemic stroke (RR 1.30; $P = 0.007$), MI (RR 1.56; $P < 0.001$), and vascular death (RR 1.51; $P < 0.001$). A summary statement on CRP was published in 2005 [81].

Homocysteine

Bos et al. [82] found that high homocysteine levels were associated with recurrent vascular events in 161 young patients aged 18–45 years with cerebral infarction or TIA.

Hormone replacement therapy

Bath and Gray [83] analysed 28 trials with 39 769 subjects and the effect of hormone replacement therapy on total stroke, and found that those who took such therapy had a worse outcome.

MANAGEMENT OF RISK FACTORS

Patients with established CVD are already at high risk. Patients usually want to receive as much information as possible from physicians, and often prefer to receive assistance from them in order to change behaviours such as smoking, nutrition and diet, and physical activity, rather than attend special programmes elsewhere.

A friendly and positive physician–patient interaction is a powerful tool to enhance a patient's ability to cope with stress and illness and to adhere to the recommended lifestyle change(s) and medication.

A crucial step in changing negative experiences to positive ones is to set realistic goals and goal-setting, combined with self-monitoring of the chosen behaviour, are the main tools for achieving a positive outcome. This in turn will increase self-efficacy for the chosen behaviour, and thereafter new goals should be set. Moving forward in small, consecutive steps is one of the key means of achieving long-term behavioural change.

Lifestyle recommendations [84]

- No smoking;
- Weight reduction: body mass index of less than $25 \, kg/m^2$ to avoid central obesity;
- 30 minutes of moderately vigorous exercise on most days of the week: exercise and weight reduction can prevent diabetes;
- Healthy diet.

Rigorous blood pressure and lipid control is desirable in the highest risk patients, particularly those with *'established atherosclerotic CVD'*:

- Blood pressure <130/80 mmHg;
- Total cholesterol <4.5 mmol/l (≈175 mg/dl), with an option of <4 mmol/l (≈155 mg/dl) if feasible;
- LDL cholesterol <2.5 mmol/l (≈100 mg/dl), with an option of <2.0 mmol/l (≈80 mg/dl) if feasible.

Drug treatment

- In patients with CVD: aspirin, statins for most;
- In patients with diabetes: consider glucose-lowering drugs. Fasting blood glucose <6 mmol/l (≈110 mg/dl) and HbA1c <6.5% if feasible.

SUMMARY

In addition to factors associated with the index MI, such as signs of a large MI and ventricular arrhythmias, risk factors for a recurrent MI or death are similar to conventional primary coronary risk factors such as high lipid levels, diabetes and disturbed glucose metabolism, hypertension and smoking, as well as elevated CRP, disturbed endothelial function and psychosocial factors such as depression and social isolation.

A similar risk factor pattern is seen for patients with AP, as well in patients with chest pain not regarded as classical angina pectoris. The prognostic factors after coronary bypass or percutaneous interventions also seem to be the same.

Prognostic factors after a stroke and TIA include factors associated with the index event as well as atrial fibrillation, coronary disease, hypertension, diabetes, inflammatory markers and high homocysteine levels, smoking and hormone replacement therapy.

REFERENCES

1.   Wilhelmsen L, Köster M, Harmsen P, Lappas G. Differences between coronary disease and stroke in incidence, case fatality, and risk factors, but few differences in risk factors for fatal and non-fatal events. *Eur Heart J* 2005; 18:1916–1922.
2.   Johansson S, Bergstrand R, Ulvenstam G *et al*. Sex differences in preinfarction characteristics and long-term survival among patients with myocardial infarction. *Am J Epidemiol* 1984; 119:610–623.
3.   Theres H, Maier B, Matteucci Gothe R *et al*. Influence of gender on treatment and short-term mortality of patients with acute myocardial infarction in Berlin. *Z Kardiol* 2004; 93:954–963.

4. Peterson ED, Shaw LJ, Califf RM. Risk stratification after myocardial infarction. *Ann Intern Med* 1997; 126:561–582.
5. Cantor WJ, Goodman SG, Cannon CP *et al*. Early cardiac catheterisation is associated with lower mortality only among high-risk patients with ST- and non-ST-elevation acute coronary syndromes: observation from the OPUS-TIMI 16 trial. *Am Heart J* 2005; 149:275–283.
6. Valeur N, Clemmensen P, Saunamäki K *et al*. The prognostic value of pre-discharge exercise testing after myocardial infarction treated with either primary PCI or fibrinolysis: a DANAMI-2 sub-study. *Eur Heart J* 2005; 26:119–127.
7. Ulvenstam G, Åberg A, Pennert K *et al*. Recurrent myocardial infarction. 2. Possibilities of prediction. *Eur Heart J* 1985; 6:303–311.
8. Haider AW, Davies GJ. Preinfarction angina as a major predictor of left ventricular function and long-term prognosis after a first Q wave myocardial infarction. *J Am Coll Cardiol* 1996; 27:954–955.
9. Hellermann JP, Jacobsen SJ, Redfield MM *et al*. Heart failure after myocardial infarction: clinical presentation and survival. *Eur J Heart Fail* 2005; 7:119–125.
10. Hombach V, Grebe O, Merkle N *et al*. Sequelae of acute myocardial infarction regarding cardiac structure and function and their prognostic significance as assessed by magnetic resonance imaging. *Eur Heart J* 2005; 26:549–557.
11. Goldstein S, Fagerberg B, Hjalmarson Å *et al*. Metoprolol controlled release/extended release in patients with severe heart failure: analysis of the experience in the MERIT-HF study. *J Am Coll Cardiol* 2001; 38:932–938.
12. Packer M, Coats AJ, Fowler MB *et al*. Effect of Carvedilol on survival in severe chronic heart failure. *N Engl J Med* 2001; 344:1651–1658.
13. The Cardiac Arrhythmia Suppression Trial (CAST) Investigators. Preliminary report: effect of encainide and flecainide on mortality in a randomised trial of arrhythmia suppression after myocardial infarction. *N Engl J Med* 1989; 321:406–412.
14. Makikallio TH, Barthel P, Schneider R *et al*. Prediction of sudden cardiac death after acute myocardial infarction: role of Holter monitoring in the modern treatment era. *Eur Heart J* 2005; 26:762–769.
15. Ulvenstam G, Bergstrand R, Johansson S *et al*. Prognostic importance of cholesterol levels after myocardial infarction. *Prev Med* 1984; 13:355–366.
16. Wong ND, Cupples LA, Ostfeld AM *et al*. Risk factors for long-term coronary prognosis after initial myocardial infarction: the Framingham Study. *Am J Epidemiol* 1989; 130:469–480.
17. Wilhelmsen L, Pyörälä K, Wedel H *et al*. Risk factors for a major coronary event after myocardial infarction in the Scandinavian Simvastatin Survival Study (4S). *Eur Heart J* 2001; 22:1119–1127.
18. Dobson AJ, Evans A, Ferrario M *et al*, The WHO MONICA Project. Changes in estimated coronary risk in the 1980s: data from 38 populations in the WHO MONICA Project. *Ann Med* 1998; 30:199–205.
19. Cholesterol Treatment Trialists (CTT) Collaborators. Efficacy and safety of cholesterol-lowering treatment: prospective meta-analysis of data from 90,056 participants in 14 randomised trials of statins. *Lancet* 2005; 366:1267–1278.
20. Herlitz J, Bang A, Karlsson BW. Five-year prognosis after acute myocardial infarction in relation to history of hypertension. *Am J Hypertens* 1996; 9:70–76.
21. Gustafsson F, Köber L, Torp-Pedersen C *et al*. On behalf of the TRACE study group. Long-term prognosis after acute myocardial infarction in patients with a history of arterial hypertension. *Eur Heart J* 1998; 19:588–594.
22. McCall M, Elmfeldt D, Vedin A *et al*. Influence of a myocardial infarction on blood pressure and serum cholesterol. *Acta Med Scand* 1979; 206:477–481.
23. Ridker PM, Cannon CP, Morrow D *et al*. C-reactive protein levels and outcomes after statin therapy. *N Engl J Med* 2005; 352:20–28.
24. Lagerqvist B, Diderholm E, Lindahl B *et al*. FRISC score for selection of patients for an early invasive treatment strategy in unstable coronary artery disease. *Heart* 2005; 91:1047–1052.
25. Fichtlscherer S, Breuer S, Zeiher AM. Prognostic value of systemic endothelial dysfunction in patients with acute coronary syndromes: further evidence for the existence of the 'vulnerable' patient. *Circulation* 2004; 110:1926–1932.
26. Ulvenstam G, Åberg A, Bergstrand R *et al*. Long-term prognosis after myocardial infarction in men with diabetes. *Diabetes* 1985; 34:787–792.
27. Behar S, Boyko V, Reicher-Reiss H *et al*. Ten-year survival after acute myocardial infarction: comparison of patients with and without diabetes. SPRINT Study Group, Secondary Prevention Reinfarction Israeli Nifedipine Trial. *Am Heart J* 1997; 133:290–296.

28. Franklin K, Goldberg RJ, Spencer F et al. Implications of diabetes in patients with acute coronary syndromes. The Global Registry of Acute Coronary Events. Arch Intern Med 2004; 164:1457–1463.

29. Casella G, Savonitto S, Chiarella F et al. Clinical characteristics and outcome of diabetic patients with acute myocardial infarction. Data from the BLITZ-1 study. Ital Heart J 2005; 6:374–383.

30. Weitzman S, Wang C, Rosamond WD et al. Is diabetes an independent risk factor for mortality after myocardial infarction? The ARIC (Atherosclerosis Risk in Communities) Surveillance Study. Acta Diabetol 2004; 41:77–83.

31. Bartnik M, Malmberg K, Norhammar A et al. Newly detected abnormal glucose tolerance: an important predictor of long-term outcome after myocardial infarction. Eur Heart J 2004; 25:1990–1997.

32. Kragelund C, Snorgaard O, Kober L et al. Hyperinsulinaemia is associated with increased long-term mortality following acute myocardial infarction in non-diabetic patients. Eur Heart J 2004; 25:1891–1897.

33. Zeller M, Steg PG, Ravisy J et al. Prevalence and impact of metabolic syndrome on hospital outcomes in acute myocardial infarction. Arch Intern Med 2005; 165:1192–1198.

34. Levantesi G, Macchia A, Marfisi R et al. Metabolic syndrome and risk of cardiovascular events after myocardial infarction. J Am Coll Cardiol 2005; 46:277–283.

35. Malmberg K, Norhammar A, Wedel H et al. Glycometabolic state at admission: important risk marker of mortality in conventionally treated patients with diabetes mellitus and acute myocardial infarction: long-term results from the Diabetes and Insulin-Glucose Infusion in Acute Myocardial Infarction (DIGAMI) study. Circulation 1999; 99:2626–2632.

36. Malmberg K, Ryden L, Wedel H et al. Intense metabolic control by means of insulin in patients with diabetes mellitus and acute myocardial infarction (DIGAMI 2): effects on mortality and morbidity. Eur Heart J 2005; 26:650–661.

37. Nygård O, Nordrehaug JE, Refsum H et al. Plasma homocysteine levels and mortality in patients with coronary artery disease. N Engl J Med 1997; 337:230–236.

38. Åberg A, Bergstrand R, Johansson S et al. Cessation of smoking after myocardial infarction. Effects on mortality after 10 years. Br Heart J 1983; 49:416–422.

39. Wilhelmsson C, Vedin JA, Elmfeldt D et al. Smoking and myocardial infarction. Lancet 1975; I:415–420.

40. Johansson S, Bergstrand R, Ulvenstam G et al. Cessation of smoking after myocardial infarction in women. Am J Epidemiol 1985; 121:823–831.

41. Mulcahy R, Hickey N, Graham I et al. Factors influencing long-term prognosis in male patients surviving a first coronary attack. Br Heart J 1975; 37:158–165.

42. Daly LE, Mulcahy R, Graham IM et al. Long term effect on mortality of stopping smoking after unstable angina and myocardial infarction. Br Med J 1983; 287:324–326.

43. Sparrow D, Dawber TR. The influence of cigarette smoking on prognosis after a first myocardial infarction. A report from the Framingham Study. J Chronic Dis 1978; 31:425–432.

44. Pohjola S, Siltanen P, Romo MI. Effect of stopping smoking on the long-term survival after myocardial infarction. Trans Eur Soc Cardiol 1979; 1:2.

45. Salonen JT. Stopping smoking and long-term mortality after myocardial infarction. Br Heart J 1980; 43:463–469.

46. Sato I, Nischida M, Okita K et al. Beneficial effect of stopping smoking on future cardiac events in male smokers with previous myocardial infarction. Jpn Circ J 1992; 56:217–222.

47. Greenwood DC, Muir KR, Packham et al. Stress, social support, and stopping smoking after myocardial infarction in England. J Epidemiol Community Health 1995; 49:583–587.

48. Grines CL, Topol EJ, O'Neill WW et al. Effect of cigarette smoking on outcome after thrombolytic therapy for myocardial infarction. Circulation 1995; 91:298–303.

49. Hemingway H, Marmot M. Evidence based cardiology. Psychological factors in the aetiology and prognosis of coronary heart disease: systematic review of prospective cohort studies. Br Med J 1999; 318:1460–1467.

50. Welin C, Lappas G, Wilhelmsen L. Independent importance of psychosocial factors for prognosis after myocardial infarction. J Intern Med 2000; 247:629–639.

51. van Melle JP, de Jonge P, Ormel J et al. Relationship between left ventricular dysfunction and depression following myocardial infarction: data from the MIND-IT. Eur Heart J 2005; 26:2650–2656.

52. Mookadam F, Arthur HM. Social support and its relationship to morbidity and mortality after acute myocardial infarction: systematic overview. Arch Intern Med 2004; 164:1514–1518.

53. Taylor CB, Youngblood ME, Catellier D et al. Effects of antidepressant medication on morbidity and mortality in depressed patients after myocardial infarction. Arch Gen Psychiatry 2005; 62:792–798.

54. Liu PY, Tsai WC, Chao TH *et al.* Stromelysin-1 promoter 5A/6A polymorphism is an independent genetic risk factor and interacts with smoking cessation after index premature myocardial infarction. *J Throm Haemost* 2005; 3:1998–2005.

55. Weinblatt E, Frank CW, Shapiro S *et al.* Prognostic factors in angina pectoris: a prospective study. *J Chron Dis* 1968; 21:231–245.

56. Kannel WB, Feinleib M. Natural history of angina pectoris in the Framingham study. *Am J Cardiol* 1972; 29:154–163.

57. Rose G, Reid D, Hamilton PJS *et al.* Myocardial ischaemia, risk factors and death from coronary heart disease. *Lancet* 1977; I:105–109.

58. Proudfit WL, Bruschke AWG, MacMillan JP *et al.* Fifteen year survival of patients with obstructive coronary artery disease. *Circulation* 1983; 68:986–997.

59. Hultgren HN, Penduzzi P. Relation of severity of symptoms to prognosis in stable angina pectoris. *Am J Cardiol* 1984; 54:988–993.

60. Hagman M, Wilhelmsen L, Pennert K *et al.* Factors of importance for prognosis in men with angina pectoris derived from a random population sample. The Multifactor Primary Prevention Trial, Gothenburg, Sweden. *Am J Cardiol* 1988; 61:530–535.

61. Rosengren A, Wilhelmsen L, Hagman M *et al.* Natural history of myocardial infarction and angina pectoris in a general population sample of middle-aged men: a 16-year follow-up of the Primary Prevention Study, Göteborg, Sweden. *J Intern Med* 1998; 244:495–505.

62. Clayton TC, Lubsen J, Pocock SJ *et al.* Risk score for predicting death, myocardial infarction, and stroke in patients with stable angina, based on a large randomised trial cohort of patients. *Br Med J* 2005; 331:869–872.

63. Yusuf S, Zucker D, Peduzzi P *et al.* Effect of coronary artery bypass graft surgery on survival: overview of 10-year results from randomised trials by the Coronary Artery Bypass Graft Surgery Trialists Collaboration. *Lancet* 1994; 344:563–570.

64. Domanski MJ, Borkowf CB, Campeau L *et al.* Prognostic factors for atherosclerosis progression in saphenous vein grafts: the postcoronary artery bypass graft (Post-CABG) trial. Post-CABG Trial Investigators. *J Am Coll Cardiol* 2000; 36:1877–1883.

65. Herlitz J, Brandrup-Wognsen G, Haglid M *et al.* Prediction of death during 5 years after coronary artery bypass grafting. *Int J Cardiol* 1998; 64:15–23.

66. Bradshaw PJ, Jamrozik K, Le M *et al.* Mortality and recurrent cardiac events after coronary artery bypass graft: long-term outcome in a population study. *Heart* 2002; 88:488–494.

67. Aronson S, Boisvert D, Lapp W. Isolated systolic hypertension is associated with adverse outcomes from coronary artery bypass grafting surgery. *Anesth Analg* 2002; 94:1079–1084.

68. Cavender JB, Rogers WJ, Fischer LD *et al.* Effects of smoking on survival and morbidity in patients randomised to medical or surgical therapy in the Coronary Artery Surgery Study (CASS). 10-year follow-up. *J Am Coll Cardiol* 1992; 20:287–294.

69. Voors AA, van Brussel BL, Plokker T *et al.* Smoking and cardiac events after venous coronary bypass surgery. A 15-year follow-up study. *Circulation* 1996; 93:42–44.

70. Wilhelmsen L, Rosengren A, Hagman M *et al.* 'Non-specific' chest pain associated with high long-term mortality. Results from the Primary Prevention Study in Göteborg, Sweden. *Clin Cardiol* 1998; 21:477–482.

71. Heuschmann PU, Kolominsky-Rabas PL, Misselwitz B *et al.* Predictors of in-hospital mortality and attributable risks of death after ischemic stroke: the German Stroke Registers stroke Study Group. *Arch Intern Med* 2004; 164:1761–1768.

72. Hankey GJ. Long-term outcome after ischaemic stroke/transient ischaemic attack. *Cerebrovasc Dis* 2003; 16(suppl 1):14–19.

73. Yokota C, Minematsu K, Hasegawa Y *et al.* Long-term prognosis, by stroke subtypes, after a first-ever stroke: a hospital-based study over a 20-year period. *Cerebrovasc Dis* 2004; 18:111–116.

74. Varona JF, Bermejo F, Guerra *et al.* Long-term prognosis of ischemic stroke in young adults. Study of 272 cases. *J Neurol* 2004; 251:1507–1514.

75. Okumura K, Ohya Y, Maehara A *et al.* Effects of blood pressure levels on case fatality after acute stroke. *J Hypertens* 2005; 23:1135–1136.

76. Berthet K, Neal BC, Chalmers JP *et al.* Reductions in the risks of recurrent stroke in patients with and without diabetes: the PROGRESS Trial. *Blood Press* 2004; 13:7–13.

77. Kaarisalo MM, Raiha I, Sivenius J *et al.* Diabetes worsens the outcome of acute ischemic stroke. *Diabetes Res Clin Pract* 2005; 69:293–298.

78. van Wijk I, Kapelle LJ, van Gijn J *et al*. Long-term survival and vascular event risk after transient ischaemic attack or minor ischaemic stroke: a cohort study. *Lancet* 2005; 365:2098–2104.

79. Prospective Studies Collaboration. Cholesterol, diastolic blood pressure, and stroke: 13,000 strokes in 450,000 people in 45 prospective cohorts. *Lancet* 1995; 346:1647–1653.

80. Grau AJ, Weimar C, Buggle F *et al*. Risk factors, outcome, and treatment in subtypes of ischemic stroke: the German stroke data bank. *Stroke* 2001; 32:2559–2566.

81. Di NM, Schwaninger M, Capelli R *et al*. Evaluation of C-reactive protein measurement for assessing the risk and prognosis in ischaemic stroke: a statement for health care professionals from the CRP Pooling Project members. *Stroke* 2005; 36:1316–1329.

82. Bos MJ, van Goor ML, Koudstaal PJ *et al*. Plasma homocysteine is a risk factor for recurrent vascular events in young patients with an ischaemic stroke or TIA. *J Neurol* 2005; 252:332–337.

83. Bath PMW, Gray LJ. Association between hormone replacement therapy and subsequent stroke: a meta-analysis. *Br Med J* 2005; 330:345.

84. Graham I, Atar D, Borch-Johnsen K *et al*. Fourth Joint Task of European Society of Cardiology and other Societies on Cardiovascular Disease Prevention in Clinical Practice. European Guidelines on Cardiovascular Disease Prevention in Clinical Practice. *Eur J Cardiovasc Prev Rehabil* 2007; 14(suppl 2).

10

Socioeconomic aspects of risk estimation

G. De Backer

It is interesting to see how many articles and chapters in books on epidemiology and prevention of cardiovascular diseases (CVD) begin by indicating that *'cardiovascular diseases are the main cause of death in the world'*. This may well be true, but is it an argument to emphasize the need for more prevention of CVD? It is not, or at least not for this generation of mankind. On the contrary, the more cardiovascular events can be prevented at an early age, the larger the number of subjects who will grow old and die at an advanced age from CVD since, in the very old, death is attributed to CVD in the vast majority. If the prevention of premature cardiovascular mortality is successful, one must accept that *overall* cardiovascular mortality will actually increase.

It should be clear, therefore, that the objectives of preventive cardiology are:

- To prevent premature mortality from CVD.
- To reduce the number of patients with chronic disabilities as a result of CVD.
- To constrain the healthcare costs associated with CVD.

In this chapter, particular attention has been paid to the socioeconomic aspects of CVD and of cardiovascular risk prediction. In the first part of the chapter, this is looked at from a population perspective and in the second part from the individual's viewpoint.

SOCIOECONOMIC ASPECTS OF CVD AT THE POPULATION LEVEL

REGIONAL DIFFERENCES IN MORTALITY FROM CORONARY HEART DISEASE

In Europe, CVD is the main cause of premature death (death before the age of 75 years) in 38% of men and 44% of women [1].

The age-standardized death rates from coronary heart disease (CHD) in the population aged 35–74 years are very different between European countries [1]. The rates vary by a factor of 4–5, with the lowest rates in the Southwest and the highest in the East of Europe.

In Figure 10.1, the death rates from CHD are given for men aged 35–74 years from 1968 to 2001 in a number of European countries. The time trends are very heterogeneous; low rates remained low in countries such as France but increased from low to high in Romania; high rates dropped significantly in some countries, such as the UK, but increased to even higher levels in countries such as Ukraine. A similar picture was observed in the female population of the same countries [1]. These observations, based on official mortality statistics, have been confirmed by more rigorous register data collected in the World Health Organization's (WHO) MONItoring trends and determinants in CArdiovascular disease (MONICA) project [2].

Guy de Backer, MD, PhD, Director, Department of Public Health, Ghent University; Director, Cardiac Rehabilitation Centre, University Hospital, Ghent, Belgium

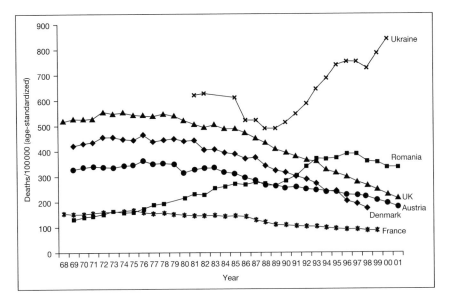

Figure 10.1 Death rates from CHD: men aged 35–74, 1968–2001, selected European countries (with permission from [1]).

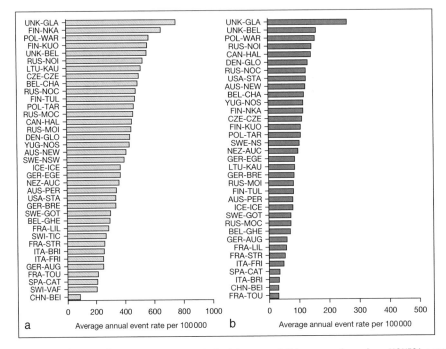

Figure 10.2 Attack rates of acute coronary events in (a) men and (b) women, in various MONICA centres.

REGIONAL DIFFERENCES IN ATTACK RATES OF ACUTE CORONARY EVENTS

In Figure 10.2, attack rates of acute coronary events are presented for populations aged 35–64 years in different parts of the world: in this figure, the age-standardized average annual event rate per 100 000 has been averaged over the last 3 years of registration (in general in the early 1990s). The attack rates demonstrate a 5:1 and a 10:1 variation in event rates between populations of the same gender and age living in different surroundings.

REGIONAL DIFFERENCES IN CHANGE OF CORONARY EVENT RATES

In Figure 10.3, the average annual change in coronary event rates in the same MONICA centres for both men and women is shown. The horizontal bars show the 95% confidence intervals around the estimated annual trend. The data cover the years from the mid 1980s to the early 1990s. The tendency in the majority of the centres is towards a decline, but in approximately one-third of centres no change or a trend towards an increase was observed.

HOW WELL CAN THESE REGIONAL DIFFERENCES BE EXPLAINED?

In the MONICA project, information was also collected on trends in the prevalence of risk factors in the community. These results show that while the levels of risk factors tended to be higher in the East of Europe, the differences between Eastern and Western Europe in terms of risk factors was far less clear-cut than for CHD rates. An ecological analysis of results from the MONICA study found that only a part (23% in men and 14% in women) of the variation in

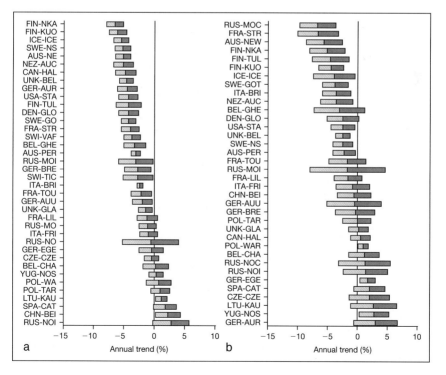

Figure 10.3   Annual change in coronary event rates in (a) men and (b) women in various MONICA centres.

CHD mortality between centres in the late 1980s could be explained by the four main cardio-vascular risk factors (smoking, elevated cholesterol, blood pressure and body mass index) [3]. More recent analyses of the MONICA data [4] from the early 1990s indicate that these four main risk factors explained 30% of CHD mortality variation in men and 45% in women.

It is generally believed that the underlying causes of the change in total and CHD death rates in Eastern Europe are social. However, there is less consensus as to the factors medi-ating these changes: health behaviour, poverty and stress have been suggested. However, regional differences in CHD mortality and morbidity have also been observed *within* coun-tries. The Belgian MONICA centre consisted of two urban areas in the country (the cities of Ghent and Charleroi). The difference in coronary event rates between the two communities was startling and the differences in change in event rates from the 1980s to the 1990s even more so [5]. These differences could partially be explained by classical risk factors, but the most striking correlate was the trend over time in the unemployment rate.

The lesson from all this is that socioeconomic differences in CVD at the population level are important. This should have implications for the development of population strategies to prevent premature CVD at the community level. All risk factors, whether conventional, dietary or psychosocial are strongly influenced by social conditions. They have to be taken into account by health policy-makers both in the development and implementation of CVD prevention strategies at the population level.

SOCIOECONOMIC ASPECTS OF CVD AND RISK ESTIMATION AT THE INDIVIDUAL LEVEL

SOCIOECONOMIC DIFFERENCES IN CHD

In the UK at the end of the 1980s, premature death rates from CHD for male manual work-ers were 58% higher than for male non-manual workers [6]. Premature death rates from CHD for female manual workers were more than twice as high as for female non-manual workers. During the 1980s, the premature death rates fell across all social groups in the UK for both men and women. However, for men, the death rates fell faster in non-manual work-ers than in manual workers and the difference in death rates between social classes increased [6]. In England and Wales during 1991–93 in the male population aged 20–64 years, it was estimated that 28% of all deaths from CHD were due to social class inequalities [6].

The social class gradient is also reflected in morbidity rates, with the incidence of myocardial infarction being more common in lower social classes. For instance, in British civil servants [7], in Finnish men [8] and in Swedish women [9], CHD mortality and mor-bidity were inversely related to socioeconomic status in a graded fashion with a four-fold difference between the highest and lowest occupational categories.

Low socioeconomic status, lack of social support, social isolation, stress at work and out-side work, negative emotions including depression and hostility have been shown to influ-ence both the risk of developing a first cardiovascular event and the prognosis in patients with established CVD. People who are isolated are at increased risk of dying prematurely from CHD [10–13]. Similarly, a lack of social support leads to decreased survival and poorer prognosis among patients with CVD [14–17]. Several aspects of low social support have been associated with poor outcome in patients with CHD even after adjustment for other factors [14, 16–19].

Several other psychosocial factors have also been associated with CVD. Stress at work predicts CHD [20], but so do long-term stressful conditions in family life [21]. The hostility component of Type A behaviour has been associated with CHD independently from other risk factors [22]. Clinical depression is also associated with an increased risk of recurrent events in patients with established CHD [23].

PSYCHOSOCIAL FACTORS AND CORONARY RISK ESTIMATION

Thus, the question whether psychosocial factors should be included in estimations of total cardiovascular risk is a relevant one. Estimating total cardiovascular risk for developing a cardiovascular event has everything to do with priority setting and is of great importance for the 'high-risk' strategy in preventive cardiology.

The healthcare costs related to CVD are enormous. Most of the healthcare systems in Europe are care driven – little support is given to preventive medicine – therefore the limited resources available should be used as efficiently as possible. Priorities have to be set, and interventions that focus on high-risk patients will be more effective in terms of 'number needed to treat'. High-risk subjects can be identified on the basis of personal antecedents of CVD or diabetes; however, in the large group of asymptomatic apparently healthy middle-aged people, models should be used to identify those at highest risk. This is because risk factors interact with each other in a complex way.

The models that are recommended are based on the results from either the Framingham study [24] or the Systemic Coronary Risk Evaluation (SCORE) project [25], but none of these models takes socioeconomic factors into account. The SCORE project builds on results from 12 independent cohort studies in Europe: in these studies, psychosocial factors were either not included or measured in different ways, and could not, therefore, be considered in the 'CORE' of the SCORE project. This does not, however, mean that they should not be considered in risk predictions and in risk factor management. However, in the European guidelines on CVD prevention in clinical practice [26], special attention was paid to psychosocial factors.

When estimating total CV risk, it is arguable as to whether or not psychosocial factors add anything to what is predicted by examining classical risk factors alone. Are the effects of psychosocial factors on CVD risk mainly mediated by the classical risk factors? If this is so, then the effects of psychosocial factors are indeed indirectly reflected in the risk levels estimated by the Framingham or SCORE models.

There is currently no firm consensus as to the mediating effects of the main risk factors in explaining socioeconomic differences in CVD. In the Whitehall II study [7], controlling for standard risk factors reduced the size of the gradient of CHD by occupational class but a significant proportion of the variance according to socioeconomic status was left unexplained.

More recently, it was suggested that more than 50% of the difference in overall mortality between the top and bottom social strata in the male populations aged 35–69 years in four countries could be explained by differences in the risk of being killed by smoking [27]. Classical risk factors, particularly smoking, make a sizeable contribution to the East–West gap in CHD mortality in Europe. Besides smoking, inappropriate dietary habits and lack of physical exercise during leisure time also exhibit social gradients.

It is difficult to estimate precisely how much of the increasing incidence of CVD with decreasing socioeconomic status is a reflection of the similar gradient in lifestyle-related risk factors. It would appear that behavioural risk factors contribute to the explanation of the social gradient in CVD incidence, but substantial differences remain even after adjustment for these factors. Therefore, the question remains as to how best to incorporate socioeconomic factors into risk prediction, whilst accepting that classical risk factors have a large part to play.

One of the reasons for using an estimate of total CV risk as a guide to adjust the intensity of the preventive approach in a given subject is because the whole person should always be considered, not just isolated risk factors. This is now generally accepted for the main CV risk factors, but it is also important for psychosocial factors. Psychosocial factors do not occur in isolation but tend to cluster in the same subjects. Women who reported high job stress were also more hostile, depressed and socially isolated [28]. These subjects are also more likely to engage in unhealthy behaviours that contribute to the socioeconomic gradient of CVD risk.

PSYCHOSOCIAL FACTORS AND RISK MANAGEMENT

This tendency of psychosocial risk factors to cluster in the same subjects has implications for strategies aimed at modifying cardiovascular risk profiles. For instance, because subjects with high levels of hostility and depression are more likely to smoke, attempts to help them to quit smoking may be more successful if they also include elements designed to reduce this hostility and depression. Behavioural interventions that reduce levels of psychosocial risk factors are likely to have broad benefits in terms of enabling people to be more successful in modifying their lifestyles.

Psychosocial factors should be considered in risk prediction and should be included in the list of qualifiers that clinicians should consider, in addition to those already provided by the standard risk models. Socioeconomic factors should also be taken into account in the implementation of risk factor management strategies.

Reducing exposure to classical risk factors in the low-educated groups of society requires another approach. One should look for points of entry for action to tackle root causes. It could well be that a combination of multiple risk factors interact differently in different social classes. Those in the lower social class may be more vulnerable to the health-damaging effects of a cluster of risk factors. The metabolic syndrome may be a good example: obesity (including abdominal obesity), low high-density lipoprotein-cholesterol, elevated blood pressure and impaired fasting glycaemia together with smoking is a profile that is more frequently encountered in the lower social classes of society. This cluster reflects an important risk for developing diabetes and CVD. It may already be present at a young age and is cumulative over the subject's lifetime. Reducing these inequalities requires particular strategies adapted to the needs of lower social classes.

Socioeconomic factors may also act as barriers to efforts to improve lifestyles and risk factor management. Early detection, treatment and control of elevated blood pressure, elevated cholesterol and fasting glycaemia are examples where, at each level of management plans, socioeconomic differences exist. Low socioeconomic status is not amenable to change. However, the mechanisms mediating the effects of low social class on CVD risk can be modified. Therefore, preventive efforts need to focus particularly on individuals and patients with low education, low job position and in poor-quality residential areas.

REFERENCES

1. British Heart Foundation. European cardiovascular disease statistics. www.heartstats.org 2005
2. Tunstall-Pedoe H, for the WHO-MONICA project. *MONICA: Monograph and Multimedia Sourcebook.* WHO, Geneva, 2003.
3. Tunstall-Pedoe H, Kuulasmaa K, Amouyel P, Arveiler D, Rajakangas AM, Pajak A. Myocardial infarction and coronary deaths in the World Health Organization MONICA project: registration procedures, event rates and case fatality rates in 38 populations from 21 countries in four continents. *Circulation* 1994; 90:583–612.
4. Kuulasmaa K, Tunstall-Pedoe H, Dobson A *et al*. Estimation of contribution of changes in classical risk factors to trends in coronary-event rates across the WHO-MONICA project populations. *Lancet* 2000; 335:675–687.
5. De Henauw S, De Bacquer D, de Smet P, Kornitzer M, De Backer G. Trends in coronary heart disease in two Belgian areas: results from the MONICA Ghent-Charleroi study. *J Epidemiol Community Health* 1999; 52:89–98.
6. British Heart Foundation. 2006 Coronary heart disease statistics. www.heartstats.org
7. Marmot MG, Smith GD, Stansfeld S *et al*. Health inequalities among British civil servants: the Whitehall II study. *Lancet* 1991; 337:1387–1393.
8. Lynch JW, Kaplan GA, Cohen RD, Tuomiletho J, Salonen JT. Do cardiovascular risk factors explain the relation between socioeconomic status, risk of all-cause mortality, cardiovascular mortality and acute myocardial infarction? *Am J Epidemiol* 1996; 144:934–942.

9.   Wamala SP, Mittleman MA, Schenck-Gustafsson K, Orth-Gomer K. Potential explanations for the educational gradient in coronary heart disease: a population based case-control study in Swedish women. *Am J Public Health* 1999; 89:315–321.

10. Kaplan GA, Salonen JT, Cohen RD, Brand RJ, Puska P. Social connections and mortality from all causes and from cardiovascular disease: prospective evidence from eastern Finland. *Am J Epidemiol* 1988; 128:370–380.

11. Kawachi I, Colditz GA, Ascherio A *et al*. A prospective study of social networks in relation to total mortality and cardiovascular disease in men in the US. *J Epidemiol Community Health* 1996; 50:245–251.

12. Orth-Gomer K, Rosengren A, Wilhelmsen L. Lack of social support and incidence of coronary heart disease in middle-aged Swedish men. *Psychosom Med* 1993; 55:37–43.

13. Vogt TM, Mullooly JP, Ernst D, Pope CR, Hollis JF. Social networks as predictors of ischemic heart disease, cancer, stroke and hypertension. *J Clin Epidemiol* 1992; 45:659–666.

14. Berkman LF, Leo-Summers L, Horwitz RI. Emotional support and survival after myocardial infarction. A prospective population-based study of the elderly. *Ann Intern Med* 1992; 117:1003–1009.

15. Orth-Gomer K, Unden AL, Edwards ME. Social isolation and mortality in ischemic heart disease. A 10 year follow-up study of 150 middle-aged men. *Acta Med Scand* 1988; 224:205–215.

16. Ruberman W, Weinblatt E, Goldberg JD, Chaudhary BS. Psychosocial influences on mortality after myocardial infarction. *N Engl J Med* 1984; 311:552–559.

17. Williams RB, Barefoot JC, Califf RM *et al*. Prognostic importance of social and economic resources among medically treated patients with angiographically documented coronary artery disease. *JAMA* 1992; 267:520–524.

18. Case RB, Moss AJ, Case N, McDermott M, Eberly S. Living alone after myocardial infarction. Impact on prognosis. *JAMA* 1992; 267:515–519.

19. Frasure-Smith N, Lesperance F, Gravel G *et al*. Social support, depression, and mortality during the first year after myocardial infarction. *Circulation* 2000; 101:1919–1924.

20. De Bacquer D, Pelfrene E, Clays E *et al*. Perceived job stress and incidence of coronary events: 3 yr follow up of the Belgian job stress cohort. *Am J Epidemiol* 2005; 161:434–441.

21. Orth-Gomer K, Wamala SP, Horsten M, Schenck-Gustafsson K, Schneidermann N, Mittelman MA. Marital stress worsens prognosis in women with coronary heart disease; the Stockholm Female Coronary Risk study. *JAMA* 2000; 284:3008–3014.

22. Miller TQ, Smith TW, Turner CW, Guijarro ML, Hallet AJ. A meta-analytic review of research on hostility and physical health. *Psychol Bull* 1996; 119:322–348.

23. Hermann-Lingen C, Buss U. *Angst and Depressivitat im Verlauf der koronaren Herzkrankheit*. VAS Verlag, Frankfurt/Main, 2003.

24. Anderson KM, Wilson PW, Odell PM, Kannel WB. An updated coronary risk profile. A statement for health professionals. *Circulation* 1991; 83:356–362.

25. Conroy R, Pyörälä K, Fitzgerald A *et al*. Prediction of ten-year risk of fatal cardiovascular disease in Europe: the SCORE project. *Eur Heart J* 2003; 24:987–1003.

26. Graham I, Atar D, Borch-Johnsen K *et al*. Fourth Joint Task of European Society of Cardiology and other Societies on Cardiovascular Disease Prevention in Clinical Practice. European Guidelines on Cardiovascular Disease Prevention in Clinical Practice. *Eur J Cardiovasc Prev Rehabil* 2007;14(suppl 2).

27. Jha P, Peto R, Zatonski W, Boreham J, Jarvis MJ, Lopez A. Social inequalities in male mortality, and in male mortality from smoking: indirect estimation from national death rates in England and Wales, Poland and North America. *Lancet* 2006; 368:367–370.

28. Williams RB, Barefoot JC, Blumenthal JA *et al*. Psychosocial correlates of job strain in a sample of working women. *Arch Gen Psychiatry* 1997; 54:543–548.

11

Risk estimation systems in clinical use: SCORE, HeartScore and the Framingham system

C. McGorrian, T. Leong, R. B. D'Agostino, Sr, I. M. Graham

INTRODUCTION

Since atherosclerosis, and hence cardiovascular disease (CVD), is the product of multiple risk factors, it is clear that a comprehensive risk factor evaluation is the cornerstone of primary prevention. The challenges for the busy health professional are as follows:

- How do I identify people who are at increased risk of a cardiovascular event?
- How do I weigh the individual effects of all the causative risk factors, when assessing a person's risk?
- How do I stratify that risk, to determine who needs lifesyle advice and who needs additional medical therapy?
- How do I ensure I am not overmedicalising those persons who are at low risk of an event?

There are two important concepts here, which are stressed by both the American College of Cardiology's 27th Bethesda conference [1], and the 1994 [2], 1998 [3], 2003 [4] and 2007 [5] Joint Task Force of European and other Societies on cardiovascular disease prevention in clinical practice: the use of a multiple risk factor equation in estimating total risk of a person developing a cardiovascular event, and the need to tailor patient management to overall risk instead of considering single risk factors in isolation.

RISK ESTIMATION SYSTEMS

Cardiovascular risk estimation systems are widely recommended for use in the primary prevention of cardiovascular diseases. They provide a scientific method for healthcare

Catherine McGorrian, MRCPI, Senior Research Fellow, Department of Cardiology, The Adelaide and Meath Hospital, Dublin, Ireland

Tora Leong, MB, MRCPI, Senior Reseach Fellow, Department of Cardiology, The Adelaide and Meath Hospital, Dublin, Ireland

Ralph B. D'Agostino, Sr, PhD, Professor of Mathematics/Statistics and Public Health, Director of Data Management and Statistical Analysis of Framingham Study, Mathematics and Statistics Department, Framingham Study, Boston University, Boston, Massachusetts, USA

Ian M. Graham, FRCPI, FESC, Consultant Cardiologist; Professor of Cardiovascular Medicine, Trinity College, Dublin; Professor of Preventive Cardiology, Royal College of Surgeons in Ireland

professionals to stratify risk, to ensure that those persons at high risk of developing cardio-vascular diseases are identified. Then, appropriate management steps can be undertaken for this group. For the lower risk patients, lifestyle advice is usually appropriate, without recourse to pharmacological therapy.

It should be noted that these risk factor equations are not formulated for use in sec-ondary prevention. Persons with pre-existing CVD, in particular coronary heart diseases (CHD), have already identified themselves as being at risk for future events. Therefore, their need for optimum risk factor control is already evident. Furthermore, some subgroups of individuals are also deemed 'high risk' automatically: these include patients with severe, often familial hypercholesterolaemia, with severe hypertension, particularly if target organ damage is present, and with diabetes mellitus. Diabetes is often quoted as being a 'CVD equivalent' [6], but this is an oversimplification, given the spectrum of disease ranging from the young, well-controlled type 1 diabetic, to the older type 2 diabetic with other risk factors such as the metabolic syndrome.

It is also important to note that many of these risk equations do not include risk factors such as a family history of premature CHD (which in the Framingham data [7], was found to have an odds ratio for CVD events of 1.3), raised triglyceride levels or reduced high-density lipoprotein (HDL) cholesterol levels. Neither do many of them include newer risk markers, such as C-reactive protein (CRP). In both Framingham [8] and Systematic Coronary Risk Evaluation (SCORE) [9], caveats are added that features such as the metabolic syndrome and its components will add to total risk, and must be considered when evaluating the results of the risk assessment. Whilst this means that the professional using the scoring system has to keep these caveats in mind, it is probably fair to say that a risk scoring system which included all possible risk factors would be unwieldy to use, and might not be substantially better at identifying high-risk subjects than the existing, simpler scores.

A number of cardiovascular risk estimation systems have been proposed to date, the most well-known being those based on the Framingham function [8], which has been used to construct the risk estimation system advised for use by the National Cholesterol Education Program (NCEP) Adult Treatment Panel III [6]. The Framingham function also formed the basis of a number of other systems [10, 11]. Independent systems include Prospective Cardiovascular Münster (PROCAM) [12], the Dundee risk disk [13], and a risk estimation system published by Pocock *et al.* [14]. SCORE [9] is the European cardio-vascular risk estimation tool which is endorsed by the European Society of Cardiology (ESC) and the Third and Fourth Joint Task Force recommendations on Cardiovascular Prevention [4, 5].

PROSPECTIVE CARDIOVASCULAR MÜNSTER (PROCAM) STUDY

The investigators in the PROCAM study [12] in Europe took a cohort of 5389 men aged 35–65 years without evidence of CVD, and followed them for 10 years. They used a Cox model to construct a risk algorithm [15], examining age, low-density lipoprotein (LDL) cholesterol, smoking, HDL cholesterol, systolic blood pressure, family history of premature myocardial infarction, diabetes mellitus and triglyceride levels. The endpoints were cardiac death or non-fatal myocardial infarction. An integer score was given to each level of risk fac-tor, to give an absolute risk score. Usefully, this score includes such parameters as lipid sub-fractions and family history. Limitations are the small sample size, that it was based on volunteers rather than a representative population sample, and that no data on women were used in the construction of the initial scoring system. The International Task Force for Prevention of Coronary Heart Disease later published a formula to calculate 10-year risk of myocardial infarction and sudden cardiac death in women based on PROCAM data [16], but as there were only 32 events in 2810 women, the authors themselves advise using this formula with caution.

SCORE AND HEARTSCORE

The development of the SCORE project is discussed in detail in chapter 2. In brief, the European Society of Cardiology, the European Atherosclerosis Society and the European Society of Hypertension came together to publish the first Joint Recommendations on the Prevention of Cardiovascular Disease and Clinical Practice in 1994 [2]. These recommendations, and the Second Joint Task Force recommendations in 1998 [3], published a chart to predict 10-year risk of fatal and non-fatal coronary heart disease using age, sex, cholesterol, smoking status and blood pressure. This chart was based on a risk function which was derived from the Framingham project.

However, there were some concerns about this approach. Framingham data are from a small, homogenous population in North America, and this was being applied to a large, culturally diverse European population. Secondly, the endpoints used in the Framingham study included angina pectoris – not an endpoint that is commonly used in most cohorts, which therefore makes the charts difficult to validate. Thirdly, although the Framingham function has been validated in one study in the UK [17], it has also been shown to overpredict risk in a number of European cohorts [18–20]. In response to these concerns, and at the request of the ESC, the SCORE investigators developed an independent cardiovascular risk prediction system using European data. Data on 216 000 subjects were pooled from eleven countries in Europe, and mean follow-up was 13 years. Charts were developed for areas with high and low incidences of cardiovascular diseases (Figure 11.1). They were published in the Third Joint Task Force recommendations, and also in a paper discussing methods [9]. Tables 11.1 and 11.2 show the qualifiers for correct use of the charts.

It is worth considering the endpoints used in SCORE. Given the heterogeneity of the datasets used, data collection methods could not be standard between the cohorts. Some of the studies only collected follow-up data on fatal events. Furthermore, since some of the studies commenced their recruitment and surveys as long ago as the 1970s, the demographics, hospital admission rates, treatment, and even the very definition of endpoints such as myocardial infarction would have differed significantly from what we see today. Therefore, it was evident that the most appropriate endpoint was the 'hard' endpoint of cardiovascular death. This means that, in contrast to the original Framingham endpoints, and the charts published in the Second Joint Task Force Guidelines, SCORE estimates 10-year risk of *fatal* cardiovascular events. Therefore, from a 10-year risk of any cardiovascular event of 20% indicating a subject deemed to be at 'high' cardiovascular risk in the Framingham equation, the emphasis now was on those subjects with a 10-year risk of a fatal event of 5%. Although this change of endpoint was a considered one, and was carefully highlighted in the guidelines, nevertheless it has almost inevitably caused some confusion. Furthermore, some clinicians are uncomfortable with only being able to estimate fatal events, even though a high risk of cardiovascular death would intuitively indicate a higher risk of a non-fatal event. SCORE Plus, a function which estimates total cardiovascular risk, fatal and non-fatal, for high-risk countries, based on FINRISK, will be released shortly. Preliminary results suggest that the equivalent of a 5% 10-year risk of fatal CVD is about 10%, more in younger men and less in women and the elderly.

One problem with all risk charts is that a low absolute risk in a young person may conceal large relative risk that would mandate intensive lifestyle advice and perhaps drug therapy as the person ages. For this reason, the European Fourth Joint Task Force recommendations [5] include a chart that illustrates relative risk (Figure 11.2).

One strength of the SCORE system is that it is paper-based, and the risk levels are read directly off it. There is no calculation required on the part of the clinician. Furthermore, it is free to disseminate without copyright. This is highly advantageous when it comes to making the charts available in the public forum. The downside of this paper chart, however, is that other risk factors cannot be added without making the system many pages longer, and

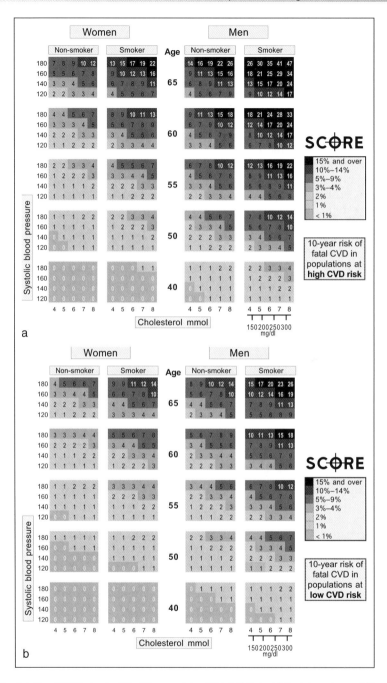

Figure 11.1 (a) The SCORE charts [9]. 10-year risk of fatal CVD in high risk regions of Europe by gender, age, systolic blood pressure, total cholesterol and smoking status. (b) The SCORE charts [9]. 10-year risk of fatal CVD in low risk regions of Europe by gender, age, systolic blood pressure, total cholesterol and smoking status.

Table 11.1 Instructions on how to use the charts (From the Third Joint Task Force Recommendations [4])

- The low risk chart should be used in Belgium, France, Greece, Italy, Luxembourg, Spain, Switzerland and Portugal; the high risk chart should be used in all other countries of Europe.
- To estimate a person's total 10-year risk of CVD death, find the table for their gender, smoking status and age. Within the table find the cell nearest to the person's systolic blood pressure (mmHg) and total cholesterol (mmol/l or mg/dl).
- The effect of lifetime exposure to risk factors can be seen by following the table upwards. This can be used when advising younger people.
- Low risk individuals should be offered advice to maintain their low risk status. Those who are at 5% risk or higher, or will reach this level in middle age, should be given maximal attention.
- To define a person's relative risk, compare their risk category with that of a non-smoking person of the same age and gender, blood pressure <140/90 mmHg and total cholesterol <5 mmol/l (190 mg/dl).
- The chart can be used to give some indications of the effect of changes from one risk category to another, for example, when the subject stops smoking or reduces other risk factors.

Table 11.2 Qualifiers (From the Third Joint Task Force Recommendations [4])

Note that total CVD risk may be higher than indicated in the chart:
- as the person approaches the next age category
- in asymptomatic subjects with pre-clinical evidence of atherosclerosis (e.g. CT scan, ultrasonography)
- in subjects with a strong family history of premature CVD
- in subjects with low HDL cholesterol levels, with raised triglyceride levels, with impaired glucose tolerance, and with raised levels of C-reactive protein, fibrinogen, homocysteine, apolipoprotein B or Lp(a)
- in obese and sedentary subjects.

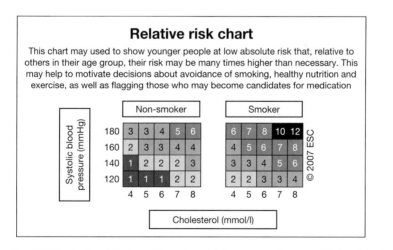

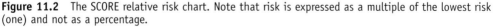

Figure 11.2 The SCORE relative risk chart. Note that risk is expressed as a multiple of the lowest risk (one) and not as a percentage.

therefore much more unwieldy. The potential solution to this is in the electronic version of SCORE: HeartScore [21]. This web-based tool is based on the SCORE function, and allows for country-specific recalibration using national mortality data. To date, country-specific risk estimation systems have been published for Belgium, Germany, Greece, The

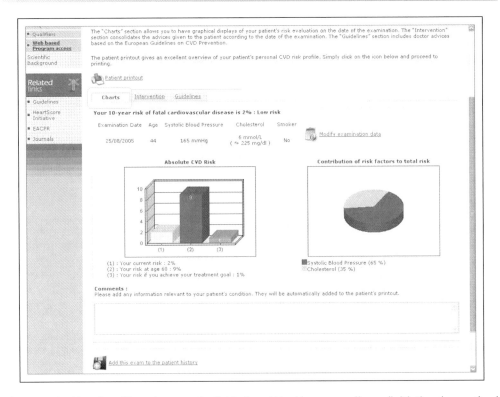

Figure 11.3   HeartScore™ results page. Available from http://www.escardio.org/initiatives/prevention/ HeartScore.html.

Netherlands, Poland, Spain and Sweden, with others in production or pending publication. Forthcoming projects seek to include other risk factors such as HDL cholesterol, body mass index and family history of CVD.

The first version of HeartScore was based on the Danish PRECARD™ computer-based risk estimation and management system, as developed by Troels Thomsen and colleagues [22, 23]. HeartScore is based on the SCORE function, and uses the same risk factors and algorithms. It was initially available as a Windows program, launched in 2004; however, this was a little cumbersome, and sometimes proved difficult to download. With the increasing availability of broadband technology and higher internet connection speeds, it has become possible to have a web-based HeartScore, and this is the form taken by the current version. It is available through the European Society of Cardiology website, www.escardio.org, and high risk, low risk and country-specific versions are available. Thanks in particular to the recent work of Sylvain Boyer and others at the European Heart House in Nice, France, this application is easily accessible and enjoyable to use. Once the risk factors for a particular patient are inputted, absolute risk at current and ideal risk factor levels are displayed, and these graphs can be printed and given to the patient for his or her own reference (Figure 11.3). Details inputted on a particular patient can also be saved under the doctor's personal login code, and referred to during future consultations.

Score and HeartScore also provide risk factor management advice, and tailor it to the level of total risk estimated. There are also management strategies described for situations when individual risk factors are markedly elevated. HeartScore, in particular, is geared towards provision of management advice, as links lead to pages with advice taken from the

Pocket Guidelines of the Fourth Joint Task Force. This is acknowledged to be a particular strength of the program. Given that best risk factor management changes as more evidence is published, there are clear benefits to this adaptable web-based system. In addition, in response to requests from countries in which clinicians do not always have ready access to broadband in their day-to-day practices, a stand-alone, desktop version of HeartScore is currently in test phase and due for release in 2008.

THE FRAMINGHAM STUDY

The Framingham Study is a classic prospective epidemiological cohort study. It began in 1948 when 5209 residents aged 28 to 62 in the town of Framingham, Massachusetts, were enrolled, and subsequently reassessed with surveys every 2 years. From 1971 onwards, 5124 of the original cohort's offspring and offspring's spouses were enrolled [24]. More recently, a third generation cohort has been added. Prior to Framingham, the prevailing concept was that a single cause of CVD would be found. However this, of course, was not found to be the case: rather, a number of predisposing 'risk factors' were identified [25], including increasing age, male gender, hypertension, high serum cholesterol and LDL subfraction, low HDL cholesterol, cigarette smoking, glucose intolerance and diabetes mellitus, obesity, physical inactivity and left ventricular hypertrophy. It is no exaggeration to say that the Framingham Study has fundamentally shaped our understanding of both the aetiology of atherosclerotic cardiovascular diseases and their prevention.

In 1973, the Framingham investigators published CHD risk equations [26]. In 1991, this risk system was updated using data from both the original Framingham cohort and the Framingham Offspring cohort [27]. It included the data on those persons aged 30–74, who were free of stroke, transient ischaemic attack, heart failure, intermittent claudication, and CHD (angina pectoris, coronary insufficiency, myocardial infarction and sudden death) at the beginning of the study. A Cox proportional hazards model was used, and a chart was devised where each risk factor is given a weighting in points, including age, sex, total cholesterol, HDL cholesterol, systolic and diastolic blood pressure, diabetes, smoking status and left ventricular hypertrophy on ECG. From the sum of these points, the absolute 5-year and 10-year CHD risks can be calculated, and these can then be compared to the baseline risk in the community (Figure 11.4).

However, the endpoints used in this 1991 risk equation included the 'soft' endpoint of angina pectoris, which is not commonly used as an endpoint in other studies. Therefore, an updated coronary prediction model was published in 1998 [8], which also used the Joint National Committee (JNC-V) [28] and NCEP [6] cholesterol, LDL cholesterol and blood pressure categories. In this project, Framingham subjects who had evidence of CHD at baseline were again excluded, and the remainder were followed up for a mean of 12 years. CHD endpoint events were angina pectoris, recognised and unrecognised myocardial infarction, coronary insufficiency and CHD death. 'Hard' events include all the above, except angina pectoris. These updated charts are available on the world wide web at http://www.nhlbi.nih.gov/about/framingham/index.html, and there are charts for men and women, and for LDL cholesterol and total cholesterol, as well as a stroke risk estimation function. They allow the estimation of 10-year risk of CHD events, which includes the 'soft' endpoint of angina pectoris, but the charts published in *Circulation* also permit comparison between 'hard' CHD risk, and CHD risk including angina pectoris.

For the most recent NCEP Adult Treatment Panel III guidelines, the NCEP have updated the Framingham risk score to use only 'hard' endpoints (Figure 11.5). They recommend the use of this equation for risk estimation in primary prevention in persons with more than two risk factors, and 'high risk' individuals are deemed to be those with a 10-year risk of CHD events of >20%. As already stated, this contrasts markedly with SCORE, where high-risk individuals were those with a 10-year risk of >5%, but it must be

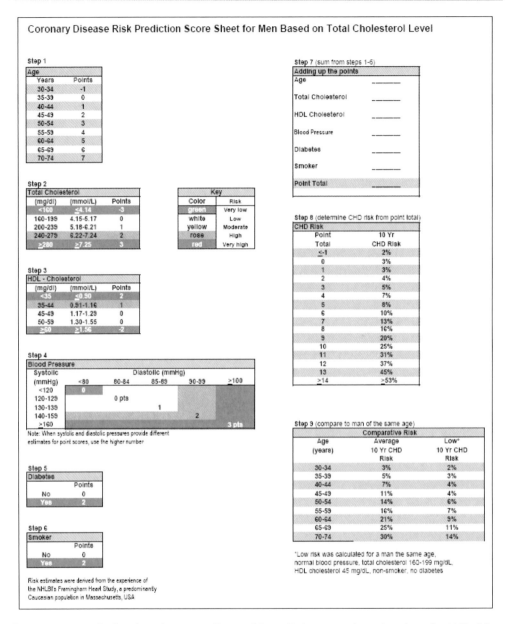

Figure 11.4 Framingham based coronary disease risk prediction score sheet, based on the 1998 risk tables [8] and available from http://www.nhlbi.nih.gov/about/framingham/index.html.

remembered that SCORE deals with fatal events in contrast to Framingham's wider endpoint definitions. The NCEP have a web-based risk calculator at http://www.nhlbi.nih.gov/guidelines/cholesterol/. Also available from the NCEP guidelines are summaries of specific management advice for those persons at high risk, including an 'At-a-glance' desk reference.

The Framingham study data were also used in the development of the Joint British Societies risk assessment charts. These are published in the most recent JBS2 guidelines [11], and an electronic form is available at http://www.bnf.org/BNF/extra/current/450024.html.

ASSIGN AND QRISK

Recently, two other cardiovascular risk estimation systems were introduced: ASSIGN [29] in Scotland and QRISK [30] in England. ASSIGN (Assessing cardiovascular risk using SIGN

Estimate of 10-Year Risk for Men (Framingham Point Scores)

Age	Points
20–34	-9
35–39	-4
40–44	0
45–49	3
50–54	6
55–59	8
60–64	10
65–69	11
70–74	12
75–79	13

Total Cholesterol	Points at Ages 20–39	Points at Ages 40–49	Points at Ages 50–59	Points at Ages 60–69	Points at Ages 70–79
<160	0	0	0	0	0
160–199	4	3	2	1	0
200–239	7	5	3	1	0
240–279	9	6	4	2	1
≥280	11	8	5	3	1

	Points at Ages 20–39	Points at Ages 40–49	Points at Ages 50–59	Points at Ages 60–69	Points at Ages 70–79
Nonsmoker	0	0	0	0	0
Smoker	8	5	3	1	1

HDL	Points
≥60	-1
50–59	0
40–49	1
<40	2

Systolic BP	If Untreated	If Treated
<120	0	0
120–129	0	1
130–139	1	2
140–159	1	2
≥160	2	3

Point Total	10-Year Risk	Point Total	10-Year Risk
<0	<1%	11	8%
0	1%	12	10%
1	1%	13	12%
2	1%	14	16%
3	1%	15	20%
4	1%	16	25%
5	2%	≥17	≥30%
6	2%		
7	3%		
8	4%		
9	5%		
10	6%		

Figure 11.5   Framingham-based coronary risk score for 'hard' endpoints, from the National Cholesterol Education Program guidelines [6].

10-Year Risk Estimates for Women (Framingham Point Scores)

Age	Points
20–34	-7
35–39	-3
40–44	0
45–49	3
50–54	6
55–59	8
60–64	10
65–69	12
70–74	14
75–79	16

Total Cholesterol	Points at Ages 20–39	Points at Ages 40–49	Points at Ages 50–59	Points at Ages 60–69	Points at Ages 70–79
<160	0	0	0	0	0
160–199	4	3	2	1	1
200–239	8	6	4	2	1
240–279	11	8	5	3	2
≥280	13	10	7	4	2

	Points at Ages 20–39	Points at Ages 40–49	Points at Ages 50–59	Points at Ages 60–69	Points at Ages 70–79
Nonsmoker	0	0	0	0	0
Smoker	9	7	4	2	1

HDL	Points
≥60	-1
50–59	0
40–49	1
<40	2

Systolic BP	If Untreated	If Treated
<120	0	0
120–129	1	3
130–139	2	4
140–159	3	5
≥160	4	6

Point Total	10-Year Risk	Point Total	10-Year Risk
<9	<1%	20	11%
9	1%	21	14%
10	1%	22	17%
11	1%	23	22%
12	1%	24	27%
13	2%	≥25	≥30%
14	2%		

Figure 11.5 (contd)   Framingham-based coronary risk score for 'hard' endpoints, from the National Cholesterol Education Program guidelines [6].

guidelines to ASSIGN preventive treatment) includes two additional risk factors, family history and an area measure of social deprivation. It was developed to take into account the effect of social deprivation on cardiovascular risk. Those in the highest 20% of social deprivation in Scotland were shown to have an increased risk comparable with being 10 years older or having diabetes [31]. The risk function was derived using the Scottish Heart Health Extended Cohort (SHHEC) study, a cohort study containing 6419 men and 6618 women, and it is available on the internet; www.assign-score.com. While the inclusion of social deprivation as a risk factor is important, because it is based on Scottish postal code this risk score may be difficult to apply to other populations.

QRISK, is a risk estimation system derived from and validated on a large dataset containing pooled medical records from 318 UK general practices, including 1.28 million patients [30]. The function is based on follow-up of general practice patients in contrast to other risk scores which are based on prospective population studies with randomly selected participants.

Again, this function contains information on social deprivation based on postal code. Data were not available on lipid measures for up to 70% of the participants; these values were generated using the multiple imputation method. Additionally, no allowance was made for usage of lipid-lowering therapy. This resulted in a trivial and insignificant hazard ratio for total cholesterol/HDL cholesterol as a continuous variable (1.001 [95% confidence interval: 0.999–1.002]). The score risk has been criticised for these reasons, amongst others [32, 33]. The authors have since revised the function in an attempt to correct for these limitations [34]. However, whether this risk score is generalizable to other populations remains in question.

A validation study of QRISK has recently been published [35] suggesting that it is better calibrated to the UK population than Framingham. This study also reported better summary discrimination, but threshold discrimination in terms of who will or will not reach a given threshold for treatment was not examined.

SUMMARY

A number of risk functions are available to the healthcare professional, and all have their own strengths and weaknesses. Framingham is the most widely used system, and has the advantage of uniform data collection methodologies. SCORE is a European system, with a more ethnically heterogenous pan-European mix, but only predicts fatal CVD events. A new model which will predict fatal cardiovascular and non-fatal 'hard' CHD and stroke events is currently being produced. Web-based applications are accessible and convenient, and can produce printable results which may be given to the patient to aid compliance. Web-based risk scoring is likely to be the most commonly used method of risk stratification in the future, given the increasing penetration of internet access, and also the flexibility of these systems. Such fast moving technologies will allow us to update the scores as more evidence on cardiovascular risk appears. Our goal must be to ensure the accuracy and to promote the use of these tools in day-to-day clinical practice.

REFERENCES

1. 27th Bethesda Conference. Matching the intensity of risk factor management with the hazard for coronary disease events. *J Am Coll Cardiol* 1996; 27:957–1047.
2. Pyörälä K, DeBacker G, Graham I *et al*. Prevention of coronary heart disease in clinical practice: recommendations of the Second Joint Task Force of the European Society of Cardiology, European Atherosclerosis Society and European Society of Hypertension. *Atherosclerosis* 1994; 110:121–161.
3. Wood D, DeBacker G, Faergeman O, Graham I, Mancia G, Pyörälä K. Prevention of coronary heart disease in clinical practice: recommendations of the Task Force of the European and other Societies on Coronary Prevention. *Eur Heart J* 1998; 19:1434–1503.
4. De Backer G, Ambrosioni E, Borch-Johnsen K *et al*. Third Joint Task Force of the European and other Societies on Cardiovascular Disease Prevention in clinical practice. European Guidelines on cardiovascular disease prevention in clinical practice. *Eur Heart J* 2003; 24:1601–1610.
5. Graham I, Atar D, Borch-Johnsen K *et al*. Fourth Joint Task Force of the European Society of Cardiology and other Societies on Cardiovascular Disease Prevention in Clinical Practice. European Guidelines on Cardiovascular Disease Prevention in Clinical Practice. *Eur J Cardiovasc Prev Rehabil* 2007; 14(suppl 2): S1–S113.
6. NCEP (National Cholesterol Education Program) Expert panel on detection, evaluation and treatment of high blood cholesterol in adults (Adult Treatment Panel III) final report. *Circulation* 2002; 106:3143–3421.
7. Myers RH, Kiely DK, Cupples LA, Kannel WB. Parental history is an independent risk factor for coronary artery disease: the Framingham Study. *Am Heart J* 1990; 120:963–969.
8. Wilson PW, D'Agostino RB, Levy D, Belanger AM, Silbershatz H, Kannel WB. Prediction of coronary heart disease using risk factor categories. *Circulation* 1998; 97:1837–1847.
9. Conroy RM, Pyörälä K, Fitzgerald AP *et al*. Estimation of ten-year risk of fatal cardiovascular disease in Europe: the SCORE project. *Eur Heart J* 2003; 24:987–1003.
10. Haq IU, Jackson PR, Yeo WW, Ramsay LE. Sheffield risk and treatment table for cholesterol lowering for primary prevention of coronary heart disease. *Lancet* 1995; 346:1467–1471.

11. JBS2: Joint British guidelines on prevention of cardiovascular disease in clinical practice. British Cardiac Society, British Hyperlipidaemia Association, British Hypertension Society, British Diabetic Association. *Heart* 2005; 91:1–52.

12. Assmann G, Schulte H. The Prospective Cardiovascular Münster (PROCAM) study: prevalence of hyperlipidaemia in persons with hypertension and/or diabetes mellitus and the relationship to coronary heart disease. *Am Heart J* 1988; 116:1713–1724.

13. Tunstall-Pedoe H. The Dundee Risk Disc for management of change in risk factors. *Eur Heart J* 1991; 303:744–747.

14. Pocock SJ, McCormack V, Gueyffier F, Boutitie F, Fagard RH, Boissel JP. A score for predicting risk of death from cardiovascular disease in adults with raised blood pressure, based on individual patients' data from randomised controlled trials. *BMJ* 2001; 323:78–81.

15. Assmann G, Cullen P, Schulte H. Simple scoring scheme for calculating the risk of acute coronary events based on the 10-year follow-up of the prospective cardiovascular Münster (PROCAM) study. *Circulation* 2002; 105:310–315.

16. International Task Force for the Prevention of Coronary Heart Disease & International Atherosclerosis Society. Pocket Guide to Prevention of Coronary Heart Disease. Börm Bruckmeier Verlag GmbH, 2003.

17. Haq IU, Ramsay LE, Yeo WW, Jackson PR, Wallis EJ. Is the Framingham risk function valid for northern European populations? A comparison of methods for estimating absolute coronary risk in high risk men. *Heart* (Br Cardiac Soc) 1999; 81:40–46.

18. Hense HW, Schulte H, Lowel H, Assmann G, Keil U. Framingham risk function overestimates risk of coronary heart disease in men and women from Germany – results from the MONICA Augsburg and the PROCAM cohorts. *Eur Heart J* 2003; 24:937–945.

19. Menotti A, Puddu PE, Lanti M. Comparison of the Framingham risk function-based coronary chart with risk function from an Italian population study. *Eur Heart J* 2000; 21:365–370.

20. Marrugat J, D'Agostino R, Sullivan L *et al.* An adaptation of the Framingham coronary heart disease risk function to European Mediterranean areas. *J Epidemiol Commun Health* 2003; 57:634–638.

21. http://www.escardio.org/initiatives/prevention/HeartScore.html.

22. Thomsen TF, Davidsen M, Jorgensen HIT, Jensen G, Borch-Johnsen K. A new method for CHD prediction and prevention based on regional risk scores and randomized clinical trials; PRECARD and the Copenhagen Risk Score. *J Cardiovasc Risk* 2001; 8:291–297.

23. Bonnevie L, Thomsen T, Jørgensen T. The use of computerized decision support systems in preventive cardiology – principal results from the national PRECARD survey in Denmark. *Eur J Cardiovasc Prev Rehabil* 2005; 12:52–55.

24. Kannel WB, Feinleib M, McNamara PM, Garrison RJ, Castelli WP. An investigation of coronary heart disease in families: the Framingham Offspring Study. *Am J Epidemiol* 1979; 110:281–290.

25. Kannel WB, Dawber TR, Kagan A *et al.* Factors of risk in the development of coronary artery disease – six-year follow up experience; the Framingham study. *Ann Intern Med* 1961; 55:33–50.

26. American Heart Association: Coronary Risk Handbook: Estimating the Risk of Coronary Heart Disease in Daily Practice. Dallas, Texas, 1973.

27. Anderson KM, Wilson PWF, Odell PM, Kannel WB. An updated coronary risk profile. *Circulation* 1991; 83:356–362.

28. Chobanian AV, Bakris GL, Black HR *et al.* National Heart, Lung, and Blood Institute Joint National Committee on Prevention, Detection, Evaluation, and Treatment of High Blood Pressure. National High Blood Pressure Education Program Co-ordinating Committee. The Seventh Report of the Joint National Committee on Prevention, Detection, Evaluation, and Treatment of High Blood Pressure: the JNC 7 report. *JAMA* 2003; 289:2560–2572.

29. Woodward M, Brindle P, Tunstall-Pedoe H; for the SIGN group on risk estimation. Adding social deprivation and family history to cardiovascular risk assessment: the ASSIGN score from the Scottish Heart Health Extended Cohort (SHHEC). *Heart* 2007; 93:172–176.

30. Hippisley-Cox J, Coupland C, Vinogradova Y, Robson J, May M, Brindle P. Derivation and validation of QRISK, a new cardiovascular disease risk score for the United Kingdom: prospective open cohort study. *BMJ* 2007; 335:136–147.

31. Tunstall-Pedoe H, Woodward M. By neglecting deprivation, cardiovascular risk scoring will exacerbate the social gradients in disease. *Heart* 2006; 92:307–310.

32. Tunstall-Pedoe H, Woodward M. FRAMINGHAM, ASSIGN and QRISK cardiovascular risk scores. www.bmj.com/cgi/eletters/335/7611/136#172180, accessed 9th October 2007.

33. Cooney MT, Dudina AL, Graham IM. QRISK – Methodological limitations? www.bmj.com/cgi/eletters/335/7611/136#172411, accessed 9th October 2007.
34. Hippisley-Cox J, Coupland C, Vinogradova Y, May M, Brindle P. QRISK – authors response. www.bmj.com/cgi/eletters/335/7611/136#174181, accessed 9th October 2007.
35. Hippisley-Cox J, Coupland C, Vinogradova Y, Robson J, Brindle P. Performance of the QRISK cardiovascular risk prediction algorithm in an independent UK sample of patients from general practice: a validation study. *Heart* 2008; 94:34–39.

12

Epidemiological research and preventive cardiology: lessons from Framingham

W. B. Kannel, R. B. D'Agostino, Sr

INTRODUCTION

CONTRIBUTIONS TO PREVENTIVE CARDIOLOGY

Six decades of Framingham Study research have prospectively investigated the prevalence, incidence, clinical manifestations, lifetime risk, prognosis, secular trends and predisposing factors for the development of atherosclerotic cardiovascular disease (CVD). By maintaining continuous constant participant contact and intensive surveillance, this population research illuminated the full clinical spectrum of CVD including not only standard outcomes such as recognized myocardial infarction and completed documented strokes, but also sudden coronary deaths, unrecognized myocardial infarctions, silent strokes and presymptomatic peripheral artery disease.

The Framingham Study provided early evidence that CVD is preceded by biologically plausible and correctable predisposing independent risk factors impacting on atherogenic mechanisms [1], making it one of the most cited references in the cardiovascular medical literature [2]. It helped place prevention at the forefront of cardiology by establishing the risk factor concept for the evolution of CVD, recognizing that it is unlikely that there is a single cause that is both essential and sufficient for its development. The Study alerted physicians to the ominous implications of 'benign essential' hypertension, intermittent claudication, atrial fibrillation (AF), left ventricular hypertrophy, heart failure, type 2 diabetes, small amounts of proteinuria, and reduced vital capacity [3]. It provided the first prospective population-based documented data on familial aggregation of CVD, determining its hazard based on examination and long-term follow-up of parents and their offspring.

Clinical misconceptions were corrected about systolic hypertension, arterial rigidity, pulse pressure, dyslipidaemia, diabetes, smoking, AF, obesity, physical exercise and the efficacy of hormone replacement therapy [3]. It substantiated and quantified the risk of carotid stenosis and wall thickness, high homocysteine and haemostatic factors. It delineated the important distinction between usual (average) and optimal levels of risk factors.

The Framingham Study devised multivariable CVD risk profiles for use in preventing CVD that enabled physicians to pull together relevant risk factor information on their patients, allowing a more precise assessment of their risk [4–9]. These risk assessment tools

William B. Kannel, MD, MPH, Professor of Medicine and Public Health, Boston University School of Medicine, Framingham Heart Study, Framingham, Massachusetts, USA

Ralph B. D'Agostino, Sr, PhD, Professor of Mathematics/Statistics and Public Health, Director of Data Management and Statistical Analysis of Framingham Study, Mathematics and Statistics Department, Framingham Study, Boston University, Boston, Massachusetts, USA

Table 12.1 Framingham risk assessment: a cholesterol management implementation tool based on ATP III (Available on: http:/hin.nhlbi.nih.gov/atpiii/calculator.asp)

NATIONAL CHOLESTEROL EDUCATION PROGRAM
Third Report of the Expert Panel on
Detection, Evaluation, and Treatment of High Blood Cholesterol in Adults (Adult Treatment Panel III)

**Risk Assessment Toll for Estimating 10-year Risk of Developing Hard CHD
(Myocardial Infarction and Coronary Death)**

The risk assessment tool below uses recent data from the Framingham Heart Study to estimate 10-year risk for 'hard' coronary heart disease outcomes (myocardial infarction and coronary death). This tool is designed to estimate risk in adults aged 20 and older who do not have heart disease or diabetes. Use the calculator below to estimate 10-year risk.

Age:	[____] years
Gender:	○ Female ○ Male
Total Cholesterol:	[____] mg/dl
HDL Cholesterol:	[____] mg/dl
Smoker:	○ No ○ Yes
Systolic Blood Pressure:	[____] mm/Hg
Currently on any medication to treat high blood pressure:	○ No ○ Yes

Calculate 10-Year Risk

have been validated and shown to be transportable (with calibration) to culturally diverse populations [10].

Identification of major *risk factors*, a term coined by the Framingham Study [11], stimulated a greater interest in preventive cardiology and made cardiovascular epidemiology its basic science. It established the utility of the risk factor concept for gaining valuable insights into the development and prevention of chronic diseases making it a prototype for other epidemiological studies around the world. It exerted a major influence on cohort study design using the risk factor concept. In evaluating predisposing factors for CVD, epidemiologists were motivated to conceptualize disease as an outcome of multiple forces, now an important doctrine of modern epidemiology. This concept has had clinical, public health, preventive and therapeutic applications.

Multivariable assessment

The Framingham Study pioneered the concept of multivariable risk assessment, and analysis [5]. Framingham Study multivariable risk formulations, requiring only input of ordinary office procedures and readily available blood tests, are now procurable to facilitate office estimation of the risk of coronary heart disease (CHD) (Table 12.1), stroke, peripheral artery disease, and heart failure outcomes [4–9]. Framingham Study risk profiles have been tested in a variety of population samples and found to be reasonably accurate, except for populations with very low coronary disease rates [12, 13, 14]. However, even in these areas, high-risk persons can be distinguished from those at low risk and after calibration the true absolute risk can be estimated [10]. The homogenous nature of the Framingham population sample prevents simple extrapolation of Framingham multivariable risk assessment instruments to other populations. However, by calibrating the Framingham Study multivariable risk function, it was possible to adapt the Framingham risk profile for use in European

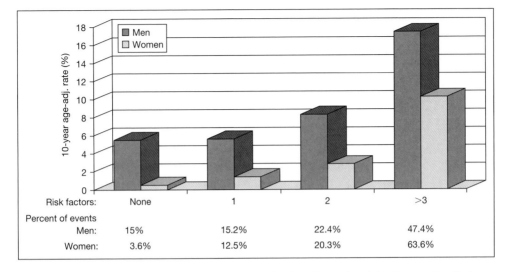

Figure 12.1   Risk of coronary attacks in the obese by burden of associated risk factors (Framingham Study subjects aged 30–74 years: associated risk factors: age, SBP, cholesterol, diabetes, smoking, heart rate ECG-LVH).

Mediterranean and Asian areas [15, 16]. Risk factors relate to CVD occurrence in a continuous graded fashion, extending down into the perceived 'normal' range, without indication of a critical value. For each defined risk factor, CVD risk varies widely in accordance with the burden of accompanying risk factors [17]. National guidelines are now linking treatment goals to global CHD risk [18]. CVD risk factors seldom occur in isolation from each other and it is postulated that an insulin resistance syndrome may be the metabolic basis for the tendency of atherogenic risk factors to cluster [19]. Weight gain leading to visceral adiposity promotes a cluster of risk factors that have been characterized as an insulin resistant *metabolic syndrome* and the hazard associated with obesity increases with the burden of atherogenic risk factors that accompany it (Figure 12.1). When confronted with a patient with any particular CVD risk factor, it is essential to test for the others that coexist with it 80% of the time. Now that guidelines for dyslipidaemia, hypertension and diabetes recommend treating modest abnormality, candidates for treatment are best targeted by global risk assessment so that the number needed to treat to prevent one event can be minimized.

Because of shared modifiable risk factors, the CHD risk profile also predicts other atherosclerotic CVD outcomes and measures taken to prevent any one outcome can be expected to also benefit the others. Novel risk factors under investigation at Framingham and elsewhere deserve attention, but the standard CVD risk factors identified by the Framingham Study appear to account for as much as 90% of the coronary disease arising within the population [20].

DELINEATION OF THE FULL CVD CLINICAL SPECTRUM

Population appraisal of the total constellation of atherosclerotic CVD by the Framingham Study revealed that CHD is an extremely common and highly lethal disease that attacks one in five persons before they attain 60 years of age, that women lag men in incidence by 10 years, and that sudden death is a prominent feature of coronary mortality. One in every six coronary attacks was found to present with sudden death as the first, last, and only symptom of the presence of coronary disease [21].

It also became evident that coronary disease can be asymptomatic in its most severe form, with one in three myocardial infarctions going unrecognized because it is either silent

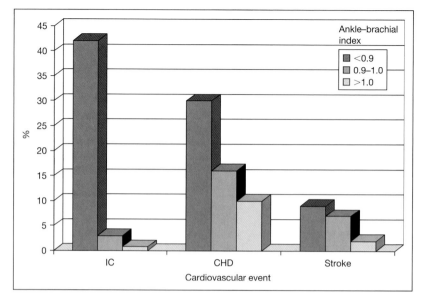

Figure 12.2 CVD prevalence by ankle-brachial index (Framingham Offspring Study). With permission from [24]. IC = intermittent claudication.

or atypical and, similarly, that strokes can be silent [22, 23]. Among persons with initial strokes, 10% were found to have computed tomography evidence of prior silent strokes and that, as with silent myocardial infarction, glucose intolerance was a strong risk factor for their occurrence [23]. The Study also confirmed that silent peripheral artery disease is common and detectable by the ankle-brachial index which, when abnormal, carries a substantial risk of overt peripheral artery disease and CVD in general [24] (Figure 12.2). Because of the clandestine nature of potentially lethal CVD, a preventive approach is essential.

MAGNITUDE OF THE PROBLEM

For decades, national statistics on CVD were largely confined to mortality derived from death certificate data. Population data from the Framingham Study for a long time provided the only information available on the incidence of non-fatal CVD. Despite identification of major modifiable predisposing risk factors for its development, CHD remains the largest single killer of Americans, accounting for one of every five deaths in 2001 [25]. Stroke also remains a major cause of death and disability [25].

CVD imposes a $300 billion/year economic burden. In the US, heart attacks occur every 20 seconds. Each year 1.2 million Americans have a new (700 000) or recurrent (500 000) coronary event, with 40% dying of it. There are 13.2 million Americans who have a history of myocardial infarction and angina or both. During 2001, there were 922 000 deaths from CVD (38.5% of all deaths) and 6.2 million hospitalizations, constituting more than for any other disease group. About 60% of cardiac deaths occur before the victims reach a hospital underscoring the need for a preventive approach [26].

LIFETIME RISK

More than five decades of surveillance of the Framingham Study cohort has enabled ascertainment of lifetime risk of cardiovascular events. The remaining lifetime risk of coronary

Table 12.2 Lifetime risk of coronary disease according to Framingham Multivariable Risk Score: Framingham Study, 1971–1996

Tertiles of Framingham Multivariable Risk Score	Lifetime risk for CHD			
	At age 40 years		At age 80 years	
	Men (%)	Women (%)	Men (%)	Women (%)
Tertile 1	38.4	12.2	16.4	12.8
Tertile 2	41.7	25.5	17.4	22.4
Tertile 3	50.7	33.2	38.8	27.4
With permission from [29].				

disease for 40-year-old men was found to be about 49% and for women 32% [27]. This lifetime risk was shown to increase stepwise with the serum cholesterol [28], and with the total risk factor burden [28]. Subjects with two or more risk factors had substantially higher lifetime coronary disease risks than those with optimal risk factors (5.2% vs. 68.9% for men and 8.2% vs. 50.2% for women). Lifetime risk increases progressively with tertiles of multivariable risk [29] (Table 12.2). These data are useful for communicating risk to patients and support the need for intensive preventive therapy linked to the level of risk.

Based on Framingham Study surveillance, the lifetime chance of a stroke was found to be one in six for men and one in five for women. This was equal to the risk for Alzheimer Disease in women and greater than the Alzheimer risk for men. Hypertension doubled the lifetime stroke risk compared to normotensive persons [30].

The Framingham Study also estimated lifetime risks for AF. At age 40 years, lifetime risks for AF were 26.0% for men and 23.0% for women, which did not change substantially with increasing index age despite decreasing remaining years of life. Even when unassociated with heart failure or myocardial infarction, lifetime risk of AF was approximately 16%. These substantial lifetime risks indicate the major public health burden posed by AF and the need for further investigation into predisposing conditions, preventive strategies, and more effective therapies [31]. The Framingham Study also found an astonishingly high lifetime risk of developing hypertension, estimating that as many as nine out of every ten Americans are at risk of developing high blood pressure (BP) at some point in their lives [32].

The population long-term risks for development of overweight and obesity were not known until the Framingham Study investigation in 2005. For persons of 50 years of age, the lifetime risk for overweight (body mass index [BMI] $>25 \, kg/m^2$) was found to be 50% and for obesity (BMI $>30 \, kg/m^2$) 25%, and for gross obesity (BMI $>35 \, kg/m^2$) 10% [33].

The Framingham Study was the first to make known the highly lethal nature of heart failure, pointing out that its survival rate was no better than that for cancer [34]. Recent determination of the lifetime risk of this end-stage cardiovascular condition revealed that persons aged 40 or older have a one in five chance of developing heart failure. Hypertension was the most important risk factor in women and a coronary attack an important contributor to lifetime heart failure risk in men [35].

CLINICAL MISCONCEPTIONS CORRECTED

Hypertension

Prior to the Framingham Study, there was a concept of *benign essential hypertension* and a lack of effective and tolerable means for lowering BP, so that emphasis was placed on identifying correctable causes of hypertension. Because of population research at Framingham

Table 12.3   Risk of CVD by systolic vs. diastolic BP: Framingham Study 38-year follow-up

Risk factor adjusted increment per standard deviation increase				
	BP			
	Systolic		*Diastolic*	
Age	*Men*	*Women*	*Men*	*Women*
35–64	40%	38%	37%	29%
65–94	41%	25%	25%	15%
	Type of hypertension			
	Age-adjusted risk ratio			
Age	*Isolated systolic*		*Isolated diastolic*	
35–64	2.4***	1.9**	1.8*	1.2
65–94	1.9**	1.4**	1.2*	1.6***

Covariates: cholesterol, glucose, cigarettes, ECG-left ventricular hypertrophy. All differences in incremental risk significant at $P < 0.001$. For risk ratios: *$P < 0.05$; **$P < 0.01$; ***$P < 0.001$.

With permission from [36].

and elsewhere, routine testing to identify causes of hypertension is no longer recommended unless there are history or physical findings suggestive of secondary hypertension or BP control cannot be achieved. Identifiable underlying causes were found to be responsible for only a small percentage of the hypertension encountered in clinical practice. One common possible cause now being considered is obesity-induced *insulin resistance or the metabolic syndrome* which may be responsible for a substantial amount of hypertension.

Before Framingham Study investigation, it was believed that the common variety of hypertension was benign and that it was essential for the BP to rise with age to ensure adequate perfusion of vital organs. Its cardiovascular sequelae were believed to derive chiefly from the diastolic pressure component and it was held that the disproportionate rise in systolic BP with age was an innocuous accompaniment of arterial stiffening. Hence it was believed that treatment of isolated systolic hypertension would not only be fruitless but also intolerable and dangerous. The tenaciously held belief in the prime importance of the diastolic pressure was convincingly refuted by Framingham Study data and later confirmed by other prospective data, demonstrating that the impact of systolic pressure is actually greater than the diastolic component [37, 38]. Examination of the increment in CVD risk per standard deviation increment in systolic vs. diastolic BP, to take into account the different range of values for each, indicated a consistently greater impact for the systolic BP (Table 12.3).

Women were thought to tolerate hypertension well, and it was believed that *normal* BPs in both sexes were substantially higher in the elderly than in the middle-aged. Regarding hypertensive cardiovascular hazards, it was held that there were age-related critical thresholds for BP. As indicated in Table 12.4, Framingham Study data indicate that while the hypertensive risk ratios for all the major atherosclerotic CVD events are larger for those under than over age 65 years of age, the incidence of disease is clearly greater in the elderly. Systolic BPs formerly regarded as *normal* for the elderly (100 plus age mmHg) were shown to impose a substantial CVD risk. Also, while the incidence of all events except stroke in the

Table 12.4   Risk of cardiovascular events in hypertension according to age and sex: Framingham Study 36-year follow-up

	Age 35–64 years				Age 65–94 years			
	Rate		Risk ratio		Rate		Risk ratio	
Events	Men	Women	Men	Women	Men	Women	Men	Women
CHD	45	21	2.0	2.2	72	44	1.6	1.9
Stroke	12	6	3.8	2.6	36	38	1.9	2.3
PAD	10	7	2.0	3.7	17	10	1.6	2.0
CHF	14	6	4.0	3.0	33	24	1.9	1.9

All biennial rates per 1000 at risk and risk ratios are age-adjusted and statistically significant at $P < 0.0001$. CHD = coronary heart disease; CHF = congestive heart failure; PAD = peripheral artery disease.

elderly are lower in women than men, the risk ratios in women are similar to those in men. Thus, neither the elderly nor women tolerate hypertension well.

Initiation of antihypertensive treatment was often delayed until there was evidence of target organ involvement. Framingham Study data indicated that this practice was imprudent because 40–50% of hypertensive persons developed overt CVD prior to evidence of proteinuria, cardiomegaly or electrocardiograph (ECG) abnormalities.

Medical concepts about the hazards of hypertension were preoccupied with the diastolic BP component from the beginning of the 20th century and, even today, there appears to be lingering uncertainty about the CVD impact of the various components of the BP. Influenced by Framingham Study findings, the focus has shifted to the systolic BP and, most recently, to the pulse pressure [39]. An increased pulse pressure in advanced age was considered an innocuous accompaniment of progressive arterial rigidity. However, assessment of pressure components in the Framingham Study indicated that increments of pulse pressure at particular systolic pressures are associated with increased CHD incidence. Framingham Study investigation found that with increasing age there is a shift in importance from diastolic to systolic and finally to pulse pressure for prediction of CHD [40].

Based on Framingham Study data, the current concept of an *acceptable* BP is now based on what is *optimal* for avoiding hypertension-related CVD rather than on what is *usual*. Epidemiological data from the Framingham Study clearly indicate that at all ages and in both sexes, CVD risk increases incrementally with the BP even within the 'normal' range. Similar graded relationships of BP to CHD and all-cause mortality have been reported in several other cohorts [41–43]. There is no threshold for BP risk as claimed by some and in the Framingham cohort 45% of the CVD events in men occurred at a systolic BP <140 mmHg, the value recently claimed by some to be the threshold of risk [41, 44]. Large data sets are available that precisely estimate CVD incidence trends in the lower BP range. Both the Multiple Risk Factor Intervention Trial (MRFIT) data on over 350 000 men screened and followed for CVD mortality, and the Prospective Studies Collaboration involving almost one million participants and 56 000 vascular deaths found no indication of a threshold of risk down to 115/75 mmHg [42, 43]. Persons aged 40–69 years had a doubling of stroke or CHD mortality with every 20/10 mmHg increment of BP throughout its entire range. Recent examination of the relation of non-hypertensive BP to the rate of development of CVD in the Framingham Study found a significant graded influence of BP from optimal (<120/80 mmHg) to normal (120–129/80–84 mmHg) to high-normal (130–139/85–89 mmHg)

Table 12.5 Relation of non-hypertensive BP categories to development of CVD

Framingham Study subjects ages 35–90 years 10-year cumulative incidence	Women		Men	
BP category (mmHg)	Age-adj rate	HR	Age-adj rate	HR
Optimal (120/80)	1.9%	1.0	5.8%	1.0
Normal (120–129/80–84)	2.8%	1.1 (0.6–3.1)	7.6%	1.3 (0.8–1.9)
High-normal (130–139/85–89)	4.4%	1.8 (1.0–3.1)	10.1%	1.6 (1.1–2.3)
P for trend across categories:	<0.001		<0.001	

Stratified by examination. HR = hazard ratio adjusted for age, BMI, cholesterol, diabetes, cigarette smoking.

With permission from [45].

Table 12.6 Control of systolic vs. diastolic BP: Framingham Study participants 1990–1995

	All hypertensives	On treatment
Control of:	(n = 1995)	(n = 1189)
Systolic BP (<140 mmHg)	33%	49%
Diastolic BP (<90 mmHg)	83%	90%
Both (<140/90 mmHg)	30%	48%

Covariates associated with poor systolic BP control: older age, obesity, left ventricular hypertrophy.

With permission from [46].

among untreated men and women [45]. Compared with optimal, high-normal BP conferred a 1.6- to 2.5- fold age- and risk factor-adjusted risk of a CVD event (Table 12.5).

The chief hazard of hypertension was believed to be a stroke. Framingham Study established that although its risk ratios are no larger than for other cardiovascular events, the most common hazard for hypertensive patients of all ages is coronary disease, equalling in incidence all the other hypertensive atherosclerotic consequences combined (Table 12.4). Hypertension was shown to predispose to all clinical manifestations of CHD including myocardial infarction, angina pectoris and sudden death, imposing a two- to three-fold increased risk.

Despite the demonstrated efficacy of treating *systolic* hypertension, poor BP control is overwhelmingly due to failure to control the systolic pressure component [46] (Table 12.6). Guidelines now place greater emphasis on achieving specified *systolic* BP goals.

It has been alleged that there is an increased CVD risk at low as well as at high diastolic BP (a so-called J-curve) causing fear of lowering the diastolic BP too much. The Framingham Study tested prospectively the hypothesis that the upturn in CVD incidence at low diastolic BP is largely confined to persons with increased systolic pressure and hence reflecting risk from an increased pulse pressure [47]. The ten-year risk associated with 951 non-fatal CVD events and 205 CVD deaths was estimated at diastolic pressures of <80, 80–90, and >90 mmHg, according to concomitant systolic BP. An increasing tendency for a J-curve relation

Table 12.7 Incidence of non-fatal cardiovascular events by diastolic pressure at specified levels of systolic BP. Framingham Study cohorts: subjects: men and women aged 35–80 years

10-year incidence rate (%)			
	Systolic BP		
Diastolic BP	*<140 mmHg*	*140–159 mmHg*	*≥160 mmHg*
<80 mmHg	7.2	29.8	36.0
80–89 mmHg	9.2	16.7	29.0
>90 mmHg	16.2	17.2	27.9
With permission from [47].			

of CVD incidence to diastolic BP was observed with successive increments in accompanying systolic BP (Table 12.7). In both sexes, a statistically significant excess of CVD events was observed at diastolic BPs <80 mmHg only when accompanied by a systolic pressure >140 mmHg, and this persisted after adjustment for age and associated CVD risk factors [46]. Persons with this condition of isolated systolic hypertension have been shown to benefit from antihypertensive treatment [48, 49].

Left ventricular hypertrophy

Hypertrophy of the left ventricle was originally considered compensatory, helping the heart deal with a pressure overload. Left ventricular hypertrophy was shown by the Framingham Study to be an ominous harbinger of CVD rather than an incidental compensatory response to hypertension, CHD, and heart valve deformity. The Framingham Study showed that left ventricular hypertrophy is an ominous feature of hypertension that independently escalates the risk of future CVD, equivalent to that of persons who already have overt atherosclerotic CVD [50].

Atrial fibrillation (AF)

AF is the most common cardiac dysrhythmia and a source of considerable morbidity and mortality. Before the Framingham Study report on the significance of non-rheumatic AF in 1982, its prognosis was believed to depend chiefly on the CVD with which it was associated. AF unassociated with CVD was considered benign and unassociated with excess mortality. Further, the risk of embolism was not considered excessive unless the fibrillation was paroxysmal, or associated with mitral stenosis. Framingham Study data showed that chronic sustained AF was actually more dangerous than the intermittent variety and further increased the stroke risk associated with coronary disease and cardiac failure [51]. Wolf *et al.* [52] in 1987 summarized insights of the Framingham Study concerning the stroke risk imposed. AF was found to increase stroke risk five-fold, causing strokes that are 70% fatal, or at least moderately severe [52]. These revelations stimulated trials resulting in effective therapies for AF.

Dyslipidaemia

The role of dietary and plasma cholesterol in the evolution of coronary disease was for a long time in dispute. It took epidemiological research to convince skeptics that serum cholesterol was a true risk factor for coronary disease, and that the lipoprotein-cholesterol fractions were fundamental to atherogenesis. Diets rich in saturated fat and cholesterol presumed to be healthy, were shown to promote dyslipidaemia and its cardiovascular sequelae [53]. Population research, including Framingham, also established that high-density

Table 12.8   Relation of blood lipids and their ratios to CHD occurrence: 20-year follow-up of Framingham offspring cohort

Relative risk				
	Age-adj Q_5/Q_1		Multivariable adj Q_5/Q_1	
Lipid parameter	Men	Women	Men	Women
Total cholesterol	2.4 (1.8–3.2)	4.1 (2.4–7.1)	2.3 (1.7–3.1)	3.7 (2.2–6.5)
HDL-c	2.2 (1.7–2.9)	2.4 (1.7–3.4)	2.1 (1.6–2.7)	1.8 (1.2–2.6)
LDL-c	1.9 (1.4–2.4)	4.6 (2.8–7.7)	1.8 (1.4–2.4)	3.9 (2.3–6.5)
Total/HDL ratio	2.9 (2.2–3.9)	4.8 (3.0–7.8)	2.8 (2.1–3.8)	3.8 (2.3–6.1)
LDL/HDL-c	2.7 (2.1–3.6)	4.4 (2.8–6.9)	2.7 (2.0–3.6)	3.5 (2.2–5.5)

lipoprotein cholesterol (HDL-c) was actually a strong independent risk factor inversely related to the development of coronary disease [54, 55].

Lipid risk of CHD was initially designated categorically as a cholesterol value greater than two standard deviations over the mean (>310 mg/dl). However, the average cholesterol value at which coronary cases occurred in the Framingham Study was found to be well within what was designated as the *normal* range of 200–310 mg/dl. Risk of CHD in the Framingham Study was found to increase incrementally over a five-fold range with the serum cholesterol and this included the purported normal range.

As early as 1979, the Framingham Study reported that cholesterol was a powerful independent risk factor for coronary disease with an impact that is augmented by the presence of other risk factors and influenced by its partition in lipoprotein fractions. It concluded that the widely held belief 'that all lipid information pertaining to CHD resides in the total cholesterol' must be modified [56]. Further investigation revealed that the serum total cholesterol reflected a two-way traffic of cholesterol in the low-density lipoprotein (LDL) and HDL and that the joint effect of these components is indicated by the total/HDL-c ratio. The total/HDL-c ratio was found to be the best lipid profile for estimating the dyslipidaemic risk of CHD (Table 12.8) [57]. This total/HDL-c ratio predicted coronary disease occurrence whether or not the total cholesterol was elevated.

Diabetes

When the Framingham Study began investigating factors predisposing to CVD, proper control of diabetes was deemed advisable but there was uncertainty as to whether coronary atherosclerosis is more frequent or severe in the uncontrolled diabetic. It was held that diabetics, including type 2 diabetics, were subject to microvascular but not macrovascular disease. The Framingham Study provided data that type 2 diabetes was a powerful independent risk for all the major atherosclerotic CVD outcomes [58]. Diabetes was shown to operate more powerfully in women, eliminating their advantage over men for most atherosclerotic cardiovascular events [58].

Increased risk of CHD has now been reported in persons with impaired glucose tolerance, in the metabolic syndrome and in type 2 diabetes [59]. The Framingham Study established that the CVD risk of type 2 diabetes varies depending on the amount of clustering with other metabolically linked risk factors [60]. This insight prompted the Framingham Study to suggest that there is more to be gained by correcting the associated risk factors than by tightly controlling the hyperglycaemia. The cluster of risk factors commonly accompanying diabetes is chiefly what is now designated as the *metabolic syndrome*. For type 2 diabetics more emphasis should be placed on correcting the components of the metabolic insulin resistance syndrome than on controlling the blood sugar; which has not been consistently shown to reduce CVD risk. The CVD risk factors that comprise the syndrome (obesity, glucose, triglycerides, HDL-c and BP are each predictors of diabetes itself, so that the metabolic syndrome composed of three or more of them imposes a five-fold increased risk of type 2 diabetes [61].

Smoking

Epidemiological research at the Framingham Study in collaboration with others was required to demonstrate that cigarette smoking was not only a carcinogen for lung cancer but also a substantial risk for atherosclerotic CVD. The Framingham Study provided valuable information about the relation of cigarette smoking to CVD [62]. Its population research established that smoking is a major risk factor for CHD, precipitating coronary attacks and sudden deaths, especially in high-risk coronary candidates. It showed that risk of coronary attacks could be promptly halved in smokers who quit, regardless of how long or how much they previously smoked [63, 64]. Smoking cessation led within two years to a reduction of CVD risk almost equivalent to non-smokers, except for the occurrence of intermittent claudication [65]. Smoking was also shown to be a hazard for stroke and peripheral artery disease [66, 67].

Exercise

Before its epidemiological investigation, physical exercise was considered dangerous for cardiac candidates. Population research established that physical activity is actually protective, but in a study of civil servants Morris *et al.* [68] claimed that only vigorous aerobic exercise in men actively participating in sports led to a lower heart attack incidence. However, the Framingham Study established that only moderate amounts of exercise were required, the position now adopted by the American Heart Association [69].

Obesity

There was much scepticism about the importance of obesity as a risk factor for CVD [70–72]. This was dispelled by Framingham epidemiological research demonstrating that obesity and weight gain promote all the major cardiovascular risk factors [73]. Abdominal obesity was shown to be particularly important because it promotes insulin resistance and the *metabolic syndrome* recently defined by the Third Report of the Adult Treatment Panel (ATP III) guidelines [59]. The average number of cardiovascular risk factors acquired by Framingham Study participants of both sexes was found to increase in relation to their body mass index and among the obese the risk of coronary attacks was found to increase with the associated burden of these acquired cardiovascular risk factors (Figure 12.1). There was dispute about whether variability in weight (usually resulting from repeated unsuccessful attempts at weight reduction) was hazardous. The Framingham Study data suggested that variability in weight may carry an excess CVD risk [74].

Proteinuria

Small amounts of protein or albumin in the urine were largely ignored as inconsequential prior to Framingham Study evaluation of its significance in 1984. Investigation of the prognostic significance of proteinuria as it occurs in the general population indicated that even a trace of proteinuria, in casual urine specimens, carries a three-fold excess mortality rate, and that its prevalence was three times more common in hypertensive persons and also occurred in excess in diabetics and persons with cardiac enlargement [75]. Among men, proteinuria was associated with increased overall and CVD mortality rates even when other contributing risk factors were taken into account. It concluded that proteinuria in the ambulatory general population is not benign, carries a serious prognosis and appears to reflect widespread vascular damage. Proteinuria and microalbuminuria are now accepted as important *new* risk factors for CVD.

Menopause

Women in affluent countries have lower coronary disease rates than men, but their risk abruptly increases three-fold once they become post-menopausal compared to women of the same age who remain pre-menopausal. The escalation of risk was largely attributed to loss of the cardioprotective effects of oestrogen [76]. The Framingham Study, based on long-term surveillance, routine collection of information preceding post-menopausal oestrogen treatment, accurate information on the age of menopause, and confirmed details about the nature of surgical menopause, provided a critical appraisal of the consequences of undergoing the menopause and post-menopausal use of oestrogen in relation to risk of coronary disease. These data indicated an abrupt three-fold increase in CVD risk on undergoing the menopause compared to women the same age remaining pre-menopausal. There was no difference depending on whether the menopause was natural or surgical and, surprisingly, no difference in the adverse effect of surgical menopause in relation to whether the ovaries were or were not removed. The clinical manifestations of CHD shifted from a predominance of angina pectoris to that of myocardial infarction and sudden death [77, 78]. The rapid escalation of the risk, the shift to development of the more serious forms of coronary disease, and the adverse effect of surgical menopause independent of removal of the ovaries, suggested something more than oestrogen deficiency at work. A loss of protection against arterial thrombogenesis seemed a likely possibility.

A study by Ritterband *et al.* [79] comparing coronary disease experience of women with hysterectomy including bilateral oophorectomy with that of those having only hysterectomy found, like the Framingham Study, no difference in CHD risk, leading them, because of the lack of a control group, to the erroneous conclusion that surgical menopause did not increase CHD risk. Not all investigations of the relation of surgical menopause to CVD have found an increased CVD risk independent of whether the ovaries were removed or not. Bush *et al.* [80] reported that oophorectomized women not taking oestrogen had high rates of CVD, whereas women who only had a hysterectomy had no increased risk of a CVD death. In fact, they reported that hysterectomized women had *lower* CVD rates than women who were intact, leading them to conclude that women selected for hysterectomy were actually healthier.

Observational data concerning benefits of hormone replacement therapy, while not definitive because of the inherent possibility of selection bias, can be useful by observing unanticipated hazards needing further investigation. Reviewing the epidemiological evidence in 1991, Stampfer and Colditz [81] pointed out that of 16 *prospective* studies, 15 found decreased relative risks, statistically significant in most instances. They concluded that, overall, the bulk of evidence strongly supports a protective effect of oestrogens that is unlikely to be explained by confounding factors. Taking all the studies together, they estimated a relative risk of 0.50–0.56. The Framingham Study alone showed no benefit and possible increased risk for stroke.

Recent trials examining the efficacy of hormone replacement therapy question our understanding of the influence of the menopause and the alleged protective role of oestrogen for atherosclerotic CVD. It surprised many when large randomized clinical trials reported that hormone replacement therapy in women with or without coronary disease did not reduce their risk of future events [82, 83], causing the American Heart Association to recommend that hormone replacement therapy not be initiated solely for *secondary prevention* of CVD [84]. The Women's Health Initiative Randomized Controlled Trial of the risks and benefits of a combined oestrogen-progestin hormone preparation for *primary* prevention was stopped after 5.2 years of follow-up because of excessive occurrence of breast cancer and evidence of risks exceeding benefits. For vascular endpoints, there was a 29% *excess* of coronary disease,

41% excess of stroke, and two-fold excess of pulmonary embolism. It was concluded that this hormone regimen should not be initiated or continued for *primary* prevention of CHD [82].

Consistent with this recent finding, Wilson *et al.* [85] reported in 1985 the results of an observational study of the effect of oestrogen use on morbidity and mortality from CVD in a Framingham Study sample of post-menopausal women aged 50–80 years. Despite a more favourable risk profile to begin with and control for the major cardiovascular risk factors, women reporting oestrogen use had more than a 50% *increased* cardiovascular morbidity and two-fold greater risk for stroke in particular ($P < 0.01$). Increased myocardial infarction rates were observed, especially in oestrogen users who smoked. CVD mortality did not differ in relation to oestrogen use. Thus, the Framingham Study data did not show any benefit, and it was concluded that *'the potential drawbacks of post-menopausal oestrogen therapy should be considered carefully before recommending its widespread use'*.

SOME MORE RECENT ACCOMPLISHMENTS

From the 1980s to the present the Framingham study has been engaged in the study of subclinical manifestations of CVD such as carotid stenosis and wall thickness, the role of novel CVD markers such as haemostatic, inflammatory and biomarkers and the investigation of secular trends in CVD and its risk factors. C-reactive protein (CRP) is currently considered the best indicator of vascular inflammation that can be reliably measured. Consistent with most investigations of clinical and subclinical vascular disease in relation to CRP, the Framingham Study found that CRP alone is an effective discriminator of coronary and CVD cases. However, from the Framingham experience, inclusion of CRP testing did not appear to provide great benefit for multivariable CVD risk assessment because the C-statistic, that measures the ability of a multivariate risk assessment function to discriminate those who will develop CVD from those who will not, did not improve significantly when CRP is added to the traditional multivariable risk factor assessment [86].

Haemostatic factors associated with development of CVD include fibrinogen, tissue plasminogen activator antigen, plasminogen activator inhibitor-1, factor VII, and von Willebrand factor. Each standard deviation increment in these increases the association with CVD occurrence 24–30%. Most haemostatic factors are inter-correlated with inflammatory markers and LDL cholesterol. Fibrinogen seems the most fundamental haemostatic CVD risk factor. The Framingham Study reaffirmed its association with all the major risk factors showing linear risk factor trends across fibrinogen tertiles. Fibrinogen may also directly increase CVD risk because of its role in platelet aggregation, plasma viscosity and fibrin formation. Fibrinogen is an acute phase reactant that is elevated in inflammatory states and it may mediate the thrombogenic effect of other risk factors. Framingham Study data indicate that each standard deviation increase in fibrinogen imposes a 20% independent increment in CVD risk. It appears likely that fibrinogen and CRP may be useful for detecting persons at added risk for thrombotic CVD events [87].

SUMMARY

Risk factor alteration significantly reduces risk of initial and recurrent atherosclerotic CVD. Hypertension, dyslipidaemia and diabetes are best regarded as ingredients of a CVD multivariable risk profile comprised of metabolically linked risk factors because the hazard of each varies widely, contingent upon the associated burden of other risk factors. Maximum CVD risk reduction, even in diabetics, is best achieved by concomitant control of the accompanying burden of risk factors.

Evaluation and treatment of dyslipidaemia can be guided by the total/HDL-c ratio, and the aggressiveness of therapy linked to the global risk. In evaluation and treatment of hypertension there is no justification for reliance on the diastolic component of the BP. Isolated systolic hypertension and a widened pulse pressure auger ill and need to be treated at all ages. Antihypertensive therapy is safe, well tolerated and efficacious for CVD without any penalty of overall mortality. Physicians treating high-risk hypertension, dyslipidaemia, or diabetes can seek out more aggressive therapy in pre-clinical atherosclerotic disease signified by an abnormal ankle-brachial index, arterial vascular bruits, coronary artery calcification, left ventricular hypertrophy, a low ejection fraction, silent myocardial infarction, or protein-uria, among others. High-risk candidates with an ominous multivariable risk profile indi-cating a ten-year risk of a CVD event exceeding, for example, 20% require more aggressive risk factor modification. The goal of therapy of dyslipidaemia, diabetes and hypertension should be linked to the global level of risk. Framingham Study multivariable risk formula-tions, requiring input of ordinary office procedures and readily available blood tests, are procurable to facilitate office estimation of the risk of coronary disease, stroke, peripheral artery disease, and heart failure outcomes [4–9]. Because CVD risk factors usually cluster, and the risk imposed by each of them varies widely in relation to this, multivariable CVD risk assessment is a necessity, especially now that near average risk factor levels are recom-mended for treatment. Measures taken to prevent any one CVD outcome can be expected to also benefit the others. Novel risk factors deserve attention, but the standard CVD risk fac-tors appear to account for as much as 85% of the CVD arising within the population.

Just as the cardiovascular risk factors identified by the Framingham Study have been found to apply universally, the multivariable risk functions have been validated and found to have transportability in culturally diverse populations around the world, such as the Chinese and Spanish populations [15, 16]. Healthcare providers should undertake a multi-variable risk assessment whenever a patient is evaluated or treated for obesity, diabetes, dyslipidaemia, or hypertension. The laboratory being sent blood samples for testing of blood sugar, or blood lipids, should be encouraged to request the other ingredients of the CVD risk profile, including BP and cigarette smoking and provide a multivariable estimate of risk along with the requested lipid or glucose determination. Serial assessment of global risk should be used to monitor progress of patients on treatment and improvement in their multivariable risk score can motivate patients to comply with the recommended programme.

The CVD epidemic cannot be conquered solely by cardiologists caring for referred patients. The entire healthcare system has to be mobilized. Unfortunately, our healthcare system rewards doing procedures more than preventive services. Despite means available to identify high-risk candidates and proof of the efficacy of modifying predisposing risk fac-tors, goals for prevention of CVD are not often met. Physicians need to implement estab-lished guideline goals for management of dyslipidaemic, hypertensive and diabetic patients at risk of atherosclerotic CVD more aggressively.

ACKNOWLDEGEMENTS

Framingham Heart Study research is supported by NIH/NHLBI Contract No. N01-HC-25195 and the Visiting Scientist Program which is supported by AstraZeneca.

REFERENCES

1.   Cupples LA, D'Agostino RB. In: Kannel WB, Wolf PA, Garrison RJ (eds). Section 34: Some risk factors related to the annual incidence of cardiovascular disease and death using pooled repeated biennial measurements. Framingham Heart Study, 30-year follow-up. National Technical Information Service, Springfield, 1987.

2.   Mehta NJ, Kahn IA. Cardiology's 10 greatest discoveries of the 20th century. *Tex Heart Instit* 2002; 29:164–171.

3.   Kannel WB. Clinical misconceptions dispelled by epidemiological research. *Circulation* 1995; 92:3350–3360.

4.   Kannel WB, D'Agostino RB, Silbershatz H *et al*. Profile for estimating risk of heart failure. *Arch Intern Med* 1999; 159:1197–1204.

5.   Kannel WB, McGee DL, Gordon T. A general cardiovascular risk profile. The Framingham Study. *Am J Cardiol* 1976; 38:46–51.

6.   Anderson KM, Wilson PWF, Odell PM *et al*. An updated coronary risk profile: a statement for health professionals. *Circulation* 1991; 83:357–363.

7.   Wolf PA, D'Agostino RB, Belanger AJ *et al*. Probability of stroke: a risk profile from the Framingham Study. *Stroke* 1991; 3:312–318.

8.   Murabito JM, D'Agostino RB, Silberschatz H, Wilson PWF. Intermittent claudication: a risk profile from the Framingham Heart Study. *Circulation* 1997; 96:44–49.

9.   Wilson PWF, D'Agostino RB, Levy D *et al*. Prediction of coronary heart disease using risk factor categories. *Circulation* 1998; 97:1837–1847.

10.   D'Agostino RB, Grundy S, Sullivan LM, Wilson P, for the CHD Risk Prediction Group. Validation of the Framingham risk prediction scores. Results of a multiple ethnic group investigation. *JAMA* 2001; 286:180–187.

11.   Kannel WB, Dawber TR, Kagan A, Revotskie N, Stokes J III. Factors of risk in the development of coronary heart disease – six-year follow-up experience. The Framingham Study. *Ann Intern Med* 1961; 55:33–50.

12.   Brand RJ, Rosenman RH, Sholz RI, Friedman M. Multivariate prediction of coronary heart disease in the Western Collaborative Group Study compared to the findings of the Framingham Study. *Circulation* 1976; 53:348–355.

13.   Leaverton PE, Sorlie PD, Kleinman JC *et al*. Representativeness of the Framingham risk model for coronary heart disease mortality: a comparison with a National Cohort Study. *J Chronic Dis* 1987; 40:775–784.

14.   McGee D, Gordon T. The results of the Framingham Study applied to four other U.S.-based studies of cardiovascular disease. In: Kannel WB, Gordon T (eds). *The Framingham Study: An Epidemiological Investigation of Cardiovascular Disease, Section 31*. US Dept of Health Education and Welfare publication No. 76–1083. US Government Printing Office, Bethesda MD, 1976.

15.   Marrugat J, D'Agostino RB, Sullivan L *et al*. An adaptation of the Framingham coronary heart disease risk function to European Mediterranean Areas. *J Epidemiol Community Health* 2003; 57:634–638.

16.   Liu J, Hong Y, D'Agostino RB, Wu Z *et al*. Predictive value for the Chinese of the Framingham CHD risk assessment tool compared with the Chinese Multi-Provincial Cohort Study. *JAMA* 2004; 291:2591–2566.

17.   Kannel WB, Castelli WP, Gordon T. Cholesterol in the prediction of atherosclerotic disease. New perspectives based on the Framingham Study. *Ann Intern Med* 1979; 90:85–91.

18.   Grundy SM. United States Cholesterol Guidelines 2001: expanded scope of intensive low-density lipoprotein lowering therapy. *Am J Cardiol* 2001; 88:23J–27J.

19.   DeFronzo RA, Ferrannini E. Insulin resistance: a multifaceted syndrome responsible for NIDDM, obesity, dyslipidemia, and atherosclerotic cardiovascular disease. *Diabetes Care* 1991; 14:173–194.

20.   Yusuf S, Hawken S, Ounpuu S, on behalf of the INTERHEART Study Investigators. Effect of potentially modifiable risk factors associated with myocardial infarction in 52 countries (the INTERHEART study): case-control study. *Lancet* 2004; 364:937–952.

21.   Gordon T, Kannel WB. Premature mortality from coronary heart disease. The Framingham Study. *JAMA* 1971; 215:1617–1625.

22.   Kannel WB, Abbott RD. Incidence and prognosis of unrecognized myocardial infarction: an update on the Framingham Study. *N Engl J Med* 1984; 311:1144–1147.

23.   Kase C, Wolf PA, Chodos EH *et al*. Prevalence of silent strokes in patients presenting with initial stroke. The Framingham Study. *Stroke* 1989; 20:850–852.

24.   Murabito JM, Evans JC, Nieto K *et al*. Prevalence and clinical correlates of peripheral arterial disease in the Framingham Offspring Study. *Am Heart J* 2002; 143:961–965.

25.   American Heart Association. Heart disease and stroke statistics, 2004 update. American Heart Association, Dallas Texas, 2003.

26.   Chartbook on Cardiovascular, Lung and Blood Disease: NIH, NHLBI, 1999; US Dept. HHS. PHS.

27.   Lloyd-Jones DM, Larson MG, Beiser A, Levy D. Lifetime risk of developing coronary heart disease. *Lancet* 1999; 353:89–92.

28.   Lloyd-Jones DM, Wilson PWF, Larson MG *et al*. Lifetime risk for coronary heart disease by cholesterol levels at selected ages. *Arch Intern Med* 2003; 163:1966–1972.

29. Lloyd-Jones DM, Wilson PW, Larson MG *et al*. Framingham risk score and prediction of lifetime risk for coronary heart disease. *Am J Cardiol* 2004; 94:20–24.

30. Seshadri S, Beiser A, Margaret Kelly-Hayes RN *et al*. The lifetime risk of stroke estimates from the Framingham Study. *Stroke* 2006; 37:345–350.

31. Lloyd-Jones DM, Wang TJ, Leip EP *et al*. Lifetime risk for development of atrial fibrillation. The Framingham Study. *Circulation* 2004; 110:1042–1046.

32. Vasan RS, Beiser A, Seshadri M *et al*. Residual lifetime risk for developing hypertension in middle-aged women and men. *JAMA* 2002; 287:1003–1010.

33. Vasan R, Pencina MJ, Cobain M, Freiberg MS, D'Agostino RB. Estimated risks for development of obesity in the Framingham Study. *Ann Intern Med* 2005; 143:437–480.

34. McKee PA, Castelli WP, McNamara PM, Kannel WB. The natural history of congestive heart failure. The Framingham Study. *N Engl J Med* 1971; 285:1441–1446.

35. Lloyd-Jones DM, Larson MG, Leip EP *et al*. Lifetime risk for developing congestive heart failure. The Framingham Heart Study. *Circulation* 2002; 106:2997–2998.

36. Kannel WB. Elevated systolic blood pressure as a cardiovascular risk factor. *Am J Cardiol* 2000; 15:251–255.

37. Kannel WB, Gordon T, Schwartz MJ. Systolic versus diastolic blood pressure and risk of coronary heart disease. The Framingham Study. *Am J Cardiol* 1971; 27:335–345.

38. Kannel WB, Dawber TR, McGee DL *et al*. Perspectives on systolic hypertension. The Framingham Study. *Circulation* 1980; 61:1179–1182.

39. Chobanian A, Bakris JL, Black HR *et al*. The seventh report of the joint national committee on prevention, detection, evaluation and treatment of high blood pressure: The JNC 7 Report. *JAMA* 2003; 289:2560–2572.

40. Franklin SS, Kahn SA, Wong ND, Larson MG, Levy D. Is pulse pressure useful in predicting risk for coronary heart disease? The Framingham Study. *Circulation* 1999; 100:354–360.

41. Kannel WB, Vasan RS, Levy D. Is the relation of systolic blood pressure to risk of cardiovascular disease continuous and graded, or are there critical values? *Hypertension* 2003; 42:453–456.

42. Neaton JD, Kuller L, Stamler J, Wentworth DN. Impact of systolic and diastolic blood pressure on cardiovascular mortality. In: Laragh JH, Brenner BM (eds). *Hypertension: Pathophysiology, Diagnosis and Management*, 2nd edition. NY Raven Press Ltd, New York, 1995, pp 127–144.

43. Prospective Studies Collaboration. Age-specific relevance of usual blood pressure to vascular mortality: a meta-analysis of individual data for one million adults in 61 prospective studies. *Lancet* 2002; 360:1903–1913.

44. Port S, Demer L, Jennrich R, Walter D, Garfinkel A. Systolic blood pressure and mortality. *Lancet* 2000; 355:175–180.

45. Vasan RS, Larson MG, Leip EP *et al*. Impact of high-normal blood pressure on the risk of cardiovascular disease. *N Engl J Med* 2001; 345:1291–1297.

46. Lloyd-Jones DM, Evans JC, Larson MG *et al*. Differential control of systolic and diastolic blood pressure. Factors associated with lack of blood pressure control in the community. *Hypertension* 2000; 36:594–599.

47. Kannel WB, Wilson PWF, Nam B-Ho, D'Agostino RB. A likely explanation for the J-curve of blood pressure cardiovascular risk. *Am J Cardiol* 2004; 94:380–384.

48. SHEP Cooperative Research Group. Prevention of stroke by antihypertensive drug treatment in older persons with isolated systolic hypertension. *JAMA* 1991; 265:3255–3264.

49. Staessen JA, Fagard R, Thijs L *et al*. Randomized double blind comparison of placebo and active treatment for older patients with isolated systolic hypertension. *Lancet* 1997; 350:757–764.

50. Kannel WB, Dannenberg AL, Levy D. Population implications of left ventricular hypertrophy. *Am J Cardiol* 1987; 60:851–931.

51. Kannel WB, Abott RD, Savage DD, Mcnamara P. Epidemiologic features of chronic atrial fibrillation. The Framingham Study. *N Engl J Med* 1982; 306:1018–1022.

52. Wolf PA, Abbott RD, Kannel WB. Atrial fibrillation: a major contributor to stroke. The Framingham Study. *Arch intern Med* 1987; 147:1561–1564.

53. Gotto AM Jr, LaRosa JC, Hunninghake D *et al*. The cholesterol facts: a summary of the evidence relating dietary fats, serum cholesterol and coronary heart disease. A joint statement by the American Heart Association and the National Heart, Lung and Blood Institute. *Circulation* 1990; 81:1721–1733.

54. Grundy SM, Goodman DS, Rifkind BM *et al*. The place of HDL in cholesterol management: a perspective from the National Cholesterol Education Program. *Arch Intern Med* 1989; 149:505–510.

55. Castelli WP, Garrison RJ, Wilson PWF *et al*. Coronary heart disease incidence and lipoprotein levels. The Framingham Study. *JAMA* 1986; 256:2835–2838.

56. Kannel WB *et al*. Cholesterol for prediction of atherosclerotic disease; new perspectives from the Framingham Study. *Ann Intern Med* 1979; 90:85–89.

57. Kannel WB, Wilson PWF. Efficacy of lipid profiles in prediction of coronary disease. *Am Heart J* 1992; 124:768–774.

58. Kannel WB, McGee DL. Diabetes and glucose tolerance as risk factors for cardiovascular disease. The Framingham Study. *Diabetes Care* 1979; 2:120–126.

59. Expert Panel on Detection, Evaluation and Treatment of High Blood Cholesterol in Adults. Executive summary of the third report of the National Cholesterol Education Program (NCEP) expert panel on detection, evaluation and treatment of high blood cholesterol in adults (Adult Treatment Panel III). *JAMA* 2001; 285:2486–2497.

60. Wilson PWF, Anderson KM, Kannel WB. Epidemiology of diabetes mellitus in the elderly. The Framingham Study. *Am J Med* 1986; 80(suppl 5A):3–9.

61. Wilson PW, McGee DL, Kannel WB. Obesity, very low density lipoproteins and glucose intolerance over 14 years. The Framingham Study. *Am J Epidemiol* 1981; 114:697–704.

62. Freund K, D'Agostino RB, Belanger AJ, Kannel WB, Stokes J. The health risks of smoking: 34 years of follow-up. *Annals of Epidemiology* 1993; 3:417–424.

63. Rosenberg L, Kaufman DW, Helmrich SP *et al*. The risk of myocardial infarction after quitting smoking in men under 55 years of age. *N Engl J Med* 1985; 313:1511–1514.

64. Kannel WB, McGee DL, Castelli WP. Latest perspectives on cigarette smoking and cardiovascular disease. The Framingham Study. *J Cardiac Rehab* 1984; 4:267–277.

65. Kannel WB, D'Agostino RB. Risk reduction after quitting smoking. *Quality of Life and Cardiovasc Care* 1990; 84–85.

66. Wolf PA, D'Agostino RB, Kannel WB, Bonita R, Belanger AJ. Cigarette smoking as a risk factor for stroke. *JAMA* 1988; 259:1025–1029.

67. Kannel WB, McGee DL. Update on some epidemiologic features of intermittent claudication. The Framingham Study. *J Amer Geriatric Society* 1985; 33:13–18.

68. Paffenbarger RS. Jerry Morris: pathfinder for health through an active way of life. *Br J Sports Medicine* 2000; 34:217.

69. Kannel WB. Habitual level of physical activity and risk of coronary heart disease. The Framingham Study. *Can Med Assoc J* 1967; 96:811–812.

70. Keys A. Overweight, obesity, coronary heart disease and mortality. *Nutr Rev* 1980; 38:297–307.

71. Mann GV. The influence of body weight on health (second of 2 parts). *N Engl J Med* 1974; 291:226–232.

72. Barrett-Conner EL. Obesity, atherosclerosis and cardiovascular disease. *Ann Intern Med* 1985; 103:1010–1019.

73. Ashley FW Jr, Kannel WB. Relation of weight change to changes in atherogenic traits. The Framingham Study. *J Chronic Dis* 1974; 27:103–114.

74. Lissner L, Odell PM, D'Agostino RB *et al*. Variability in weight and health outcomes in the Framingham population. *N Engl J Med* 1991; 324:1839–1844.

75. Kannel WB, Stampfer MJ, Castelli WP, Verter J. The prognostic significance of proteinuria. The Framingham Study. *Am Heart J* 1984; 108:1347–1352.

76. Mendelsohn ME. Protective effects of estrogen on the cardiovascular system. *Am J Cardiol* 2002; 89(suppl):12E–18E.

77. Kannel WB, Hjortland MC, McNamara PM, Gordon T. Menopause and risk of cardiovascular disease. The Framingham Study. *Ann Intern Med* 1976; 85:447–452.

78. Gordon T, Kannel WB, Hjortland MC, McNamara PM. Menopause and coronary heart disease. The Framingham Study. *Ann Intern Med* 1978; 89:157–161.

79. Ritterband AB, Jaffe IA, Densen PM, Magagna JF, Reed E. Gonadal function and the development of coronary heart disease. *Circulation* 1963; 27:237–251.

80. Bush TL, Barrett-Conner E, Cowen LD *et al*. Cardiovascular mortality and non-contraceptive use of estrogen in women: results from the Lipid Research Program Follow-up Study. *Circulation* 1987; 75:1102–1109.

81. Stampfer M, Colditz G. Estrogen replacement therapy for coronary heart disease: a quantitative assessment of the epidemiologic evidence. *Prev Med* 1991; 20:47–63.

82. Risks and benefits of estrogen plus progestin in healthy postmenopausal women. Principal results from the Women's Health Initiative Randomized Controlled Trial. Writing Group for the Women's Health Initiative Investigators. *JAMA* 2002; 288:321–333.

83. Hulley S, Grady D, Bush T *et al.* Randomized trial of estrogen plus progestin for secondary prevention of coronary heart disease in postmenopausal women. For the Heart and Estrogen/progestin Replacement Study (HERS) Research Group. *JAMA* 1998; 280:605–613.

84. Mosca L, Collins P, Heerington DM *et al.* Hormone replacement therapy and cardiovascular disease. A Statement for Health Care Professionals from the America Heart Association. *Circulation* 2001; 104:499–503.

85. Wilson PWF, Garrison RJ, Castelli WP. Postmenopaual estrogen use, cigarette smoking, and cardiovascular disease. The Framingham Study. *N Engl J Med* 1985; 313:1038–1043.

86. Wilson PWF, Nam B-Ho, Pencina M *et al.* C-reactive protein and risk of cardiovascular disease in men and women from the Framingham Heart Study. *Arch Intern Med* 2005; 165:2473–2478.

87. Kannel WB. Overview of hemostatic factors involved in atherosclerotic cardiovascular disease. *Lipids* 2005; 40:1215–1220.

13

Electronic and interactive risk estimation

T. F. Thomsen

INTRODUCTION

In preventive cardiology, time is often of the essence. So, although a multifactorial approach is recommended, it has been proven beyond any doubt that this is far from real practice. Estimation of risk is straightforward if the patient has recently survived a coronary event, is diabetic or has markedly increased risk factors. These patients are all at high risk, and are eligible for intensive risk reduction [1]. But for the large proportion of patients the process of risk stratification is far from easy. A combination of electronic risk estimation with individual health advice to the patient and online access to the guidelines may prove to become a useful method in clinical practice.

In order to put the current situation into perspective, it could be useful to take a brief look back in history: a tale of why electronic risk estimation got off to a very bad start and why it took a couple of generations to get things right.

THE FIRST GENERATION

Electronic risk prediction was born in the beginning of the 1990s with several risk calculators, which were developed and distributed mainly by the medical industry. These initiatives were followed by a series of DOS-based computer programmes, likewise developed by the industry and, though innovative at that time, they were mainly perceived as cumbersome systems in clinical practice.

This first generation of computerized systems were characterized by being simple electronic reproductions of the paper version of the risk chart. All the programmes used the Framingham risk equation published by Anderson *et al.* [2] in 1991, but were otherwise not linked to any recommendations. They all therefore predicted the same endpoint; namely the Framingham composite coronary endpoint. None of the programmes was developed in order to be implemented in a busy clinical practice and some of the programmes were even restricted to suggest the use of certain specific pharmaceutical drugs.

Since these electronic systems offered only little advantage to the medical community, and while they were all developed by private industry, not one of these systems was ever endorsed by any scientific society. In view of the fact that programming at this point in time was still an extremely costly affair, no scientific society could afford to develop such a programme *de novo*. It is therefore obvious that this first generation of electronic risk prediction systems suffered from a rather poor reputation amongst both clinicians and scientific societies in the mid 1990s.

Troels F. Thomsen, MD, MPH, PhD, Specialist in Publisc Health Medicine, Research Centre for Prevention and Health, Glostrup University Hospital, Glostrup, Denmark

THE SECOND GENERATION

This generation was born when Windows®-based programming became available in the late 1990s. It now became possible to offer more than just simple risk prediction. The aim became computerized decision support for both the clinician as well as the high-risk patient, throughout all stages of the preventative consultation. With Windows®, the graphical component of risk estimation improved substantially. Furthermore, it was now possible to produce flexible applications containing different languages and risk models etc. This latter aspect was a consequence of several studies showing that a risk model predicting absolute risk must be derived from a population with the same incidence of the disease as the population to which it is to be applied [3]. Therefore, absolute risk prediction had to be flexible if dissemination in several populations was intended.

Soon after, the first scientific attempts were made to evaluate the effect of applying computerized decision support in clinical practice. With the obvious precaution of potential publication bias, the initial work suggested that computerized decision support in preventive cardiology was superior to normal care [4]. Some studies suggested that if the clinician had a series of methods to use in cardiovascular risk estimation, it could also improve the quality of care. Finally, it was shown that computer-generated, individually tailored health advice was superior to standard leaflets, especially in individuals with low vocational training [5]. This last finding attracted considerable attention, since almost all other preventive initiatives in cardiology had shown the opposite social gradient.

This may be one of the greatest advantages of electronic risk estimation. Often, written advice for the patient is in the form of a standard pamphlet, written for a broader audience, and usually produced by a national patient organization. This kind of pamphlet will inevitably contain irrelevant information, e.g. on antihypertensive treatment during pregnancy when you have a male patient in front of you. This kind of redundant information has been shown to dilute the relevant messages, especially in patients with low vocational training.

By tailoring the information to the patient, several benefits are gained. First of all, the information is conceived by the patient as personal advice from his/her doctor and no longer general advice to change lifestyle. Secondly, there will be a higher concordance between what is said and written to the patient, which is likely to improve compliance with the given advice. The physician can choose only to print the topics that were discussed during the consultation to the patient. And finally, this tailored advice will ideally be the same if the patient consults another doctor, since the advice is written by the National Cardiac Society. This requires of course that all doctors use the recommended tool for prevention of cardiovascular disease (CVD).

To gain further interest in the clinical world, the programmes had to offer more than just a number or a percentage that depicted the patient's risk status. A natural question evolved when the patient turned out to be at high risk, namely how to reduce the risk most efficiently. And in order to answer this question a closer link to the existing guidelines was needed. In an attempt to accommodate this need for sophistication of risk estimation, the first version in this generation using the European Guidelines on CVD prevention, called the PRECARD® programme, was developed in Denmark [6]. Figures 13.1 and 13.2 show the graphical presentation of the programme, where risk is shown both as a bar chart (absolute risk) and as a pie chart (relative risk).

This programme aimed at combining electronic risk prediction based on national data, with evidence-based tailored advice to the individual patient according to his/her risk profile. The PRECARD® programme predicted several endpoints and could be adjusted to several risk functions. It was originally published in the Nordic countries, with nine risk factors, and was available in six languages.

Four years after the PRECARD® programme was launched, an evaluation showed that approximately one-third of GPs had installed it. Nine out of ten physicians thought the

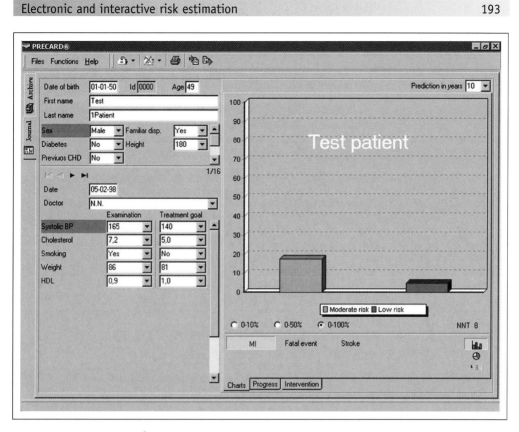

Figure 13.1 The PRECARD® programme showing the actual absolute risk (left-hand bar) and the obtainable risk if the patient reaches the treatment goals (right-hand bar). ©Research Centre for Prevention and Health, 2007.

programme improved the patient's motivation to comply with the lifestyle advice given by the physician. The evaluation also showed that the use of electronic risk prediction improved the overall quality of the consultation even though the majority of physicians stated that it prolonged the consultation [7].

THE EFFECT OF INTERVENTION

Another advantage of electronic risk estimation is the ability to develop statistical models that will calculate the effect of risk reduction. The paper version of the chart, in contrast to an electronic model, is restricted to using only epidemiological data. This means that, for example, the effect of quitting smoking cannot be calculated, since the risk chart only contains the dichotomous 'Smoking' and 'Non-smoking'. Therefore, when a smoker is advised to stop smoking, he moves, in the paper version, from a risk model based on a population of smokers to a model based on never-smokers. This may well be in conflict with the evidence showing that ex-smokers have a higher risk than never-smokers, at least for some time after they have quit smoking.

Likewise, it could be argued that a person who has had a cholesterol level of 7 mmol/l all his life but has now reached a cholesterol level of 5 mmol/l due to statin treatment, has a

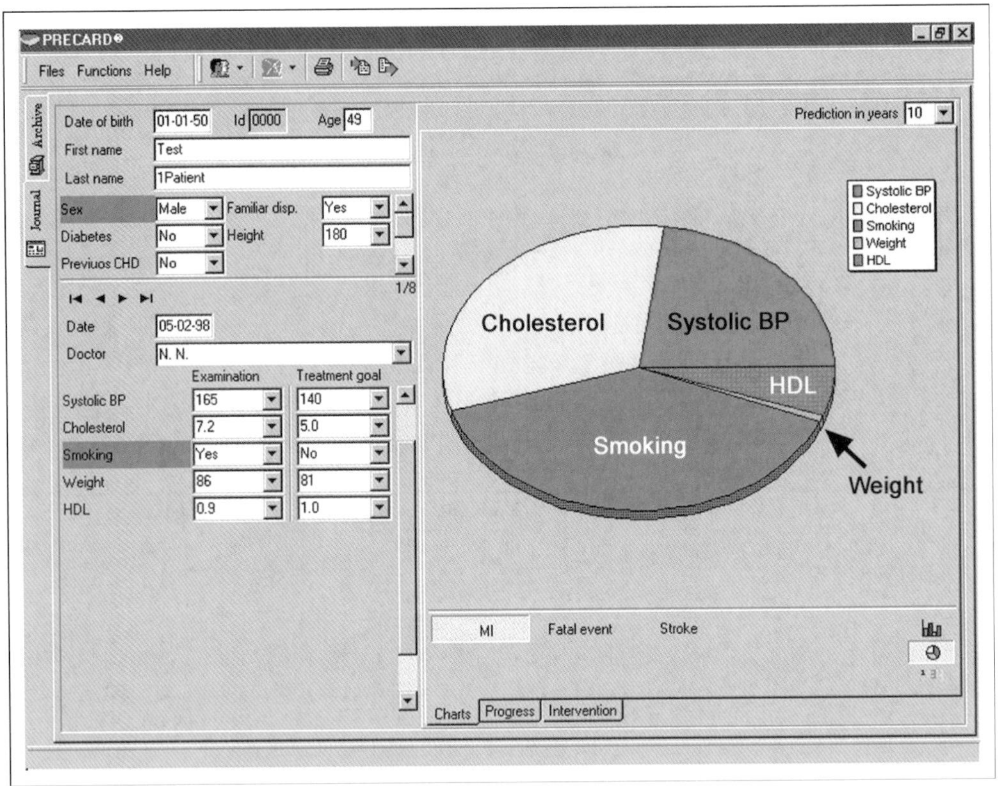

Figure 13.2   The PRECARD®-programme showing the actual absolute risk (left-hand bar) and the obtainable risk if the patient reaches the treatment goals (right-hand bar). ©Research Centre for Prevention and Health, 2007.

different risk to a person who has had a cholesterol level of 5 mmol/l all his life without any treatment. These two individuals would also be estimated in the same way by the paper version of the risk chart. However, by using electronic risk estimation it would be possible to include the effect of intervention, from randomized trials, into the estimation. The PRECARD® programme also calculated numbers needed to treat (NNT), which is another way of expressing the effect of intervention, as a novel feature.

THE SYSTEMIC CORONARY RISK EVALUATION (SCORE) RISK ESTIMATION SYSTEM

As previously mentioned, the estimation of absolute risk requires that the model used to predict is derived from a population with a similar incidence of the disease. This has been shown in numerous studies and also has its own intuitive logic. Based on the observation on the applicability of the existing Framingham function all across Europe, the Systemic Coronary Risk Evaluation (SCORE) study was initiated in 1997 by the European Society of Cardiology. The aim of the study was to assemble European population based data and prepare a risk score system optimized for assessment of risk among Europeans [8]. This work coincided with the development of the PRECARD® programme, and in 2001, when an update of the guidelines from 1998 was taking place, the European Society of Cardiology took over the PRECARD® programme and named it HeartScore® [9]. This was done in the light of a growing digitization of the physician's clinical work, and in the new guidelines of 2003 the

HeartScore® programme was the officially recommended electronic risk estimation tool. The system was still a Windows®-based application and therefore belongs to this second generation. The fourth joint task force of the European Society's guidelines for CVD prevention continue to recommend the HeartScore system [1].

In 2004, the HeartScore® programme was offered in two European versions based on the four published SCORE risk charts: 'European Low Risk' and 'European Low Risk TC/HDL Ratio' for Belgium, France, Greece, Italy, Luxembourg, Spain, Switzerland and Portugal. The other version is the 'European High Risk' and 'European High Risk TC/HDL Ratio' for all other European countries.

In the analyses of SCORE it became evident that the previous risk estimate of 20% of having a combined mortality/morbidity endpoint equalled the 5% CVD mortality endpoint. In other words, being at high risk of getting any event is the same as being at high risk of dying, i.e. almost the same population is being identified. The SCORE system was restricted to predicting CVD death, since morbidity data in many countries were not reliable. From a patient perspective however, it may be argued that interest is not purely in the risk of dying within the next ten years, but rather the risk of having to live with chronic disability. The potential of having different endpoints to predict is relevant since the evaluation of the PRECARD® programme also showed that almost two-thirds of clinicians predicted different endpoints when talking to patients. The SCORE-plus study is designed to accommodate this need.

Responding to several requests received from national cardiac societies, the European Society of Cardiology supported the development of country-specific versions of HeartScore®. This allowed two major leaps forward, namely tailored risk estimation systems based on national mortality data plus advice in local languages. By 2004, all 43 country-specific versions appeared in national European languages and were available for download at the European Society of Cardiology's website.

The next step was to tailor the risk function in the programme to national CVD mortality. A method was developed to take account of both risk factor levels and CVD mortality in each country. The SCORE risk function was calibrated to national mortality statistics (from the World Health Organization [WHO]) and to MONitoring trends and determinants in CArdiovascular disease (MONICA) data on risk factor prevalence. This would ideally mean that if the entire adult population between 30 and 60 years of age was risk-estimated, the average risk would be the exact incidence over the next ten years.

However, still being a Windows®-based programme, the users would have to download and install the entire programme in order to use it. This turned out to hamper the process for two reasons. Firstly, many clinicians were now working in networks, and were therefore not allowed to install programmes on their computers; this had to be done by the administrator of their system. Secondly, many users, especially in Eastern Europe, only had low-capacity modems, which prolonged the downloading unacceptably.

The third generation of electronic risk estimation therefore had to be entirely web-based. This would avoid the process of downloading and installing a programme. Everything would now take place within the Web-browser.

THE THIRD GENERATION

THE HEARTSCORE® PROGRAMME

In 2005 HeartScore® was reprogrammed into a Web-based application by the European Society of Cardiology, to be used in European CVD risk management based on the SCORE risk charts published in the European Guidelines on CVD Prevention. It builds on the previous experience and aims at becoming *the* interactive tool for predicting and managing the risk of heart attack and stroke in Europe with direct on-line access to the current guidelines.

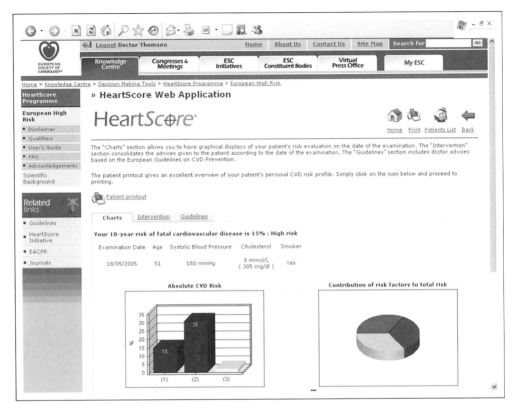

Figure 13.3   The HeartScore® programme. ©European Society of Cardiology, 2007.

The primary benefit of using HeartScore® is that no programme needs to be downloaded or installed. Everything takes place within the Web-browser. This allows quick and easy risk estimation, performed in the clinic, while the patient and the doctor discuss how to reduce risk in this patient. Furthermore, the programme, like the previous versions, offers the patient tailored and printed health advice, based on actual risk profile. But not only may the patient benefit from getting tailored advice on treatment, the doctor who is using the Web application may also obtain individual advice compiled from the current guidelines. This information is tailored to the specific patient, giving the doctor advice on potential treatment options on the basis of this patient's risk profile. This information, the risk model and all other functions can be updated regularly by the scientific societies whenever new knowledge emerges.

Finally, there is the benefit of potential surveillance of preventive cardiology by using a Web-based model. As a registered user, all data entered in to the programme are stored encrypted on a central server. From this server, specific data can be extracted and analysed. If, for example, a campaign has been launched for using the programme, the National Cardiac Society can follow the use of the programme on the Internet: what kinds of patients are exposed to the programme; for how long; what is printed for the patient etc.

The HeartScore® programme gives a graphical picture of absolute CVD risk (based on SCORE data), not just current risk but also, if the patient does not change risk profile, until the age 60 (Figure 13.3). Finally, the programme shows how much the risk is reduced if the

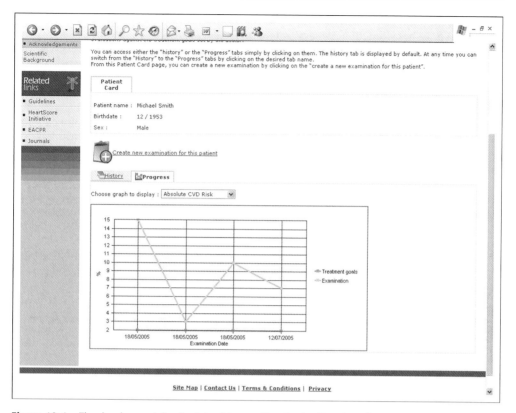

Figure 13.4 The development in absolute risk over time in the HeartScore® programme. ©European Society of Cardiology, 2007.

treatment targets are achieved. The January 2008 update of HeartScore also contains an estimate of the relative risk, in line with the recommendations of the fourth joint task force of the European societies. This is for counselling younger people, who are at low absolute risk but high relative risk [1].

Figure 13.4 shows how the development in the patient's modifiable risk factors, as well as total cardiovascular risk, has proceeded over time. This may support the patient in complying with the suggested changes in lifestyle or pharmacological treatment.

The programme is accessible from **www.heartscore.org**, use is free of charge and only requires that the user is registered at the ESC website: **www.escardio.org**. There are no operating system requirements for using the HeartScore® Web-based programme; however, a Web-browser (e.g. Internet Explorer) is needed, together with an Internet connection (a low bandwidth modem line 56 kb/s is sufficient). No software needs to be downloaded.

OTHER METHODS

The risk of CVD may, of course, be established by several other means than the recommended SCORE system. These methods of CVD assessment in Europe include risk scores such as PROCAM [10], DECODE [11] and UKPDS [12]. PROCAM is a German based worksite study which can be used for assessing cardiovascular risk in a healthy male worksite population, while

DECODE, like SCORE, is derived from pooling several European population studies. The DECODE study has strength in its registration of diabetes with the oral glucose tolerance test (OGTT) as a standard measurement of glucose tolerance.

The UKPDS risk engine is the only one derived from a population of diabetics. It estimates the risk of CHD and stroke given that the patient has diabetes. Furthermore, it is the only risk estimation programme capable of allowing for regression dilution bias, which takes account of the amount of individual measurements. This affects the risk estimation when several measurements are available on the same patient. For example, if the patient's systolic blood pressure has been measured at 170 mmHg at three consecutive consultations, the absolute risk increases, since it now is more certain that the first measurements were not due to random fluctuations.

In America, several systems are now available through the Internet, all of which are based on Framingham data. The American Heart Association has developed a risk assessment tool with the possibility of comparing a person's risk with the risk estimates for someone of the same age group and gender with very low or low levels of risk factors. There is no link to the guidelines and it is not possible to store the data entered.

It must be further emphasized that the main difference between the existing electronic risk estimation programmes is from which population the risk score has been developed. In general, the method of estimating risk should be derived from a population as similar as the one to which it is to be applied. Applying the Framingham function to a British, Danish, Spanish or Italian population will result in various degrees of overestimation, simply due to the fact that the incidence of the disease is lower in these countries. This is, as mentioned, the basic rationale for the national adaptation proposed by the SCORE study, which resulted in a more precise prediction of CVD in each region in Europe.

STRENGTHS AND LIMITATIONS IN ELECTRONIC RISK ESTIMATION

In general, the main strength of risk estimation is that it identifies patients at actual risk and should be used as a guide throughout the treatment. There is a direct association between absolute risk and the benefit of intervention; the higher the absolute risk, the higher the benefit. This relationship does not exist for relative risk reduction, which is usually the same for a high-risk as for a low-risk individual.

Having said that, there is indeed some added value in performing risk estimation electronically. The graphics in the electronic version can be used to motivate the patient for lifestyle changes. Both types of risk communication have been shown to increase the patient's motivation for lifestyle changes and it seems reasonable to extend this benefit to drug compliance.

A physician estimating risk without any tool has a very low discriminatory ability. Likewise, high relative risk is often confused with high absolute risk. This emphasizes the need for an assessment tool. The additional effect of assessing risk by computer programmes as compared with using paper risk charts has only been analysed in a few studies. Those evaluated have all belonged to the second generation of programmes and the results have been rather inconsistent. In general, the uptake of these Windows® programmes has been relatively poor, especially in countries with high CVD incidence (i.e. mainly the Eastern European countries). Also, the use of these programmes has been reported as rather time-consuming. There has, however, been a tendency for the more sophisticated, and officially-recommended, programmes to be more successful than previous programmes.

There are certain limitations in electronic risk estimation and some pitfalls that have to be taken into account. Firstly it requires not only a computer, but also that the screen is visible to the patient; a simple requirement, but often difficult to accommodate in clinical practice.

Secondly, it requires a steady online connections, or at least a stable computer if a Windows®-based solution is to be used.

Another obstacle is the entering of risk factor data which is already stored in the physician's computer. It would aid the process if these data (i.e. cholesterol, smoking etc.) could be automatically transferred to the risk calculation programme. However, this integration is technically difficult since the amount of systems operating in clinical practice is vast. And for each of these systems, a special application has to be made to transfer data automatically. For this reason, almost no attempts have been made to solve this problem.

The greatest pitfall, however, is an unrealistic expectation as to what electronic risk prediction can do. The problems, such as doctor's compliance with current recommendations in preventive cardiology, will never be solved by introducing electronic risk prediction methods. They are not time-saving and will require some maintenance from time to time. Experience from use of the Danish PRECARD® programme showed that electronic risk estimation indeed prolongs the preventive consultation to some degree, but also that it improves both the patient's understanding of CVD and motivation for following the doctor's advice. So the argument for using electronic risk estimation is not to make the estimation easier; the argument is that electronic risk estimation will improve the quality of risk estimation as well as the patient's compliance with the advice on risk reduction given.

SUMMARY

Cardiovascular risk estimation represents a cornerstone in preventive cardiology. If not properly stratified by their risk, the treatment of patients will be subject to unjustified variability, many risk factors may be left untreated and our focus will not be reserved for those at the highest actual risk. This being said, total risk estimation is associated with numerous difficulties and pitfalls. The risk score used for assessment should be derived from a population with similar incidence, and the programme should be linked to current guidelines and easy to work with in clinical practice.

Electronic risk evaluation may be efficient in some practices and may extend the concept of risk assessment to actual risk management. This practice does, on the other hand, require more time spent with the patient, and electronic risk estimation is never better than the physician performing it. The greatest challenge facing electronic risk estimation is therefore unrealistic expectations as to what problems can be solved by electronic means. Electronic risk estimation may improve CVD risk reduction, but it will never make it perfect.

REFERENCES

1. Graham I, Atar D, Borch-Johnsen K *et al.*, Fourth Joint Task Force of the European Society of Cardiology and other Societies on Cardiovascular Disease Prevention in Clinical Practice, European Guidelines on Cardiovascular Disease Prevention in Clinical Practice. *Eur J Cardiovasc Prev Rehabil* 2007; 14(suppl 2):S1–S113.
2. Anderson KM, Odell PM, Wilson PW, Kannel WB. Cardiovascular disease risk profiles. *Am Heart J* 1991; 121:293–298.
3. Thomsen TF, McGee D, Davidsen M, Jorgensen T. A cross-validation of risk-scores for coronary heart disease mortality based on data from the Glostrup Population Studies and Framingham Heart Study. *Int J Epidemiol* 2002; 31:817–822.
4. Lowensteyn I, Joseph L, Levinton C, Abrahamowicz M, Steinert Y, Grover S. Can computerized risk profiles help patients improve their coronary risk? The results of the Coronary Health Assessment Study (CHAS). *Prev Med* 1998; 27:730–737.
5. Dijkstra A, De Vries H, Roijackers J. Long-term effectiveness of computer-generated tailored feedback in smoking cessation. *Health Educ Res* 1998; 13:207–214.
6. Thomsen TF, Davidsen M, Ibsen H, Jorgensen T, Jensen G, Borch-Johnsen K. A new method for CHD prediction and prevention based on regional risk scores and randomized clinical trials; PRECARD and the Copenhagen Risk Score. *J Cardiovasc Risk* 2001; 8:291–297.

7. Bonnevie L, Thomsen TF, Jorgensen T. The use of computerized decision support systems in preventive cardiology – principal results from the national PRECARD survey in Denmark. *Eur J Cardiovasc Prev Rehabil* 2005; 12:52–55.

8. Conroy RM, Pyörälä K, Fitzgerald AP *et al.*, SCORE project group. Estimation of ten-year risk of fatal cardiovascular disease in Europe: the SCORE project. *Eur Heart J* 2003; 24:987–1003.

9. Thomsen TF. HeartScore®: a new web-based approach to European cardiovascular disease risk management. *Eur J Cardiovasc Prev Rehabil* 2005; 12:424–426.

10. **www.chd-taskforce.com**

11. Balkau B, Hu G, Qiao Q *et al.*, DECODE Study Group, European Diabetes Epidemiology Group. Prediction of the risk of cardiovascular mortality using a score that includes glucose as a risk factor. The DECODE Study. *Diabetologia* 2004; 47:2118–2128. Epub 2004 Dec 15.

12. Stevens RJ, Kothari V, Adler AI, Stratton IM, United Kingdom Prospective Diabetes Study (UKPDS) Group, The UKPDS risk engine: a model for the risk of coronary heart disease in Type II diabetes (UKPDS 56). *Clin Sci* 2001; 101:671–679.

14

Management of specific behavioural risk factors – exercise, obesity and smoking

G. Burell, B. Lindahl

INTRODUCTION

A few weeks ago J.P., a 52-year-old man, after a particularly stressful day, suffered an attack of severe chest pain. Although very reluctant to seek medical help, he let his wife drive him to the hospital. He spent a night and the next day in the coronary care unit (CCU), but tests showed no evidence of acute myocardial infarction (MI).

However, follow-up examinations confirmed angina pectoris, although not to the degree that demanded invasive treatment. He was prescribed the usual medications, and told to 'watch his lifestyle habits'.

J.P. is a section supervisor in a middle-sized industry. He is married and the father of two teenagers. His wife is in full-time employment and the children are engaged in many activities away from home, so the family rarely eats their meals together. J.P. never cooks for himself – his diet is mainly take-away fast food, or just coffee and a sandwich. He often skips breakfast, and sometimes lunch too. To 'get some energy back' in the afternoon he may resort to cookies and candy. J.P.'s body mass index (BMI) is 29, and before the event he smoked a pack of cigarettes per day. For some months, he says, he had 'thought about' getting more physically active, but says he was under such stress at work that he just did not have the energy for it. He felt very tired when he got home from work in the evening but had difficulty relaxing because he felt tense and irritable. He habitually had some beers or drinks in order to relax, which 'may or may not help'. He did not sleep well, woke up early and rarely felt refreshed. His sleep has deteriorated even more after his event. He still smokes about 10 cigarettes a day, and his diet is basically unchanged.

J.P. is reporting feeling depressed and 'out of control'. His physician has advised him to stop smoking, start exercizing, and try to lose some weight. But J.P. is not very confident in his own ability to achieve these changes.

- Can smoking cessation, weight loss, and increased physical exercise decrease cardiac symptoms and improve prognosis in this patient?
- How can behaviour change be achieved?
- How can the physician improve compliance with and long-term maintenance of lifestyle change?

Gunilla Burell, PhD, Lecturer and Assistant Professor, Department of Public Health and Caring Sciences, Uppsala University, Uppsala, Sweden

Bernt Lindahl, MD, PhD, Associate Professor and Senior Physician, Behavioural Medicine, Department of Public Health and Clinical Medicine, Umeå University, Umeå, Sweden

EXERCISE

There is a strong inverse relationship between physical activity and cardiovascular disease (CVD), and the evidence for this relationship must be considered as solid. However, most of our knowledge is built on epidemiological studies. Thousands of person-years observed in different studies over the years have consistently shown this inverse dose–response relationship. Low levels of physical activity (physical inactivity) increase the risk of CVD [1]. To date no randomized controlled trials (RCTs) have been done in primary prevention to verify the effects of physical activity on cardiovascular morbidity or mortality. However, RCT studies in secondary prevention have shown increased physical activity to reduce cardiovascular mortality [2]. A large body of evidence examining the effects of physical activity on intermediary cardiovascular risk factor variables has also documented risk factor reduction due to increased physical activity [1], mainly a lowering of blood pressure [3] and a less atherogenic lipid profile [4]. Later studies have also indicated effects on endothelial dysfunction and inflammatory reaction in blood vessels, at least in high-risk individuals for CVD or in CVD patients [5, 6].

Despite all this evidence for the beneficial effects of physical activity on CVD, the majority of people in most industrialized countries is physically less active than recommended and about 25% of the population is not active at all [1]. The reason for this discrepancy is not clear-cut, but at least it indicates that pure information on the beneficial effects of physical activity is not enough to change individuals' behaviours. An important shift in the view of physical activity was introduced in the middle of the 1990s. Large epidemiological studies demonstrated that even less intensive physical activity and shorter bouts of activity had health-promoting effects. It was shown that a dose of physical activity corresponding to 1000 kcal per week significantly lowered all-cause mortality by 20–30% [7], and CVD mortality possibly even more [8]. This level of weekly energy expenditure corresponds to about 30 min of moderately intensive physical activity each day, i.e. brisk walks, bicycling and swimming. Hence, the concept of lifestyle physical activity, i.e. to incorporate 30 min of moderate physical activity a day into everyday life, was born. The importance of this new type of message about physical activity is the greater flexibility it brings for the individual to become physically active, and this is of paramount interest since the primary obstacle reported for physical activity is lack of time [9, 10].

A crucial step in adopting long-term behaviour change, e.g. increased physical activity, is to believe in one's own inborn capacity to perform the new chosen behaviour. In social cognitive theory (SCT), this self-confidence in performing an activity is named self-efficacy, and is considered a prerequisite for long-term behaviour change [11]. Self-efficacy may in this respect be seen as a mediating factor between the intervention efforts and an outcome such as physical activity. In a RCT in healthy, sedentary older subjects, increase in self-efficacy during the first 6 months of the study was positively associated with exercise adherence during the following 6 months [12].

The most important factor in controlling self-efficacy is one's own past experiences. Previous failure to change behaviour will result in a lower self-efficacy for future change in that behaviour, and will probably lead to another failure. A crucial step in changing negative experiences into positive ones is to set realistic goals, and goal-setting combined with self-monitoring of the chosen behaviour are the main tools in achieving a positive outcome. This in turn will increase self-efficacy for the chosen behaviour, and thereafter new goals can be set. Moving forward in small consecutive steps is one of the key points in long-term behaviour change. Behavioural therapy based on SCT has also been used in a large study of sedentary primary care patients and was found to be more effective than advice, at least in females [13]. Furthermore, using goal-setting and self-regulation techniques, in a study of sedentary older individuals with a high risk for CVD, significantly increased physical fitness at 12 months' follow-up compared to a structured exercise programme [14]. The same kind of results were also found in similar behavioural approaches compared with usual care in type 2 diabetes patients [15] and in patients with earlier acute myocardial infarction [16]. A study in cardiac patients comparing a traditional cardiac rehabilitation programme (supervised exercise) and a modified programme based upon Bandura's self-efficacy theory, showed a higher level of self-efficacy for exercise without continuous electrocardiograph (ECG) monitoring in the modified programme, which in turn might facilitate future independent exercise [17].

Much still needs to be done within this area of research, especially to explore the mechanisms behind health behaviour change. What mediates the change? It is also vital that more research is done into how to translate research results into regular working routines in the clinic.

OBESITY

Obesity is often defined as a condition of excessive fat accumulation in adipose tissue to the extent that health may be impaired. The underlying mechanism is a process of undesirable positive energy balance and weight gain. Obesity is associated with many other diseases or risk conditions such as type 2 diabetes, CVD, osteoarthritis and joint pain, sleep apnoea, cancer (colon, breast, endometrium, prostate, and pancreas), poor health-related quality of life (HRQL) and physical inactivity. In the clinic, obesity is often measured by calculating BMI, which is body weight (kg) divided by height (m) squared. According to the World Health Organization (WHO), normal weight is defined as having a BMI between 18.5 and 24.9 kg/m^2, overweight as having a BMI between 25 and 29.9, and obesity a BMI of 30 kg/m^2 or more.

Another important measure, especially in respect to obesity-related diseases, is the distribution of body fat. Already in the late 1940s, the French scientist Jean Vague presented data of an increased risk for diabetes among individuals having android fat accumulation, i.e. central or abdominal obesity. Several epidemiological studies have later confirmed these findings. Waist circumference, a proxy measure for abdominal obesity, is more closely associated with diabetes and CVD and also total mortality than adipose tissue in other regions of the body [18, 19]. On the contrary, hip circumference, as a measure of peripheral or gynoid fat accumulation, has been found to be associated with lower insulin resistance, lower prevalence and incidence of diabetes and lower total mortality [20].

The relation in the population between BMI and mortality has often been described as J- or U-shaped, indicating that there is an excess death rate among those having underweight (BMI <18.5 kg/m^2) and those having overweight/obesity. There has been a discrepancy between different studies concerning where on the BMI scale mortality starts to rise. In the Cancer Prevention Study II the lowest rates of death from all causes was between BMI of 22–24.9 [21], but in the National Health and Nutrition Examination Survey (NHANES) studies, the whole area of overweight (BMI 25–29.9) had a lower mortality than the reference group of normal weight (BMI 18.5–24.9) [22]. A majority of studies examining the effect of weight loss and weight gain in the population has found increased mortality among those losing weight [23]. In a study among Harvard alumni, those in whom weight did not change during a 10–15-year period seemed to have both the lowest all-cause and coronary heart disease mortality [24].

Obesity predisposes an individual to several cardiovascular risk factors including hypertension, dyslipidaemia, impaired glucose tolerance and type 2 diabetes. Moreover, these risk factors tend to cluster in the same individual and form the metabolic syndrome. Other risk indicators often mentioned in this context are markers of endothelial dysfunction, inflammation and hypercoagulability. At the moment, there are several working definitions of the metabolic syndrome with varying constellations and cut-off values of the principal components [25]. There is also an ongoing debate on the overall value of using the syndrome, especially since the syndrome does not seem to predict CVD better than the single risk factors comprised in the syndrome. Furthermore, an underlying pathophysiologial cause of the metabolic syndrome has not clearly been elucidated and no specific treatment that targets the syndrome beyond the usual treatments of its individual components is available [26, 27].

However, the metabolic syndrome may facilitate the clinician's focus on individuals at high risk of both CVD and diabetes [28]. In a recent publication based on 11 prospective

European cohort studies, the prevalence of the metabolic syndrome was 15.7% in men and 14.2% in women. Individuals with the metabolic syndrome vs. individuals without the syndrome had a 1.4-fold increase in the risk for all-cause mortality in both men and women, and a 2.3-fold increase in the risk of cardiovascular mortality for men and 2.8-fold increase in women [29]. Taken together, obesity is an important risk factor for CVD [30], and was declared by the International Obesity Task Force to be among the top five leading risk factors for both morbidity and mortality [31].

Behaviour modification inducing long-term lifestyle change leading to a gradual weight loss is the basis of all obesity treatment. The behaviour change process is facilitated by the use of goal-setting, self-monitoring and problem-solving techniques [32]. Studies using this approach often achieve a weight loss of 8–10% of the initial body weight at 6 months follow-up [33]. One key feature of such a programme is to discuss with the patient, in an empathic manner, both short- and long-term goals. Furthermore, the goals should be realistic, measurable, concrete and engaging. Another key feature is self-monitoring, where the patient keeps a detailed record of his behaviours such as food intake and physical activity. Using goal-setting and self-monitoring together, individuals may easily experience satisfaction by looking at their recordings and find out that their goals have been attained. This will boost the self-efficacy for the behaviour in question.

Pharmacological treatment of obesity is mainly recommended as an adjunct to lifestyle modification. Today, two different obesity medications are used for long-term treatment of obesity. Orlistat induces weight loss by blocking the absorption of fat in the diet, and sibutramine causes weight loss by suppressing the appetite. In a recent systemic review and meta-analysis using eleven studies on orlistat and three studies on sibutramine, patients using orlistat displayed a 2.9% greater weight loss than those on a placebo after 1 year of follow-up, and patients using sibutramine a 4.6% greater weight loss than placebo. The conclusion was that the pharmacological agents were modestly effective in promoting weight loss and that long-term studies are needed [34].

Rimonabant is an endocannabinoid receptor inhibitor that appears capable of inducing a modest but sustained weight loss in combination with a calorie controlled diet. It may improve glucose tolerance, beneficially affect lipid metabolism and is associated with a modest reduction in blood pressure. Possible adverse effects on depression are being monitored.

A randomized trial examining the combined effects of lifestyle modification and pharmacological treatment (using sibutramine), showed that the combination gave a significantly greater weight loss than sibutramine alone at 1 year follow-up [35]. The notion that pharmacotherapy works well in conjunction with lifestyle modification is important and supports the view that obesity medications should never be used alone.

In severe obesity (BMI ≥40) bariatric surgery may be the method of choice, especially if other treatments have been unsuccessful. Surgery may even be considered at lower body weight (BMI ≥35) in patients with many obesity-related risk factors. For those severely obese, bariatric surgery produces larger and more sustained weight losses than any other method for obesity treatment. In the Swedish Obese Subjects study, which is a large prospective controlled study comparing surgery with conventional treatment, body weight had increased by 1.6% in the control group after 10 years and decreased in the surgery group by 16.1%. After 10 years, the surgery group also had a significantly lower rate of diabetes and hypertriglyceridaemia; however, there was no difference in hypertension [36]. Based on these results surgery is probably underutilized in severe obesity.

The importance of weight loss vs. health behaviour change

The knowledge that even smaller weight losses, in the order of 8–10%, may have substantial positive effects on an individual's metabolism and risk of getting type 2 diabetes [37, 38], induces a discussion of the relative merits of weight loss vs. lifestyle change in producing health and in lowering the risk for disease. Since these two factors are also closely related to each other, problems will arise when trying to separate the one effect from the other. From a behavioural perspective, especially in respect to long-term results, it may be an advantage to position behaviour change (i.e. more physical activity and healthier food) as a first priority and weight loss as a second. Weight loss would in that case be seen as an important consequence of health behaviour change. Moreover, a lifestyle change induces a multitude of effects that protect against both CVD and type 2 diabetes. Adjusting the lifestyle change to an individual's everyday life would also increase the possibility of sustained weight loss.

SMOKING

Smoking is a major risk factor for cardiovascular disease. With regard to coronary heart disease (CHD), it relates to both first and recurrent events. Smoking cessation therefore plays a major role in prevention of CHD and reducing risk among post-MI patients. In a Cochrane Review 2006 [39] it is concluded that the crude relative risk of all-cause mortality for smokers who quit compared with those who continued to smoke varied from 0.34 to 0.93.

Research suggests that, despite the widespread knowledge about the health hazards of smoking, about half of smokers continue to smoke after an acute MI [40]. About 70% of smoking patients say they would like to quit [41], but only about 8% manage to do so without help. Patients with coronary artery disease who stop smoking have reduced their risk for recurrent coronary events to the level of healthy non-smokers within 3 years [42]. Active interventions to help patients quit smoking would therefore be of major importance for prevention of CHD. The reviewed evidence suggests that interventions to help patients with CHD stop smoking can be effective (Cochrane Review 2006).

Nicotine replacement therapies

Meta-analyses examining the efficacy of nicotine patches on smoking cessation showed that the 6-month abstinence rate was 12.9% vs. 6.9% in the placebo group, and the 12-month rates were 11.2% vs. 5.5%, thus a statistically significant but clinically fairly modest effect [43]. However, caution should be observed with post-MI patients who could be affected by adverse nicotine effects, and severe arrhythmias, unstable angina, and a recent cerebral vascular event are contraindications.

The nicotine gum is an effective treatment for heavy smokers; however, it is associated with low patient compliance [43] and requires careful monitoring. The same contraindications as for the patch apply to nicotine gum.

A review of several trials reported a 6-month abstinence rate for nicotine inhalers of 22.2% vs. 10.5% for placebo, and 16.9% abstinence rate for the active group at 12 months, compared to 9.1% for placebo [43]. However, because of its rapid delivery of high concentrations of nicotine it is contraindicated in most patients with coronary artery disease.

Bupropion

This is an antidepressant drug that may be an appropriate treatment for patients for whom nicotine replacement therapies do not work and/or who suffer withdrawal symptoms such as depressive mood [43]. Bupropion can accomplish an abstinence rate of 18.2% at 12 months. Some concerns have been raised that it may affect blood pressure. Thus, even if there is no clear evidence supporting this notion, it might be wise to check the patient's blood pressure regularly. Nevertheless the Cochrance reviewers conclude that bupropion is a safe method for patients with CVD. Other antidepressants, however, do not seem to achieve smoking cessation [44].

Another new pharmacological agent that may be of help in smoking cessation is varenicline, a nicotine acetylcholine receptor agonist. Among long-term smokers treatment with varenicline was associated with a smoking cessation rate of 23% at one year as compared to 15% and 10.3% in the groups treated with bupropion and placebo respectively [45, 46]. Reports that it may be more effective than bupropion or placebo need confirmation.

Clinical implications

Ludvig *et al.* in their review [43] conclude that no difference in efficacy has been shown among the above-described smoking cessation therapies. The use of combination therapies is a promising alternative, and the combination of medication and behavioural strategies seems the most reasonable and feasible. The Cochrane Review 2006 reports main results from clinical trials on advice, individual and group counselling.

Physician advice

The effects of doctor's advice on smoking have been reviewed for CVD risk patients and unselected patient populations, mostly in primary care [47]. Pooled data revealed a small but significant effect on smoking rate, with a small advantage of intensive advice over simple advice. However, this is a measure that is very inexpensive and easy to deliver for the physician, and should therefore be routine with smoking patients.

Telephone counselling

The review of controlled trials showed that proactive telephone counselling can enhance effects of other interventions because of the personal contact [48]. It is not clear if it is equivalent to face-to-face personal contact, however with limited time resources, telephone contacts can be a feasible strategy and could preferably be done by other professionals in the team, such as nurses, physiotherapists and behavioural counsellors.

Individual behavioural counselling

Individual counselling can add to the efficacy and effectiveness of other smoking cessation methods. A review [49] could not detect a large difference between intensive and brief counselling.

The conclusion of the authors of this present chapter is that the effect is more related to *how* the counselling is performed, and we will therefore subsequently cover aspects of the communication process between the physician and the patient.

Group behaviour therapy programmes

In contrast with other behavioural change programmes where the group format seems more effective – at least for male patients – such as management of depression and stress [50], group therapy for smokers is not more effective than intense individual counselling [51]. However, group programmes are more effective than no intervention for helping patients stop smoking. Therefore, in a situation of limited time resources group programmes may be preferable, especially since they could be carried out by paramedical staff with special training for group interventions.

Conclusion

Several methods for smoking cessation have proved effective, both pharmacological treatments and behavioural counselling. Although statistically significant, the effects are often moderate from a clinical point of view. To improve outcome, attention should be paid to enhancement of the motivational process in the patient, and the quality of communication between the patient and the physician. This is true for all aspects of lifestyle intervention and long-term lifestyle change – physical activity, diet, smoking, smoking cessation and compliance with medication. Therefore, we will next turn to what is known about ways of improving the patient's compliance with long-term behaviour change.

MOTIVATION AND COMMUNICATION IN PREVENTIVE STRATEGIES

Compliance/adherence

Our patient J.P. is at risk for an acute cardiac event. He needs medication and lifestyle advice. However, he may not adopt these prescriptions, which are quite complex and may interfere with the ways of daily living that he is accustomed to. *Low compliance* is a well-known and widespread problem, and it is a *behavioural* problem [52]. Many studies have assessed the degree of compliance with, or adherence to, prescriptions in medical settings, and generally compliance is no better than about 50% [52]. For complex prescriptions, such as more than one medication, long-term or lifelong medication, and lifestyle advice, the degree of compliance is about 30% or less [52]. Furthermore, physicians' estimates of the degree to which their patients follow prescriptions show no correlation with patients' actual behaviour. Low compliance is not only a widespread problem, it is also very much underestimated. From the behavioural science point of view, information *per se* is seldom efficient in achieving behaviour change.

The WHO uses the word 'adherence' which is defined as 'the extent to which a person's behaviour – taking medication, following a diet, and/or executing lifestyle changes, corresponds with agreed recommendations from a health care provider' [53]. The WHO emphasizes the concept 'adherence' as different from 'compliance' in that adherence requires the patient's agreement to the recommendations. Recently, the concept of 'concordance' has been introduced [54]. Concordance 'is a new approach to the prescribing and taking of medicines. It is an agreement reached after negotiation between a patient and a healthcare professional that respects the beliefs and wishes of the patient in determining whether, when, and how medicines are to be taken.' [54]. The understanding of the compliance/adherence phenomenon that is implied here is that a partnership between patient and physician is needed in order to achieve long-term maintenance of behaviour change, including medication. The physician's expertise includes his or her professional knowledge, training, and experience, and the patient's expertise includes the knowledge about his or her needs, emotions, priorities, and everyday life situation.

Factors that improve compliance

Research on possible causes for low compliance has assessed several hundred potential factors. Some of them are the nature of the disease, procedures for referral, side effects of medication, the patient's age, sex, marital status, socioeconomic status (SES), or personality. None of these factors shows any consistent relationship with degree of compliance [52]. It is reasonable to assume that adequate compliance enhances the effects of treatment. However, as shown in the Multiple Risk Factor Intervention Trial (MRFIT) [55], even compliance with placebo (in this case 'usual care') was associated with an improved outcome compared with those who did not comply. While the greatest benefit was shown in those who complied with active treatment, those who were unable to comply with the active treatment advice had a higher mortality than those in the usual care group. Thus, there seems to be a benefit in complying with advice *per se* that may reflect a general benefit of high motivation. The clinical implication for the physician is to do all that he or she can to increase and sustain motivation.

Assessing motivation

The Stages of Change Model [56] is a convenient tool for assessment of the patient's motivation for change [57]. This model assumes that people go through five stages, each of which defines readiness for change: precontemplation (no interest in change), contemplation (thinking about possible change), preparation (has decided to change), action (practises new behaviour), and maintenance (long-term stability of new lifestyle). Naturally a person can go back and forth, relapse to a previous stage, and try several times before a new lifestyle acquires stability. It is important to assess the stage of the patient, because it determines which communication strategies will be the most effective. One common mistake is to give premature advice to a patient who is in a very early stage. Asking questions and offering information would be more strategic in this situation. Instead of telling the patient 'You must listen to this information', asking 'What important information can I give you about your problem and symptoms?' will increase the patient's interest. The patient is often quite ambivalent about change [58], and the physician should help the patient to verbalize pros and cons of old and new behaviour, but not put the patient under pressure to commit to a change when it is not likely to happen. Helping the patient to see pros and cons of alternatives will increase the probability that the patient will be able to develop his or her own motivation for change. Motivational interviewing strategies do not take very long to practise. It is a question of using your time with the patient differently. A few minutes of effective communication can achieve substantial reorientation in the patient.

Supporting the patient's change strategies

Hopefully, this kind of respectful communication will lead to a commitment by the patient to try out and practise new behaviours, such as good diet, exercise, and non-smoking. Three simple questions to the patient can aid in making commitment clear. (1) 'On a scale of zero to ten, how important is it for you to change behaviour (diet, physical activity, smoking)?' (2) 'On a scale of zero to ten, how confident are you that you can accomplish this?' (3) 'On a scale of zero to ten, how ready are you to start now?' The patient's ratings give a good estimate of what still needs to be done. Are they still unsure whether the change is important and needed?; do they trust their ability?; are there obstacles to starting the action? When the patient is reasonably able, willing, and ready to adopt and practise the new lifestyle, his or her own decisions about what they can do, and how, should be clarified and supported. The patient's priorities and values can be different from that of the health professional. After all, it is the patient who decides whether and how the change will be carried out in daily life, and open and respectful communication that leaves the responsibility with the patients for making such changes work will increase the chance of success.

Characteristics of successful behaviour change programmes

Behavioural science and analyses of effective lifestyle change interventions imply that the following components are of vital importance.

(1) Realism – the new behaviours should be easy to carry out and perform within ordinary daily life.
(2) Gradual changes – to overcome initial barriers.
(3) Repetition – practising the new behaviour over and over again.
(4) Long-term perspective – old habits die hard.
(5) Feedback – opportunity to check out and reflect on both successes and failures.
(6) Relapse prevention – development of built-in strategies for future threats to new lifestyle.
(7) Self-efficacy – the most important success factor in effective lifestyle interventions.
(8) Social support – provided by health professionals and significant others, to overcome delayed reward from the new behaviour *per se*. It may take a long time before it 'feels good' and natural.

Summary guidelines for clinical communication

Following here is some advice regarding how to apply such principles in clinical practice when helping patients change lifestyle.

■ Be careful and accurate when collecting information in your clinical examination. This includes information about symptoms, lifestyle, emotions, everyday life situation, personal and social resources, and it will provide a good basis for diagnosis and decisions about treatment.

■ Ask open questions that cannot be answered by a simple 'yes' or 'no'.
■ Be an emphatic listener; do not interrupt.
■ Help the patient to express their thoughts, attitudes, emotions, ambivalences and expectations on the effects of intervention.
■ Give clear and easy-to-understand explanations.
■ Make sure the patient has really understood the information given. Ask them to tell you in their own words what you have told them. Be consistent and make sure everyone within the health professional team conveys the same information.
■ Discuss and negotiate an action plan and reinforce self-efficacy.
■ Try to assess the patient's insight into possible obstacles to implementing the medication or lifestyle change. For instance, what can happen at parties, on vacations or with changes of daily routine?
■ Individualize! Find out the specific concerns and difficulties of *this* patient. Money? Language? Earlier experiences? Significant others? Depression?

For long-term maintenance of lifestyle change

■ Make sure lifestyle changes are compatible with the patient's everyday life situation.
■ Use 'reminders', for instance telephone calls, 'newsletters'.
■ Involve family to assure social support.
■ Provide specific feedback by offering opportunities for personal discussions with health professionals.
■ Agree with the patient on a structured plan for monitoring of long-term maintenance.

There is substantial evidence for the importance of lifestyle and behaviour change in the prevention of CVD. Much is also known about the mechanisms for how behaviours influence medical endpoints. It is time to move on to the development and use of clinical methods and techniques for how to make sustainable lifestyle change happen for our patients.

REFERENCES

1. US Department of Health and Human Services. Physical activity and health: a report of the Surgeon General. Atlanta, Georgia, US Department of Health and Human Services, Public Health Service, CDC, National Center for Chronic Disease Prevention and Health Promotion, 1996.
2. O'Connor GT, Buring JE, Yusuf S *et al*. An overview of randomized trials of rehabilitation with exercise after myocardial infarction. *Circulation* 1989; 80:234–244.
3. Fagard RH. Exercise characteristics and the blood pressure response to dynamic physical training. *Med Sci Sports Exerc* 2001; 33(suppl):S502–S515.
4. Leon AS, Sanchez OA. Response of blood lipids to exercise training alone or combined with dietary intervention. *Med Sci Sports Exerc* 2001; 33(suppl):S502–S515.
5. Moyna NM, Thompson PD. The effect of physical activity on endothelial function in man. *Acta Physiol Scand* 2004; 180:113–123.
6. Ford ES. Does exercise reduce inflammation? Physical activity and C-reactive protein among U.S. adults. *Epidemiology* 2002; 13:561–568.
7. Lee I-M, Skerrett PJ. Physical activity and all-cause mortality: what is the dose-response relation? *Med Sci Sports Exerc* 2001; 33(suppl):S459–S471.
8. Wannamethee SG, Shaper AG. Physical activity and cardiovascular disease. *Semin Vasc Med* 2002; 2:257–266.
9. Pate RR, Pratt M, Blair SN *et al*. Physical activity and public health. A recommendation from the Centers for Disease Control and Prevention and the American College of Sports Medicine. *JAMA* 1995; 273:402–407.

10. Haskell WL. What to look for in assessing responsiveness to exercise in a health context. *Med Sci Sports Exerc* 2001; 33(suppl):S454–S458.
11. Bandura A. Self-efficacy. The Exercise of Control. W. H. Freeman and Company, New York, 1997.
12. Brassington GS, Atienza AA, Perczek RE, DiLorenzo TM, King AC. Intervention-related cognitive versus social mediators of exercise adherence in the elderly. *Am J Prev Med* 2002; 23:80–86.
13. The Writing Group for the Activity Counseling Trial Research Group. Effects of physical activity counseling in primary care. The Activity Counseling Trial: a randomized controlled trial. *JAMA* 2001; 286:677–687.
14. Rejeski WJ, Brawley LR, Ambrosius WT *et al*. Older adults with chronic disease: benefits of group-mediated counseling in the promotion of physically active lifestyles. *Health Psychol* 2003; 22:414–423.
15. Di Loreto C, Fanelli C, Lucidi P *et al*. Validation of a counseling strategy to promote the adoption and the maintenance of physical activity by type 2 diabetic subjects. *Diabetes Care* 2003; 26:404–408.
16. DeBusk RF, Miller NH, Superko R *et al*. A case-management system for coronary risk factor modification after acute myocardial infarction. *Ann Intern Med* 1994; 120:721–730.
17. Carlson JJ, Norman GJ, Feltz DL, Franklin BA, Johnson JA, Locke SK. Self-efficacy, psychosocial factors, and exercise behaviour in traditional versus modified cardiac rehabilitation. *J Cardiopulm Rehab* 2001; 21:363–373.
18. Seidell JC, Perusse L, Despres JP, Bouchard C. Waist and hip circumferences have independent and opposite effects on cardiovascular disease risk factors: the Quebec Family Study. *Am J Clin Nutr* 2001; 74:315–321.
19. Wang Y, Rimm EB, Stampfer MJ, Willett WC, Hu FB. Comparison of abdominal adiposity and overall obesity in predicting risk of type 2 diabetes among men. *Am J Clin Nutr* 2005; 81:555–563.
20. Snijder MB, Zimmet PZ, Visser M, Dekker JM, Seidell JC, Shaw JE. Independent and opposite associations of waist and hip circumferences with diabetes, hypertension and dyslipidemia: the AusDiab Study. *Int J Obes* 2004; 28:402–409.
21. Calle EE, Thun MJ, Petrelli JM, Rodriguez C, Heath CW. Body-mass index and mortality in a prospective cohort of U.S. adults. *N Engl J Med* 1999; 341:1097–1105.
22. Flegal KM, Graubard BI, Williamson DF, Gail MH. Excess deaths associated with underweight, overweight, and obesity. *JAMA* 2005; 293:1861–1867.
23. Andres R, Muller DC, Sorkin JD. Long-term effects of change in body weight on all-cause mortality: a review. *Ann Intern Med* 1993; 119:737–743.
24. Lee IM, Paffenbarger Jr RS. Change in body weight and longevity. *JAMA* 1992; 268:2045–2049.
25. Eckel RH, Grundy SM, Zimmet PZ. The metabolic syndrome. *Lancet* 2005; 365:1415–1428.
26. Kahn R, Buse J, Ferrannini E, Stern M. The metabolic syndrome: time for a critical appraisal. *Diabetologia* 2005; 48:1684–1699.
27. Gale EAM. The myth of the metabolic syndrome. *Diabetologia* 2005; 48:1679–1683.
28. Alberti KGMM, Zimmet P, Shaw J. The metabolic syndrome – a new worldwide definition. *Lancet* 2005; 366:1059–1062.
29. Hu G, Qiao Q, Tuomilehto J, Balkau B, Borch-Johnsen K, Pyörälä K. Prevalence of the metabolic syndrome and its relation to all-cause and cardiovascular mortality in nondiabetic European men and women. *Arch Intern Med* 2004; 164:1066–1076.
30. Poirier P, Giles TD, Bray GA *et al*. Obesity and cardiovascular disease: pathophysiology, evaluation, and effect of weight loss. *Circulation* 2006; 113:[Epub ahead of print].
31. James PT, Rigby N, Leach R. The obesity epidemic, metabolic syndrome and future prevention strategies. *Eur J Cardiovasc Prev Rehab* 2004; 11:3–8.
32. Berkel LA, Poston WSC, Reeves RS, Foreyt JP. Behavioural interventions for obesity. *J Am Diet Assoc* 2005; 105:S35–S43.
33. Foster GD, Makris AP, Bailer BA. Behavioural treatment of obesity. *Am J Clin Nutr* 2005; 82(suppl):230S–235S.
34. Padwal R, Li SK, Lau DCW. Long-term pharmacotherapy for overweight and obesity: a systematic review and meta-analysis of randomized controlled trials. *Int J Obes* 2003; 27:1437–1446.
35. Wadden TA, Berkowitz RI, Sarwer DB, Prus-Wisniewski R, Steinberg C. Benefits of lifestyle modification in the pharmacologic treatment of obesity. *Arch Intern Med* 2001; 161:218–227.
36. Sjöström L, Lindroos A-K, Peltonen M *et al*. Lifestyle, diabetes, and cardiovascular risk factors 10 years after bariatric surgery. *N Engl J Med* 2004; 351:2683–2693.

37. Tuomilehto J, Lindström J, Eriksson JG *et al*. Prevention of type 2 diabetes mellitus by changes in lifestyle among subjects with impaired glucose tolerance. *N Engl J Med* 2001; 344:1343–1350.

38. Knowler WC, Barrett-Connor E, Fowler SE *et al*. Reduction in the incidence of type 2 diabetes with lifestyle intervention or metformin. *N Engl J Med* 2002; 346:393–403.

39. Critchley J, Capewell S. Smoking cessation for the secondary prevention of coronary heart disease (Review). *The Cochrane Collaboration*. John Wiley & Sons, Ltd., Chichester, 2006.

40. van Berkel TF, Boersma H, Roos-Hesselink JW, Erdman RS, Simoons ML. Impact of smoking cessation and smoking interventions in patients with coronary heart disease. *Eur Heart J* 1999; 20:1773–1782.

41. Mallin R. Smoking cessation: Integration of behavioural and drug therapies. *Am Fam Physician* 2002; 65:1107–1114.

42. Kannel WB, D'Agostino RB, Belanger AJ. Fibrinogen, cigarette smoking, and risk of cardiovascular disease – insights from the Framingham study. *Am Heart J* 1987; 113:1006–1010.

43. Ludvig J, Miner B, Eisenberg MJ. Smoking cessation in patients with coronary artery disease. *Am Heart J* 2005; 149:565–572.

44. Hughes JR, Stead LF, Lancaster T. Antidepressants for smoking cessation (Cochrane Review). *The Cochrane Library*, Issue 1, John Wiley & Sons, Ltd., Chichester, 2006.

45. Tonstad S. Smoking cessation efficacy and safety of a α4β2 nicotinic receptor partial agonist – results from varenicline in cessation therapy: optimising results. American Heart Association, Dallas, Texas, 2005.

46. Gonzales D, Rennard SI, Nides M *et al*. Varenicline, an α4β2 nicotonic acetylcholine receptor partial agonist *vs* sustained-release bupropion and placebo for smoking cessation – a randomised controlled trial. *JAMA* 2006; 296:47–55.

47. Lancaster T, Stead LF. Physician advice for smoking cessation (Cochrane Review). *The Cochrane Library*, Issue 1, John Wiley & Sons, Ltd., Chichester, 2006.

48. Stead LF, Lancaster T, Perera R. Telephone Counselling for smoking cessation (Cochrane Review). *The Cochrane Library*, Issue 1, John Wiley & Sons, Ltd., Chichester, 2006.

49. Lancaster T, Stead LF. Individual behavioural counselling for smoking cessation (Cochrane Review). *The Cochrane Library*, Issue 1, John Wiley & Sons, Ltd., Chichester, 2006.

50. Schneiderman N, Saab PG, Catellier DJ *et al*. ENRICHD Investigators. Psychosocial treatment within sex by ethnicity subgroups in the Enhancing Recovery in Coronary Heart Disease clinical trial. *Psychosom Med* 2004; 66:475–483.

51. Stead LF, Lancaster T. Group behaviour therapy programmes for smoking cessation (Cochrane Review). *The Cochrane Library*, Issue 1, John Wiley & Sons, Ltd., Chichester, 2006.

52. Vermeire E, Hearnshaw H. Patient adherence to treatment: three decades of research. A comprehensive review. *J Clin Pharm Ther* 2001; 26:331–342.

53. Sabaté E. *Adherence to long-term therapies: evidence for action*. World Health Organization, Geneva, 2003.

54. Dickinson D, Wilkie P, Harris M. Taking medicines: concordance is not compliance. *BMJ* 1999; 319:787.

55. Gump BB, Matthews KA. Special intervention reduces CVD mortality for adherent participants in the Multiple Risk Factor Intervention Trial. *Ann Behav Med* 2003; 26:61–68.

56. DiClimente CC, Prochaska JO, Fairhurst SK, Velicer WF, Velasquez MM, Rossi JS. The process of smoking cessation: an analysis of precontemplation, contemplation, and preparation stages of change. *J Consult Clin Psychol* 1991; 59:295–304.

57. Litt J. Smoking and GPs: time to cough up. Successful interventions in general practice. *Australian Family Physician* 2005; 34:425–429.

58. Miller WR, Rollnick S. Motivational Interviewing, 2nd edition. The Guilford Press, New York, 2002.

15

Management of specific risk factors – lipids

O. Faergeman

Cholesterol lowering and treatment of dyslipidaemia is only one element in the prevention of cardiovascular disease (CVD), and guidelines for the prevention of CVD in Europe and the US are based on an understanding of the multifactorial nature of risk of CVD [1, 2]. Lipid disorders are important, but so are smoking, obesity, physical inactivity, hypertension and diabetes. In emphasizing the multifactorial approach to assessment and management of risk of CVD, we may have under-emphasized some of the clinical problems that attend diagnosis and management of dyslipidaemia. Among all the risk factors, the dyslipidaemias are the most varied, and there is more to diagnosing and treating dyslipidaemia than prescribing a lipid-lowering diet and a lipid-lowering drug. It is the purpose of this chapter, which is based on an earlier publication [3], to present a broader perspective, not to focus once again on just one risk factor, but rather to enable physicians to cope a little better with some of the specific, clinical problems of dyslipidaemic patients within the overall context of preventive cardiology.

Dyslipidaemia literally means a disturbance of lipids in blood. It captures the idea of too little as well as too much lipid in blood, *hypolipidaemia* and *hyperlipidaemia*, respectively. When blood plasma contains very large amounts of triglycerides, it becomes milky or even creamy. Such visible hyperlipidaemia is called *lipaemia*. The term, dyslipidaemia, also captures the idea of rare disturbances of blood lipids that are too subtle to be detected by routine measurements of cholesterol or triglyceride. The terms, *hypercholesterolaemia* and *hypertriglyceridaemia*, are self-explanatory. Since lipids in blood are always associated with proteins in lipoproteins, hyperlipidaemia also means *hyperlipoproteinaemia*, and hypolipidaemia also means *hypolipoproteinaemia*.

The structure of lipoproteins explains some of the phenomena that seem to puzzle many physicians. Cholesterol and triglycerides are not soluble in water or watery media such as blood plasma. Cholesterol becomes even more hydrophobic when it is esterified to a fatty acid. For the purpose of transport in plasma, triglycerides and esterified cholesterol are therefore packed into the hydrophobic cores of lipoproteins, which are fairly complex macromolecules. Surrounding the hydrophobic core of a lipoprotein is a coat of unesterified cholesterol, phospholipids and various proteins called apolipoproteins. The inner surface of the coat, facing the fatty core, is hydrophobic, whereas the outer surface, facing the surrounding water, is hydrophilic. The composition of chylomicrons, very low-density lipoproteins (VLDL), low-density lipoproteins (LDL) and high-density lipoproteins (HDL) is given in Table 15.1.

Ole Faergeman, MD, DMSc, Professor, Cardiovascular Medicine, National Heart and Lung Institute, Charing Cross Campus, Imperial College, London, UK

Table 15.1   Approximate composition of plasma lipoproteins (mass percentages)

	Chylomicrons	VLDL	LDL	HDL
Triglyceride	86	55	6	4
Cholesteryl ester	3	12	42	14
Cholesterol	2	7	8	4
Phospholipid	7	18	22	33
Protein	2	8	22	45

PRACTICAL CLASSIFICATION OF DYSLIPIDAEMIA

It has seemed natural to distinguish between very severe but less common and mainly monogenetic dyslipidaemias, affecting specialty patients, on the one hand, and less severe, usually polygenic forms of dyslipidaemia, affecting people on an epidemic scale, on the other hand. As we have learned more about dyslipidaemia, however, this differentiation has become increasingly artificial. Some forms of polygenic dyslipidaemia can be severe, and some forms of monogenetic dyslipidaemia can be mild. With few exceptions, moreover, the severity of dyslipidaemia depends on interaction between genes and environment in the broadest sense: presence or absence of other conditions and diseases, dietary habits, physical activity, intake of alcohol and drugs. The biochemical and clinical pictures attending these genetically and environmentally different conditions therefore overlap substantially.

A practical, initial approach to thinking about dyslipidaemia is to consider all dyslipidaemias in terms of four broad and heterogenous categories based on routine measurements of plasma lipids.

1. Hypercholesterolaemia, almost always due to elevated LDL cholesterol.
2. Mixed dyslipidaemias. They include the combination of high triglycerides and low HDL cholesterol as well as the combination of high triglycerides and high cholesterol (LDL cholesterol).
3. Severe hypertriglyceridaemia due to chylomicronaemia and, as a rule, also to elevated VLDL.
4. Isolated low HDL cholesterol.

PRIMARY AND SECONDARY DYSLIPIDAEMIAS

Within each of these broad categories are dyslipidaemias due to primary disturbance of the metabolism of lipoproteins. Such primary dyslipidaemias are corrected by treatment specifically aimed at a step in lipoprotein metabolism.

Dyslipidaemia can also result from use of alcohol and certain drugs, or dyslipidaemia can be a part of the biochemical picture of diseases such as diabetes and hypothyroidism. These common dyslipidaemias are therefore considered secondary to abuse of alcohol, drugs or disturbances of carbohydrate or energy metabolism. Before asking the patient to embark on life-long dietary or pharmacological treatment to lower plasma lipids, secondary dyslipidaemia must be ruled out by clinical examination, a drug history, and a small battery of laboratory tests (Tables 15.2 and 15.3).

The distinction between primary and secondary dyslipidaemias is not sharp, however. It is appropriate to consider the dyslipidaemias of type 1 diabetes and hypothyroidism as secondary dyslipidaemias, because they are corrected by insulin and thyroxin. It is less

Table 15.2 Diseases and conditions causing secondary dyslipidaemia

	Cholesterol	Triglyceride	HDL cholesterol	Recommended biochemical test
Hypothyroidism	↑↑	↑		Thyroid stimulating hormone
Cushing's disease	↑	↑↑		Urinary cortisol excretion
Polycystic ovary syndrome	↑	↑↑	↓	Free testosterone index
Type 2 diabetes		↑↑	↓	Glucose in plasma and urine
Nephrotic syndrome	↑↑			Urinary protein
Chronic renal failure	↑	(↑)	↓	Creatinine
Cholestasis	↑↑			Alkaline phosphatase
Alcoholism		↑↑	↑	Alanine aminotransferease
Pregnancy		↑↑↑		
Sepsis		↑↑		

Table 15.3 Some drugs causing secondary dyslipidaemia

	Cholesterol	Triglyceride	HDL cholesterol
Isotretinoin		↑↑	↓
Corticosteroids	↑	↑	↓
Oral oestrogens		↑ (↑↑)	↑
Tamoxifen, clomiphene		↑ (↑↑)	
Cyclosporin	↑		
Protease inhibitors		↑	↓
β-blockers		↑	↓
Thiazide diuretics	↑	↑	↓
Novel antipsychotic drugs (clozapine, olanzapine)		↑	

obvious that the dyslipidaemia of type 2 diabetes is a secondary dyslipidaemia. That is partly because type 2 diabetes is a complex disorder of the metabolism of lipids as well as carbohydrates, and it is partly because type 2 diabetic dyslipidaemia is not corrected by oral hypoglycaemic drugs.

HYPERCHOLESTEROLAEMIA

When hypercholesterolaemia is not attended by high triglycerides, it is almost always due to high concentrations of LDL. Exceptions are the rare patients with very high concentrations of HDL. High concentrations of LDL and HDL are not attended by hypertriglyceridaemia, because the cores of these lipoproteins are composed of a lot of esterified cholesterol and very little triglyceride, and the surface coats of lipoproteins contain no triglyceride at all.

Moderate hypercholesterolaemia, due to elevated LDL cholesterol, affects about half of the populations of affluent societies. It is usually caused by eating too much food with a high content of saturated fat from the meat and milk of cows, pigs, and sheep. The extent to which LDL cholesterol is elevated by saturated fat depends on a background of variation in many different genes. Those patterns of genetic variation are certain to differ from person to person, and it will prove to be difficult and probably impossible to make molecular diagnoses in most people with polygenetic hypercholesterolaemia. Concentrations of LDL cholesterol are typically between 3 and 5 mmol/l (~115–190 mg/dl) in epidemic, moderate hypercholesterolaemia.

As genetic variations (polymorphisms or mutations) get more severe, fewer of them are necessary for hypercholesterolaemia to develop. Indeed, the less common and most serious form of hypercholesterolaemia, familial hypercholesterolaemia, is usually due to mutation in just one gene, typically the gene for the LDL receptor or the gene for one of the receptor's ligands, apolipoprotein B (apoB). The binding of apoB to the LDL receptor on the surface of cells in the liver and other organs is essential for the normal removal of LDL from plasma. The heterozygous form of familial hypercholesterolaemia occurs in about 1 in 500 in most populations, and the more severe homozygous form of the disease occurs in 1 in 1 million.

CLINICAL DIAGNOSIS

The more severe the hypercholesterolaemia, the higher the rates of cholesterol deposition in arteries, skin, corneas and tendons. Patients with lesser degrees of elevation of LDL cholesterol, typically with a polygenetic background, may not develop atherosclerosis rapidly enough to matter before death occurs in old age for another reason. In contrast, patients with homozygous familial hypercholesterolaemia can die of myocardial infarction in early childhood, and, untreated, most of them die before the age of 30 years. Between these extremes is a gradual, exponential increase in risk of atherosclerotic disease with increasing concentrations of LDL cholesterol.

Patients with hypercholesterolaemia develop atherosclerosis at the typical sites of predilection (bifurcations and branch points), not least in the coronary, carotid and pelvic arteries. During clinical examination, it is therefore useful to auscultate the carotid and femoral arteries. A murmur is almost certain to be due to stenotic atherosclerotic plaques, but absence of murmur does not exclude significant atherosclerosis. Patients with homozygous familial hypercholesterolaemia often have a stenosis of the ascending aorta just above the aortic valve. It produces a systolic ejection murmur, maximal in the second right intercostal space. Supravalvular aortic stenosis is an important cause of death in these patients.

Corneal arcus occurs regularly in older people without hypercholesterolaemia, but a corneal arcus in younger people, for example in their thirties, suggests familial hypercholesterolaemia. Xanthelasmata are yellow plaques in the delicate skin of the upper and lower eyelids. They are also typical of, but not specific to, patients with familial hypercholesterolaemia. In contrast, tendon xanthomata, when present, strongly suggest familial hypercholesterolaemia. They are indolent, but pain and tenderness, due to inflammation of the Achilles tendons (Achilles tendinitis), can precede development of frank xanthomata. Tendon xanthomata can be discrete, and they elude detection easily unless the physician makes it a point to look, and especially to palpate, for them in the triceps tendon of the upper arm, the extensor tendons of the third, fourth and fifth fingers just distal to the metacarpophalangeal joints, the patellar ligament, and the Achilles tendon. In general, homozygous patients have severe xanthomatosis, but at least half of patients with heterozygous familial hypercholesterolaemia do not have tendon xanthomas.

LABORATORY DIAGNOSIS

LDL cholesterol is elevated, whereas concentrations of triglycerides and HDL cholesterol are normal. The diagnosis of familial hypercholesterolaemia should be entertained when concentrations of LDL cholesterol exceed 5 mmol/l (~190 mg/dl). The family history should be queried and a pedigree drawn up. Resources permitting and family willing, first-degree relatives, in particular brothers, sisters and children, should then be examined [4]. Although it makes little difference to treatment decisions, a molecular diagnosis of a mutation in the gene for the LDL receptor or the gene for apoB is useful in tracing affected family members. The molecular diagnostic work-up in the index patient can be laborious, but when a diagnosis has been made, family members need to be tested only for the mutation identified in the index patient. This screening strategy is cost-effective, but a failure to demonstrate a mutation does not rule out the diagnosis of familial hypercholesterolaemia [5].

DIFFERENTIAL DIAGNOSIS

High HDL cholesterol
Moderate elevations of HDL cholesterol (2–4 mmol/l; ~80–160 mg/dl) are not uncommon, especially in women, and they can explain a mild hypercholesterolaemia that is associated with lower risk of CVD. It is evident that hypercholesterolaemia due to high concentrations of HDL cholesterol must not be treated, and that decisions to treat hypercholesterolaemia should not be based only on measurement of total cholesterol.

Very high concentrations of HDL cholesterol (4–6 mmol/l; ~150–230 mg/dl) are a rare cause of hypercholesterolaemia without hypertriglyceridaemia. They can be due to deficiency of cholesteryl ester transfer protein, which promotes transfer of esterified cholesterol from HDL to VLDL [5].

Secondary hypercholesterolaemia
Causes of secondary hypercholesterolaemia include hypothyroidism, cholestasis, nephrotic syndrome and treatment with cyclosporin (Tables 15.2 and 15.3).

Other diseases causing tendon xanthomata
Tendon xanthomata are characteristic of familial hypercholesterolaemia, but they also affect patients with very rare diseases with autosomal recessive inheritance: cerebrotendinous xanthomatosis, sitosterolaemia (phytosterolaemia), and, in paediatric patients, type B Niemann-Pick disease and cholesterol ester storage disease/Wolman's disease.

MIXED DYSLIPIDAEMIAS

This is a group of overlapping and heterogenous dyslipidaemias, the hallmark of which is hypertriglyceridaemia in association with another lipid abnormality. The majority of subjects with mixed dyslipidaemia have 'atherogenic dyslipidaemia', in which high triglycerides are accompanied by low concentration of HDL cholesterol. This dyslipidaemia is typical of the 'metabolic syndrome'. Other forms of mixed dyslipidaemia are characterized by various combinations of high triglycerides and high cholesterol, and in still others high triglycerides are accompanied by high HDL cholesterol.

HIGH TRIGLYCERIDES, LOW HDL CHOLESTEROL: ATHEROGENIC DYSLIPIDAEMIA

The combination of high triglycerides, low HDL cholesterol and the presence of a particular subtype of LDL (small dense LDL) is as strongly associated with atherosclerotic disease as hypercholesterolaemia. Depending on choice of cut-off points, it is also as common as hypercholesterolaemia. The combination has been called 'the lipid triad' and 'atherogenic dyslipidaemia'. It can occur as a distinct dyslipidaemia, but it is more often associated with abdominal obesity, physical inactivity, metabolic syndrome and type 2 diabetes.

Small dense LDL are a particularly atherogenic kind of LDL. Although they are characteristic of 'atherogenic dyslipidaemia', special laboratory methods are required to detect small LDL particles; hence they are not measured in routine practice. 'Atherogenic dyslipidaemia' must therefore be diagnosed on the basis of high triglycerides and low HDL cholesterol.

The production of small dense LDL and the lowering of HDL cholesterol are both closely linked to the metabolism of triglycerides. Small dense LDL tend to appear in plasma when triglycerides exceed 1.3 mmol/l (~130 mg/dl). In the range of triglycerides between 2 and 5 mmol/l (~200–500 mg/dl), VLDL as well as LDL contributes to increased risk of atherosclerotic disease. Although that contribution is reflected in the triglyceride measurements, it is taken better into account by calculating non-HDL cholesterol or by measuring concentrations of apoB, a single molecule of which is present in each particle of LDL and VLDL [6].

Like polygenetic hypercholesterolaemia, atherogenic dyslipidaemia is probably due to complex interactions between habits of diet and physical exercise on the one hand and variation in a large number of different genes on the other. The habits promoting atherogenic dyslipidaemia are simple over-eating combined with physical inactivity. Atherogeneic dyslipidaemia commonly accompanies type 2 diabetes, and it is one of the salient features of the metabolic syndrome.

METABOLIC SYNDROME

According to the current US guidelines (Adult Treatment Panel III [ATP III]), the metabolic syndrome can be diagnosed when three or more of the following features are present [2]:

1. Waist circumference >102 cm in men and >88 cm in women.
2. Serum triglycerides >1.7 mmol/l (~150 mg/dl).
3. HDL cholesterol <1 mmol/l (~40 mg/dl) in men and <1.3 mmol/l (~50 mg/dl) in women.
4. Blood pressure >130/85 mmHg.
5. Serum glucose >6.1 mmol/l (~110 mg/dl).

The World Health Organization (WHO) uses another definition:

Diabetes, impaired fasting glucose, impaired glucose tolerance or insulin resistance (assessed by clamp studies) and at least two of the following:

1. Waist-to-hip ratio >0.90 in men and >0.85 in women.
2. Serum triglycerides >1.7 mmol/l or HDL cholesterol <0.9 mmol/l in men and <1.0 mmol/l in women.
3. Blood pressure >140/90 mmHg.
4. Urinary albumin excretion rate >20 µg/min or albumin-to-creatinine ratio >30 mg/g.

About a quarter of westernized populations have the metabolic syndrome by the WHO, as well as by the ATP III, criteria. From 15% to 20% of individuals are classified as having the syndrome by one definition but not by the other, however there are other major problems with current concepts of the metabolic syndrome. The American Diabetes Association and the European Association for the Study of Diabetes, in a joint statement, have therefore recommended that physicians should avoid diagnosing patients with the metabolic syndrome, *'as this might create the impression that the metabolic syndrome denotes a greater risk than its components, or that it is more serious than other CVD risk factors, or that the underlying pathophysiology is clear'* [7].

HIGH TRIGLYCERIDES, HIGH CHOLESTEROL

Familial combined hyperlipidaemia

In some families prone to early-onset atherosclerotic disease, some members have elevated cholesterol, and some have elevated triglycerides. The patterns seem to change over time, so that in any particular person it can sometimes be cholesterol, and sometimes triglycerides that are most elevated. Observations made in the 1960s suggested that this pattern of familial combined hyperlipidaemia is a distinct, monogenetic disease with an autosomal dominant inheritance. The prevalence of familial combined hyperlipidaemia was determined to be about twice that of familial hypercholesterolaemia (1/250). Attempts to identify single genes in which mutations unambiguously cause familial combined hyperlipidaemia have been partially successful [8], but often the dyslipidaemia is probably a polygenetic disorder, and it is frequently associated with the metabolic syndrome.

Due to overproduction of VLDL from the liver, concentrations of total cholesterol are typically 6–9 mmol/l (~230–350 mg/dl), and triglycerides are typically 3–6 mmol/l (~300–600 mg/dl). The diagnosis is supported if concentrations of apoB are also elevated. In contrast to familial hypercholesterolaemia, atherosclerotic disease does not occur in the children of these families, but adults can develop atherosclerotic disease as early as patients with familial hypercholesterolaemia. Patients can have xanthelasmata and tuberous xanthomas, but tendon xanthomata occur rarely if at all. Since the relationship of the clinical syndrome to variation on the gene level has not been fully clarified, there is no way to diagnose familial combined hyperlipidaemia by molecular genetic analysis.

Dysbetalipoproteinaemia

Dysbetalipoproteinaemia is a rare cause of severe atherosclerotic disease. Atherosclerosis affects the peripheral as well as the coronary arteries, and patients can have a characteristic yellow discoloration of the creases of the palms of the hands and soles of the feet called palmar xanthomatosis ('yellow palms'). They can also have xanthelasmata and tuberous xanthomas.

Dyslipidaemia is due to accumulation of atherogenic VLDL remnant lipoproteins, which contain cholesterol as well as triglyceride. They migrate abnormally in an electrophoretic gel, in which they appear as a 'dysbeta' band (an abnormally broad beta band), hence the name. The characteristic dyslipidaemia is severe elevation of cholesterol as well as triglycerides. When measured in mmol/l, cholesterol and triglycerides are elevated to approximately the same values, e.g. 8–10 mmol/l. When measured in mg/dl, cholesterol is elevated to slightly less than half of triglyceride values, e.g. 300–400 and 600–800 mg/dl, respectively.

Dysbetalipoproteinaemia is usually the result of a complex interaction between the environment and a variation in the gene for apolipoprotein E. The patient must have inherited the apoE2 variant from both parents, i.e. the patient must be homozygous for apoE2, and the patient must also have a condition such as obesity or hypothyroidism.

Dysbetalipoproteinaemia is rare. It affects only 0.01–0.02% of the population. Molecular diagnosis of homozygosity for apoE2 is easy to do in specialized laboratories.

HIGH TRIGLYCERIDES, HIGH HDL CHOLESTEROL

Drinking alcohol is a common cause of hypertriglyceridaemia. It is due to increased production of VLDL from the liver. Alcohol also increases plasma HDL cholesterol. In postmenopausal women, hormone replacement therapy with oestrogen or oestrogen + gestagen is also a common cause of combined elevation of triglycerides and HDL cholesterol. Conjugated, equine oestrogens tend to produce a more severe hypertriglyceridaemia than

17-β oestradiol. In contrast, the gestagen component tends to mitigate the dyslipidaemia. There is no evidence that these dyslipidaemias in general do any harm, but the hope that the elevation of HDL cholesterol might benefit patients has always been doubtful in the case of alcohol, and it has been shown to be clearly wrong in the case of hormone replacement therapy [9].

In genetically susceptible people, alcohol as well as oestrogen can elicit severe hypertriglyceridaemia and acute pancreatitis.

HYPERTRIGLYCERIDAEMIA

Elevation of plasma triglycerides can be due to high VLDL, chylomicronaemia, or both. Since the cores and surface coats of VLDL and chylomicrons contain small amounts of cholesterol, hypertriglyceridaemia is also frequently attended by elevations of plasma cholesterol. Moreover, due to exchanges of lipids between lipoproteins, hypertriglyceridaemia is often attended by less conspicuous lowering of concentrations of HDL cholesterol since hypertriglyceridaemia dominates the clinical picture of the dyslipidaemias to be described in this section; however, it is easiest not to consider them still as more examples of mixed dyslipidaemias.

In fairly rare patients, hypertriglyceridaemia is almost exclusively a genetically determined and familial condition, but in most patients with moderate and severe hypertriglyceridaemia, some form of genetic susceptibility is likely to have interacted with other disturbances of metabolism or with dietary indiscretion, alcoholism, obesity, infection or drugs, to raise triglycerides in plasma.

FAMILIAL HYPERTRIGLYCERIDAEMIA

The clustering of hypertriglyceridaemia in families characterizes familial hypertriglyceridaemia. Triglycerides are usually moderately elevated by 2–5 mmol/l (~200–500 mg/dl), and they are not accompanied by severe increase of plasma cholesterol. The elevation of plasma VLDL is less ominous than in familial combined hyperlipidaemia, because it increases risk of atherosclerotic disease only slightly, if at all. That is because concentrations of LDL can be normal. Thus, if concentrations of cholesterol and LDL cholesterol are not much elevated, if apoB concentrations are normal, and if the family history does not indicate that atherosclerotic disease develops at a very early age, then therapy with drugs, especially, is not necessary. Some patients with familial hypertriglyceridaemia are obese, but many are not, and the disorder is thought to be due to defective catabolism of triglycerides, perhaps due to minor deficiency in the function of lipoprotein lipase.

In some families, the underlying metabolic problem is more severe. Severe hypertriglyceridaemia can arbitrarily be defined as triglycerides exceeding 5 mmol/l (~500 mg/dl), but sometimes patients have triglyceride concentrations that are much higher, e.g. values exceeding 100 mmol/l (~10 000 mg/dl). Such degrees of hypertriglyceridaemia always signify chylomicronaemia, often accompanied by elevation of VLDL. It can be due to deficiency of lipoprotein lipase, the enzyme in muscle and fat tissue that normally hydrolyses the triglycerides of chylomicrons and VLDL. It can also be due to the absence of cofactor for lipoprotein lipase, a small apolipoprotein called apoC-II. Finally it can be due to the high concentrations of another small apolipoprotein, apoC-III, which is an inhibitor of lipoprotein lipase.

These various genetic conditions require homozygosity, i.e. the paternal as well as the maternal alleles of the genes for the lipase, the cofactor, etc. are abnormal. They are therefore rare, but they are likely to be involved when severe hypertriglyceridaemia occurs in childhood or even in infancy.

Plasma appears milky and even creamy when triglycerides are severely elevated. Even before separation of cells from plasma, blood looks like tomato soup made with a heavy cream, and through the ophthalmoscope retinal arteries appear to be lighter than usual. A simple test can be employed to see which class of lipoproteins is the culprit. Leave a plasma sample in the refrigerator overnight. Plasma that continues to be opaque contains VLDL, whereas a creamy layer at the top is due to chylomicrons.

Severe hypertriglyceridaemia is always accompanied by some degree of elevated plasma cholesterol. This is often a source of confusion to physicians, who mistakenly believe that the hypercholesterolaemia is due to elevation of LDL. Instead it is due to the elevation of VLDL and chylomicrons. VLDL contain cholesterol in their cores and surface coats, and chylomicrons also contain cholesterol, most of it in their surface coat. It is therefore not surprising that concentrations of plasma cholesterol can be doubled or tripled when concentrations of triglycerides have been elevated to 50 times the upper limit of normal.

It is a mistake to treat hypercholesterolaemia, which is due only to chylomicronaemia, with drugs to lower LDL and VLDL. However, drugs can obviously be indicated to lower VLDL. Despite its simplicity, the refrigerator test is therefore very useful. It tells you whether plasma contains chylomicrons (creamy layer at the top), VLDL (plasma remains opaque), or both.

Chylomicronaemia syndrome

The physician must carefully question patients with hypertriglyceridaemia, especially if it is severe, about symptoms suggesting pancreatitis at some time in the past, perhaps in relatives. Acute pancreatitis is often the first manifestation of severe hypertriglyceridaemia, in children as well as adults, and it is one of the most serious consequences of this form of dyslipidaemia. Patients are protected from bouts of acute pancreatitis if triglycerides can be maintained below 10 mmol/l (~1000 mg/dl), and preferably below 5 mmol/l (~500 mg/dl), if necessary by the specialized dietary treatment described below.

There are several less serious signs and symptoms of severe hypertriglyceridaemia. Eruptive xanthomatosis is a crop of small, cutaneous nodules with a white centre and an erythematous base. They can resemble acne, but their sites of predilection are extensor surfaces of the body, i.e. the back, the posterior surface of the upper arms, the buttocks, and the anterior surface of the thighs. Less common sites are palms of the hands and soles of the feet, where these small xanthomas can be quite tender and painful. Eruptive xanthomatosis disappears in the course of a few weeks of adequate therapy.

Chylomicrons and VLDL are picked up by cells of the reticulo-endothelial system when lipoprotein lipase of muscle and fat tissue fails to remove them from the blood stream at normal rates. The result is hepatosplenomegaly, sometimes the cause of a vague abdominal discomfort, which is also rapidly alleviated by treatment.

Triglyceride can account for almost 10% of plasma volume at triglyceride concentrations of 100 mmol/l (~10 000 mg/dl). In the laboratory, severe hypertriglyceridaemia therefore interferes with routine biochemical measurements of amylase, electrolytes, etc.

Atherosclerosis

The other serious consequence of severe hypertriglyceridaemia is widespread atherosclerosis. It is associated with combined elevation of VLDL and chylomicrons, and it is due to the former, i.e. the VLDL component, because VLDL can be small enough to enter the artery wall. Unfortunately, many patients with combined elevation of VLDL and chylomicrons have diabetes as well, and it is not really possible to ascertain the relative importance of the disturbances of lipid and glucose metabolism in the development of cerebrovascular disease, coronary artery disease and intermittent claudication.

Diagnosis is based on:

1. History and clinical examination.
2. Measurements of plasma triglycerides.
3. The refrigerator test to see whether hypertriglyceridaemia is due to chylomicrons, VLDL or both.
4. Measurement of lipoprotein lipase activity, if possible.

Heparin 50 i.u./kg body weight is injected intravenously to release lipoprotein lipase from the sites of the enzyme's attachment to capillary walls. Blood is sampled 10 min later, and the activity of lipase is measured in plasma. Molecular genetic analysis of the genes for lipoprotein lipase and apolipoprotein C-II is possible but generally not useful.

SECONDARY HYPERTRIGLYCERIDAEMIAS

In Tables 15.2 and 15.3 some of the many causes of secondary hypertriglyceridaemia are listed. Some of them are rare, but taken together, secondary hypertriglyceridaemias are very common indeed, and the conditions or agents causing them must be excluded, treated or otherwise taken into consideration before prescribing drugs to lower triglycerides. Some of them can be severe, even causing the full picture of the chylomicronaemia syndrome described above.

HYPOLIPIDAEMIA

LOW HDL CHOLESTEROL AS A PRIMARY OR SOLE DYSLIPIDAEMIA

Concentrations of HDL cholesterol below 1 mmol/l (~40 mg/dl) attend hypertriglyceridaemia. Concentrations of HDL cholesterol can also be very low despite normal concentrations of VLDL, and this can be due to a primary disturbance of HDL metabolism.

LOW HDL CHOLESTEROL IN POOR COUNTRIES (EPIDEMIC LOW HDL)

In developing countries, low HDL cholesterol is common among the poor whose diet is traditionally low in fats and high in complex carbohydrates. On the other hand, atherosclerotic disease is uncommon, and low HDL cholesterol is therefore of no prognostic importance in this setting [10].

LOW HDL CHOLESTEROL IN AFFLUENT COUNTRIES

In contrast, low concentrations of HDL cholesterol are associated with high risk of atherosclerotic disease among the affluent, including, of course, the affluent parts of the population of developing countries. Thus, as a rule, low HDL cholesterol is a risk factor only if the diet is fairly rich in fats, and plasma concentrations of atherogenic lipoproteins are high.

When low HDL cholesterol nevertheless does occur as the sole dyslipidaemia, it places physicians in a quandary, especially if the patient happens to have atherosclerotic disease. That is because the data supporting drug treatment to raise HDL cholesterol are not extensive. Moreover, isolated low HDL cholesterol is associated with physical inactivity and smoking, both of which, in their own right, require non-pharmacological intervention. Finally, some people with very low HDL cholesterol must, by definition, represent the lower extreme of the normal distribution of HDL cholesterol as it is determined by interaction between environment and numerous slight variations in many different genes.

Nicotinic acid (or one of its derivatives) is the drug of first choice if the physician does elect to treat isolated low HDL cholesterol dyslipidaemia in patients with established CVD.

Alternatively, if LDL cholesterol is not already very low, a statin drug can be used to lower it to less than 1.8 mmol/l (~70 mg/dl) [11].

A small number of very rare diseases, due to mutations in genes coding for proteins directly involved in the metabolism of HDL, include low concentrations of HDL cholesterol as part of a more complex clinical picture. They are associated with other disturbances of lipids such as high triglycerides, but the primary problem is in HDL metabolism. They include lecithin-cholesterol-acyl-transferase (LCAT) deficiency, Tangier disease due to mutations in the gene for an ATP-binding-casette-transporter protein, and deficiency of apolipoprotein A1 [12].

LOW LDL CHOLESTEROL

ApoB is the major protein of VLDL and LDL, and a smaller version of apoB is necessary for chylomicrons to be secreted from the small intestine. Fat cannot be absorbed normally if the intestine is unable to make apoB. The result is abetalipoproteinaemia, a rare and serious disease beginning in childhood and becoming full-blown in the second and third decades of life.

A series of clinically innocuous conditions are due to heterozygosity for defects in the complex process of synthesis of apoB, including defects in the apoB gene itself. Concentrations of apoB are low, but physicians are more likely to run across these conditions by measurements of cholesterol. Total cholesterol is low, 2–3 mmol/l (~80–120 mg/dl), as is LDL cholesterol, 0.5–2 mmol/l (~20–80 mg/dl). Hypobetalipoproteinaemia is associated with low risk of atherosclerotic disease, and no treatment is required.

THERAPY

With few exceptions such as acute pancreatitis in the chylomicronaemia syndrome, dyslipidaemia produces no immediate symptoms. Even high concentrations of LDL cholesterol cause no immediate discomfort, and the purpose of lowering them is to prevent future discomfort due to myocardial infarction, stroke, claudication, etc.

INTERNATIONAL RECOMMENDATIONS ASSESSING RISK AND SETTING GOALS OF THERAPY

The challenge is to differentiate wisely between patients sufficiently likely, and sufficiently unlikely, to benefit adequately from long-term therapy to lower lipids, blood pressure, etc. Patients who already have atherosclerotic disease are at high risk, not only of progression of atherosclerosis, but also of the occurrence or recurrence of the consequences of atherosclerosis such as myocardial infarction and ischaemic stroke. They include patients with coronary artery disease, cerebrovascular disease and intermittent claudication, and there is broad agreement that all of these patients are at risk that is high enough to merit lipid-lowering therapy.

The risk associated with type 2 diabetes is not as well clarified. Some studies have suggested that type 2 diabetes increases risk of cardiovascular death to the same level as that in non-diabetic patients who have survived a myocardial infarction [13], and this finding gave rise to the concept of type 2 diabetes as a 'coronary risk equivalent', a concept adopted in the National Cholesterol Education Program (NCEP) Expert Panel guidelines [2]. However, not all studies support the concept of risk equivalency between diabetes and coronary artery disease [14].

In Europe, goals are for everyone to reduce cholesterol below 5 mmol/l (~190 mg/dl) and LDL cholesterol below 3 mmol/l (~115 mg/dl), but the vigour with which that effort is pursued depends on the individual's overall risk. However, the target for those with established CVD, diabetes, markedly elevated levels of single risk factors or Systemic Coronary Risk Evaluation (SCORE) risk greater than or equal to 5% is lower: total cholesterol below 4.5 mmol/l (4 mmol/l if feasible) or LDL cholesterol below 2.5 mmol/l (2 mmol/l if feasible).

The general recommendation is that drug therapy in asymptomatic people is warranted only if a combination of risk factors indicates that the absolute risk of a cardiovascular death exceeds 5% over the course of the next 10 years [1].

In the US, goals are primarily defined in terms of LDL cholesterol, and they differ as a function of an assessment of risk in a similar way to the one used in Europe. The goals are to reduce LDL cholesterol below 160 mg/dl (~4.1 mmol/l) if risk is low, below 130 mg/dl (~3.4 mmol/l) if 10-year risk is less than 20%, and below 100 mg/dl (~2.6 mmol/l) if 10-year risk of a coronary event exceeds 20% [2]. Note that there is rough correspondence between the 5% risk of cardiovascular death used in Europe and the 20% risk of a coronary event employed in the US. In an update of the US guidelines, issued in 2004, the NCEP Coordinating Committee suggested that physicians could elect to lower LDL cholesterol to <70 mg/dl (~1.8 mmol/l) if the risk is very high [15].

Neither the European nor the American recommendations provide goals of therapy to lower triglycerides or to raise HDL cholesterol. Instead, high triglycerides (>1.7 mmol/l, ~200 mg/dl) and low HDL cholesterol (<1 mmol/ l; ~40 mg/dl) are considered markers of increased risk in the European and US recommendations [1, 2]. One of the refinements of the American recommendations is the use of non-HDL cholesterol, i.e. cholesterol in LDL, VLDL and remnant lipoproteins. These lipoproteins all tend to be atherogenic, and the concentration of non-HDL cholesterol is a good predictor of risk and guide for therapy. A well-documented alternative is to measure apoB, which is an even better index of atherogenic lipoproteins in plasma [6]. Each of these lipoproteins contains just one molecule of apoB.

As we have seen, very high triglyceride concentrations can cause acute pancreatitis. A goal of therapy, always with diet and sometimes with restriction of alcohol or cessation of therapy with oestrogens, is to maintain triglycerides below 10 mmol/l (~1000 mg/dl) according to European recommendations, or below 5 mmol/l (~500 mg/dl) according to American recommendations.

Recommendations have major implications for the use of healthcare resources, and resources should be used to help those patients who need them most. In wealthy countries with low disease prevalence, it is economically realistic to prescribe expensive drugs to all patients whose 10-year risk of a cardiovascular death or a coronary event exceeds 5% and 20%, respectively. In countries with less money and more disease, higher levels of risk may be necessary before physicians prescribe drugs to lower lipids, blood pressure or glucose. This view is most widely held in Europe, because gradients of risk of CVD and gradients of economic resources are steep across Europe [16]. Goals of therapy, similar to the European or American goals, can probably be adopted elsewhere, but the therapy needed to reach them invariably depends on resources, and limited resources should be used for patients at highest risk.

HOW TO TREAT

Because of cultural traditions and explicit policies for agriculture, industry and transport, it is beyond the abilities of most physicians, and beyond the abilities even of many professional medical societies, to change circumstances enough to reduce the population risk of atherosclerotic disease [17]. However, in the consultation room, every physician must encourage his or her particular patient to make the personal choices necessary to attain or maintain a low level of risk.

DIET

The physician caring for dyslipidaemic patients should be able to use three kinds of diets. The first is a diet to lose weight. The second is a diet to lower LDL cholesterol. The purpose of the third kind of diet is to prevent pancreatitis in patients with chylomicronaemia. It is important that it is not confused with the diets to treat obesity or high LDL cholesterol.

Diets to lower risk of atherosclerotic disease by reducing body weight or
LDL cholesterol: fat modification

The diet appropriate to lowering risk of atherosclerotic disease depends on cultural context. In some developing countries, many people have only recently moved from rural to urban areas, and the challenge is to encourage them to maintain the best of traditional food patterns. In India, for example, it is a recommendation to maintain the percentage of food energy derived from fat below 21%, because it has recently been only 15% in rural areas [11]. In contrast, some Europeans and Americans eat so much fat (50% of food energy) that it is difficult to persuade them to reduce it to less than 30% of energy.

Although it may be difficult for westerners to restrict fat intake to the levels considered normal in several Asian countries, it should be restricted to about a third of total food energy according to the latest NCEP and Joint European recommendations.

The most important part of almost all dietary recommendations for lowering LDL cholesterol is restriction of intake of saturated fat to less than 7–10% of energy. This is particularly important in diets to reduce body weight, e.g. in patients with the metabolic syndrome. Although reduction of LDL cholesterol is a consequence of almost any form of intended weight loss, it lasts longer if weight reduction includes control of saturated fat.

When the primary concern is not reduction of body weight, what should replace saturated fat? Over the past two decades, recommendations have placed more emphasis on monounsaturated fats (rather than polyunsaturated fats) and carbohydrates as foods to replace saturated fat. The US recommendations, for example, allow monounsaturated fat to account for up to 20% of calories, and for complex carbohydrates to account for up to 60%. Complex carbohydrates should come from whole-grain products.

Trans fatty acids are found in dairy products and in hydrogenated industrial fats. They raise LDL cholesterol and increase the risk of atherosclerotic disease, and intake should be as low as possible. Dairy fats, bakery products (pastries, cakes, crackers, cookies, doughnuts) and potatoes (chips and French fries) and chicken deep-fried in oils should be avoided.

Cholesterol in food also raises LDL cholesterol. Since most cholesterol-rich foods are also foods containing a lot of saturated fat, however, restriction of the latter is accompanied by restriction of the former. Nevertheless, most recommendations do stipulate restrictions of dietary cholesterol.

The evidence for changing other dietary components to reduce risk is not as robust as that pertaining to fats and carbohydrates, and there is no complete agreement about recommendations for plant stanols/sterols or n-3 fatty acids from fish and plant sources (rapeseed and soya oils).

Table 15.4 provides essentials of food choice in urbanized societies.

Table 15.4   Dietary advice for most people and patients in urbanized populations

Eat more	*Eat and drink less*
Fruits, vegetables, berries, nuts, potatoes, whole-grain bread and pasta, brown rice, poultry, fish, vegetable oils	Dairy products and meat from cattle, pig, sheep and other domesticated animals Hardened fats including hardened vegetable fats. Cakes, crackers, doughnuts and pastries. Sugary foods and soft drinks, potatoes, and white (refined) bread, pasta and rice

Diet for patients with primary chylomicronaemia:
severe fat restriction

The only way to reduce the production of chylomicrons from the small intestine is to reduce the intake of long-chain fat (fatty acids with 12 or more carbon atoms). That is because long-chain fat is so insoluble in water that the intestine must package it in chylomicrons in order to forward it to the rest of the body *via* the lymphatic vessels and the left subclavian vein. In contrast, medium-chain fatty acids (10 carbon atoms or less) are soluble enough in water to be secreted directly into the blood of the portal circulation for transport to the liver.

If the chylomicronaemia syndrome is not due to diabetes, abuse of alcohol or treatment with oestrogens, patients must eat food with a very low content of long-chain fat, which includes monounsaturated and polyunsaturated fat as well as saturated fat. Vegetable oils and fish oils are therefore as dangerous to these patients as saturated fat from mammal sources. The necessary reduction of intake of fat by 75% or more to 20–40 g/day can be quite difficult, and the patient needs encouragement and often the advice of an experienced dietician. To avoid acute pancreatitis, triglyceride concentrations must be kept below 10 mmol/l (~1000 mg/dl), preferably below 5 mmol/l (~500 mg/dl), and the severity of fat restriction can be adjusted according to these measurements.

Whereas occasional departures from a fat-modified diet to reduce risk of atherosclerotic disease are perfectly acceptable, acute pancreatitis can result from a single meal with a large amount of long-chain fat. Strict adherence to this severe diet is therefore necessary. A dim ray of light is margarine made from medium-chain fat. In most countries, it can be purchased in apothecaries, drug stores or special-food stores.

ALCOHOL

In genetically susceptible persons, moderate or severe hypertriglyceridaemia can be elicited by drinking alcohol in amounts that are socially acceptable in many cultures. Unless the physician confidently can exclude alcohol as a contributor to the hypertriglyceridaemia, he should suggest to the patient a 2-week period of total abstinence. Seeing the results of repeat measurements of triglycerides, as well as of alanine aminotransferase or γ-glutamyltransferase, will then often convince the patient of the wisdom of drinking less.

DRUGS

Five classes of lipid-modifying drugs are currently available to most physicians. They are the inhibitors of HMG CoA reductase (statins), the fibrates, bile acid sequestrants (anion exchange resins), niacin (nicotinic acid) and its derivatives, and inhibitors of absorption of cholesterol from the intestine. Bile acid sequestrants, niacin and especially the statins have all been well-documented to reduce risk of coronary death and even total mortality, whereas treatment with fibrates has not been attended by the same degrees of clinical benefit. Only one inhibitor of cholesterol absorption from the intestine is as yet widely available (ezetimibe), and documentation for effects on CVD is still pending. Drug choice (Table 15.5) is important, since the benefits of pharmacologically modifying plasma lipids seem to depend on the manner by which they are lowered [11].

STATINS (HMG-COA REDUCTASE INHIBITORS)

The most convincing evidence from angiography as well as clinical endpoint trials has been obtained with the most potent of the lipid-lowering drugs, namely the statins. Statins have a good safety record, and they are easy to use. At present, therefore, they are first-line drugs for lowering LDL cholesterol. They also lower triglycerides, and they can slightly raise HDL cholesterol.

Table 15.5   Choices of drug therapy

	First choice	Second choice
Hypercholesterolaemia	Statin	Ezetimibe, anion exchange resin, niacin, fibrate
Mixed hyperlipidaemia	Statin	Niacin, fibrate
Hypertriglyceridaemia*	Niacin	Fibrate
Isolated low HDL	Niacin	Statin, fibrate

*Severe hypertriglyceridaemia responds poorly to drug therapy. Diet, abstention from alcohol, are usually more important.

Virtually all the metabolic effects of statins result from inhibition of HMG-CoA reductase, which catalyses an early step in the synthesis of cholesterol. As a result, statins not only raise the activity of LDL receptors and the rate of hepatic removal of LDL from the bloodstream; they also reduce hepatic secretion of VLDL into the bloodstream.

A meta-analysis of statin trials comprising more than 90 000 patients indicated that lowering LDL cholesterol by 1 mmol/l results in a 12% proportional reduction in all-cause mortality ($P < 0.0001$), a 19% reduction in coronary mortality ($P < 0.0001$), a 23% reduction in myocardial infarction or coronary death ($P < 0.0001$), a 24% reduction in the need for coronary revascularization ($P < 0.0001$), and a 17% reduction in fatal or non-fatal stroke ($P < 0.0001$) [18].

Doubling the dose of a statin drug lowers LDL cholesterol by an additional 6%, whereas combination therapy with low-dose anion-exchange resin or with a cholesterol absorption inhibitor provides an additional 15–20% lowering of LDL cholesterol.

Apart from potency, statins appear to differ in some ancillary properties such as antithrombotic and anti-inflammatory effects. It should be appreciated, however, that the experimental basis for these pleiotropic effects of statins is very small compared to the data that have emerged from the major trials with clinical endpoints, on which clinical practice should be based.

Clinical trials and post-marketing surveillance programmes have shown that statins are quite safe [18, 19]. Cerivastatin, nevertheless, when given in conjunction with other drugs such as mibefradil, fibrates, cyclosporin, macrolide antibiotics, warfarin, digoxin, and azole antifungals could precipitate fatal rhabdomyolysis [20]. Cerivastatin has been withdrawn from the market, but all statins should remain prescription drugs.

FIBRATES

Fibrates are also easy to use, and they lower triglycerides quite effectively. They do so by activating peroxisome-proliferator-activated receptors, which are transcription factors for several genes that encode proteins in control of the metabolism of lipoproteins. For example, the gene for lipoprotein lipase is activated in this manner. They also raise HDL concentrations in plasma, at least in part by transcriptional induction of the synthesis of apolipoproteins A-I and A-II. These, as well as other mechanisms of action of the fibrate drugs on the molecular level, would appear to be clinically beneficial, but the full spectrum of gene activation by fibrates may not be known at this point. Moreover, the apparent complexity of the mode of action of the fibrates at the level of gene activation as well as at the level of lipoprotein physiology makes it difficult if not impossible to predict what happens on the clinical level when these drugs are given to patients. In hypertriglyceridaemic patients, fibrates can sometimes increase LDL cholesterol, and it can be necessary to prescribe a low dose of a statin to accompany fibrate therapy.

The evidence from clinical trials to support the widespread use of fibrates is not as good as that supporting statins. Indeed, a conclusion of several meta-analyses has been that there is no good indication for the use of the fibrate group of drugs [21, 22]. The most recent large fibrate trial also produced equivocal results [23]. Nevertheless, fibrate therapy remains an option for selected patients, and fibrates are clearly valuable in the treatment of less common forms of hypertriglyceridaemia such as dysbetalipoproteinaemia.

Fibrates can cause myopathy, especially if combined with statins, and they increase the lithogenicity of bile and the risk of gallstones. They also potentiate the effects of warfarin, the dose of which must often be reduced.

ANION EXCHANGE RESINS

Also called bile acid sequestrant drugs, the anion exchange resins are not absorbed in the intestine. Instead they remain in the intestinal lumen where they release chloride ions in exchange for bile acids, which are removed with the drug by faecal excretion ('sequestered'). To replace the bile acids lost in this manner, the liver takes up more LDL cholesterol from blood for conversion to bile acids, and LDL concentrations in plasma are lowered. However, the liver also increases synthesis of cholesterol. The result is increased production of VLDL and, in susceptible patients, a rise in plasma triglycerides. The anion exchange resins are therefore contraindicated in hypertriglyceridaemic patients.

Treatment with anion exchange resins reduces risk of coronary artery disease [24], and the drugs have an excellent safety record. They are bulky, however, and usually they must be taken as a suspension in juice or water. They easily cause bloating, flatulence and constipation. Moreover, they can bind and decrease the absorption of other drugs (e.g. digoxin, warfarin, thyroxin, thiazide diuretics, folic acid and statins), which therefore should be taken an hour before or 4 h after the anion exchange resin. These drugs are no longer used very much as monotherapy, but they still make good combinations with statins.

Begin therapy with small doses, e.g. 4 g of cholestyramine or 5 g of colestipol, for a week or two, and use a fibre preparation to alleviate constipation. Full doses (e.g. 24 g of cholestyramine per day) are difficult to tolerate. It is often wiser to prescribe no more than 8 g of cholestyramine or 10 g of colestipol per day, and it is sometimes easiest for the patient to take the dose at bedtime, as long as he or she is not taking other medications at that time.

Colesevelam hydrochloride, a newer anion exchange resin, apparently produces fewer side-effects than cholestyramine and colestipol, and it may not interfere as much with the absorption of other drugs. In monotherapy with doses varying from 2.3 to 4.5 g/day, colesevelam reduces LDL cholesterol by up to 18%. Like cholestyramine and colestipol, colesevelam combines well with statins, and it can also be combined with ezetimibe. The usual recommended dose is 3.75 g/day.

NIACIN (NICOTINIC ACID)

Niacin is a vitamin, which, given in small doses, prevents pellagra (diarrhoea, dementia and death). Given in larger doses, niacin inhibits release of fatty acids from adipose tissue to the bloodstream, thereby reducing the availability of substrate for synthesis of triglycerides in the liver, which therefore secretes fewer VLDL into the bloodstream. The result is lowering of plasma triglycerides and LDL cholesterol, including lowering of small dense LDL. Niacin also lowers lipoprotein (a) (lp (a)), and it is the most effective drug for raising HDL cholesterol. In short, it does all the right things to lipoproteins, and treatment with combinations of niacin with other drugs is accompanied by significant reductions in angiographic progression of disease, incidence of myocardial infarction, and death [25, 26].

Like the bile acid sequestrants, niacin is difficult to use. There can be marked flushing of the skin soon after intake, and gastrointestinal symptoms include nausea, flatulence, and diarrhoea. It can also cause hepatotoxicity, hyperuricaemia, and hyperglycaemia, and rare side-effects include conjunctivitis, retinal oedema, ichthyosis and acanthosis nigricans. Cutaneous flushing can be reduced by initiating therapy with small and frequent doses (e.g. 250 mg three to four times daily, as evenly spaced as possible). Doses should then be gradually increased to 3 g/day (divided into 3–4 doses) or more over the course of a few months. Flushing can also be reduced by taking niacin at the end of a meal and, during the first days of therapy, by taking a small dose of acetylsalicylic acid (150–325 mg) 30 min before each dose of niacin. Tachyphylaxis disappears quickly, and flushing can recur if the patient has forgotten to take the previous dose. For many patients, sustained-release preparations of nicotinic acid or derivatives of nicotinic acid are easier to use than the parent drug in crystalline form, but rates of hepatotoxicity are not lower.

INHIBITION OF CHOLESTEROL ABSORPTION FROM THE GUT

Ezetimibe inhibits absorption of cholesterol from the gut [27]. The drug is well-tolerated in the recommended dose of 10 mg/24 h, and, unlike resins, it does not raise triglycerides. It lowers LDL cholesterol moderately, but combination therapy with statins is very useful [28]. Inhibition of intestinal absorption of cholesterol provides a reduction of LDL cholesterol by 15–20% in addition to that obtained already by monotherapy with statin. As yet there are no clinical endpoint data for inhibitors of cholesterol absorption.

TRIGLYCERIDE MEASUREMENTS TO GUIDE DRUG CHOICE

Anion exchange resins (bile acid sequestrants) tend to increase triglycerides, and they should only be used when triglycerides are less than 2 mmol/l (~200 mg/dl) or if given in conjunction with a triglyceride-lowering agent. Statins are usually used for patients with triglycerides up to 5 mmol/l (~500 mg/dl). When triglycerides are between 5 and 10 mmol/l (~500–1000 mg/dl), fibrates may be used, and niacin is a good drug in selected patients. When triglycerides exceed 10 mmol/l (~1000 mg/dl), drugs are generally not useful. Instead, to prevent pancreatitis, triglycerides must be reduced by restriction of alcohol, treatment of diabetes with insulin, cessation of oestrogen therapy, and, in some patients, severe restriction of long-chain fat of both animal and vegetable origin.

DRUG COMBINATIONS

In familial hypercholesterolaemia and other forms of severe hypercholesterolaemia, the combination of a statin and ezetimibe or, more traditionally, the combination of a statin and a small dose of an anion exchange resin (bile acid sequestrant), can be very useful. In the latter case, one option is for patients to take the anion exchange resin at bedtime and the statin with the evening meal. If the patient is not taking many other drugs (which must be taken an hour before or 4 h after the anion exchange resin), another option is to take the statin at bedtime and the anion exchange resin in small doses at each meal. For some patients, a triple regimen of an anion exchange resin, a statin and niacin can be necessary.

Statins can also be combined with fibrates. Since this combination has been associated with myopathy, even fatal rhabdomyolysis, patients must be carefully selected. Be especially careful if the patient is old. Renal function must be normal, and patients should not be taking other drugs that can increase systemic levels of statins or fibrates. The initial dose of statin should be low, and it should then be increased cautiously. Instruct the patient about warning symptoms (myalgia). If he or she experiences muscle pain or tenderness that cannot be explained by recent strenuous work or exercise, the drugs should be stopped, and the patient should report for measurement of creatinine kinase (CK) as soon as possible. Discontinue combination therapy if CK is more than ten times the upper limit of normal, and wait for symptoms to vanish and CK levels to return to normal before resuming therapy with lower doses of either or both drugs.

WHEN TO BEGIN LIPID-LOWERING THERAPY AFTER MYOCARDIAL INFARCTION

The Myocardial Ischaemia Reduction with Aggressive Cholesterol Lowering (MIRACL) trial in patients with acute coronary syndromes showed that treatment with atorvastatin, initiated within 4 days, can reduce the recurrence of myocardial ischaemia during the following 4 months [29], but the overall evidence is not strong enough to make early treatment mandatory [30]. In principle, therefore, drug treatment can be postponed for 3 months. The advantage of this approach is that estimation of untreated plasma lipids, and the evaluation of response to drug therapy, are more reliable, because the acute phase response of plasma lipids to myocardial infarction has passed. Moreover, it gives cardiologists and general practitioners the time and opportunity to consider whether the patient has a genetically determined dyslipidaemia requiring family investigation.

The disadvantage of postponing drug therapy is that many patients will no longer be under the care of a cardiologist when therapy should be started. In some cases, this means that drug treatment will never be considered. A pragmatic view is therefore to prescribe drug treatment in hospital on the basis of the initial cholesterol measurements. However, early drug treatment must still be combined with effective dietary intervention and the physician must still exclude secondary dyslipidaemias and consider whether the patient has a genetically determined dyslipidaemia mandating family investigation.

NON-DRUG, NON-DIETARY TREATMENT OF DYSLIPIDAEMIA

LDL apheresis

Rare patients with severe hypercholesterolaemia, especially homozygous familial hypercholesterolaemia, require a specialist to evaluate the need for LDL apheresis. By this expensive but effective technique, LDL is removed from plasma during extracorporeal circulation weekly or every other week.

Surgery

Before the advent of effective drug therapy, three forms of surgery were used to lower LDL cholesterol in patients with familial hypercholesterolaemia: creation of a shunt between the portal and inferior caval veins [31], liver transplantation [32], and partial ileal bypass [33]. The latter operation was used fairly extensively. The small intestine was transected at the transition from jejunum to ileum, and the upper end of the ileum was closed blindly. The lower end of the jejunum was then anastomosed end-to-side to the ascending colon, so that the contents of the intestine bypassed the ileum where bile acids normally are reabsorbed. The mechanism of action of the operation was therefore very similar to that of the anion exchange resins: interruption of the entero-hepatic circulation of bile acids and reduction of LDL cholesterol consequent to increased hepatic uptake of cholesterol for conversion to bile acids. The operation increased life expectancy and, in many countries, a few patients with heterozygous familial hypercholesterolaemia now attending lipid clinics will include patients whose small intestine has been rearranged in this fashion. Side-effects include steatorrhoea and, later, renal stones [34].

REFERENCES

1. Graham I, Atar D, Borch-Johnsen K *et al.*, Fourth Joint Task Force of the European Society of Cardiology and other Societies on Cardiovascular Disease Prevention in Clinical Practice. European Guidelines on Cardiovascular Disease Prevention in Clinical Practice. *Eur J Cardiovasc Prev Rehabil* 2007; 14(suppl 2):S1–S113.

2. Third Report of the National Cholesterol Education Program (NCEP) Expert Panel on Detection, Evaluation, and Treatment of High Blood Cholesterol in Adults (Adult Treatment Panel III) final report. *Circulation* 2002; 106:3143–3421.

3. Faergeman O, Grundy SM. *Dyslipidaemia*. Elsevier Science Ltd., London, 2003.

4. Hadfield SG, Humphries SE. Implementation of cascade testing for the detection of familial hypercholesterolaemia. *Curr Opin Lipidol* 2005; 16:428–433.

5. Damgaard D, Larsen ML, Nissen PH *et al.* The relationship of molecular genetic to clinical diagnosis of familial hypercholesterolemia in a Danish population. *Atherosclerosis* 2005; 180:155–160.

6. Barter PJ, Ballantyne CM, Carmena R *et al.* Apo B versus cholesterol in estimating cardiovascular risk and in guiding therapy: report of the thirty-person/ten-country panel. *J Intern Med* 2006; 259:247–258.

7. Kahn R, Buse J, Ferrannini E, Stern M. The metabolic syndrome: time for a critical appraisal: joint statement from the American Diabetes Association and the European Association for the Study of Diabetes. *Diabetes Care* 2005; 28:2289–2304.

8. Suviolahti E, Lilja HE, Pajukanta P. Unraveling the complex genetics of familial combined hyperlipidemia. *Ann Med* 2006; 38:337–351.

9. Risks and benefits of estrogen plus progestin in healthy postmenopausal women: principal results from the Women's Health Initiative randomized controlled trial. *JAMA* 2002; 288:321–333.

10. Knuiman JT, West CE, Katan MB, Hautvast JG. Total cholesterol and high-density lipoprotein cholesterol levels in populations differing in fat and carbohydrate intake. *Arteriosclerosis* 1987; 7:612–619.

11. Janus ED, Postiglione A, Singh RB, Lewis B. The modernization of Asia: implications for coronary heart disease. Council on Arteriosclerosis of the International Society and Federation of Cardiology. *Circulation* 1996; 94:2671–2673.

12. Hovingh GK, de Groot E, van der Steeg W *et al.* Inherited disorders of HDL metabolism and atherosclerosis. *Curr Opin Lipidol* 2005; 16:139–145.

13. Haffner SM, Lehto S, Ronnemaa T, Pyörälä K, Laakso M. Mortality from coronary heart disease in subjects with type 2 diabetes and in nondiabetic subjects with and without prior myocardial infarction. *N Engl J Med* 1998; 339:229–234.

14. Evans JM, Wang J, Morris AD. Comparison of cardiovascular risk between patients with type 2 diabetes and those who had had a myocardial infarction: cross sectional and cohort studies. *Br Med J* 2002; 324:939–942.

15. Grundy SM, Cleeman JI, Merz CN *et al.* Implications of recent clinical trials for the National Cholesterol Education Program Adult Treatment Panel III guidelines. *Circulation* 2004; 110:227–239.

16. Kesteloot H, Sans S, Kromhout D. Dynamics of cardiovascular and all-cause mortality in Western and Eastern Europe between 1970 and 2000. *Eur Heart J* 2006; 27:107–113.

17. Faergeman O. *Coronary Artery Disease: Genes, Drugs and the Agricultural Connection*. Elsevier, Amsterdam, 2003.

18. Baigent C, Keech A, Kearney PM *et al.* Efficacy and safety of cholesterol-lowering treatment: prospective meta-analysis of data from 90,056 participants in 14 randomised trials of statins. *Lancet* 2005; 366:1267–1278.

19. McKenney JM, Davidson MH, Jacobson TA, Guyton JR. Final conclusions and recommendations of the National Lipid Association Statin Safety Assessment Task Force. *Am J Cardiol* 2006; 97:89C–94C.

20. Omar MA, Wilson JP. FDA adverse event reports on statin-associated rhabdomyolysis. *Ann Pharmacother* 2002; 36:288–295.

21. Gould AL, Rossouw JE, Santanello NC, Heyse JF, Furberg CD. Cholesterol reduction yields clinical benefit. A new look at old data. *Circulation* 1995; 91:2274–2282.

22. Bucher HC, Griffith LE, Guyatt GH. Systematic review on the risk and benefit of different cholesterol-lowering interventions. *Arterioscler Thromb Vasc Biol* 1999; 19:187–195.

23. Keech A, Simes RJ, Barter P *et al.* Effects of long-term fenofibrate therapy on cardiovascular events in 9795 people with type 2 diabetes mellitus (the FIELD study): randomised controlled trial. *Lancet* 2005; 366:1849–1861.

24. The Lipid Research Clinics Coronary Primary Prevention Trial results. I. Reduction in incidence of coronary heart disease. *JAMA* 1984; 251:351–364.

25. Carlson LA, Rosenhamer G. Reduction of mortality in the Stockholm Ischaemic Heart Disease Secondary Prevention Study by combined treatment with clofibrate and nicotinic acid. *Acta Med Scand* 1988; 223:405–418.

26. Brown G, Albers JJ, Fisher LD *et al*. Regression of coronary artery disease as a result of intensive lipid-lowering therapy in men with high levels of apolipoprotein B. *N Engl J Med* 1990; 323:1289–1298.

27. Garcia-Calvo M, Lisnock J, Bull HG *et al*. The target of ezetimibe is Niemann-Pick C1-Like 1 (NPC1L1). *Proc Natl Acad Sci USA* 2005; 102:8132–8137.

28. Ballantyne CM, Weiss R, Moccetti T *et al*. Efficacy and safety of rosuvastatin 40 mg alone or in combination with ezetimibe in patients at high risk of cardiovascular disease (results from the EXPLORER Study). *Am J Cardiol* 2007; 99:673–680.

29. Schwartz GG, Olsson AG, Ezekowitz MD *et al*. Effects of atorvastatin on early recurrent ischemic events in acute coronary syndromes: the MIRACL study: a randomized controlled trial. *JAMA* 2001; 285:1711–1718.

30. Briel M, Schwartz GG, Thompson PL *et al*. Effects of early treatment with statins on short-term clinical outcomes in acute coronary syndromes: a meta-analysis of randomized controlled trials. *JAMA* 2006; 295:2046–2056.

31. Starzl TE, Chase HP, Ahrens EH *et al*. Portacaval shunt in patients with familial hypercholesterolemia. *Ann Surg* 1983; 198:273–283.

32. Bilheimer DW, Goldstein JL, Grundy SM, Starzl TE, Brown MS. Liver transplantation to provide low-density-lipoprotein receptors and lower plasma cholesterol in a child with homozygous familial hypercholesterolemia. *N Engl J Med* 1984; 311:1658–1664.

33. Buchwald H, Varco RL, Matts JP *et al*. Effect of partial ileal bypass surgery on mortality and morbidity from coronary heart disease in patients with hypercholesterolemia. Report of the Program on the Surgical Control of the Hyperlipidemias (POSCH). *N Engl J Med* 1990; 323:946–955.

34. Faergeman O, Meinertz H, Hylander E, Fischerman K, Jarnum S, Nielsen OV. Effects and side-effects of partial ileal by-pass surgery for familial hypercholesterolaemia. *Gut* 1982; 23:558–563.

16

Management of specific risk factors – hypertension

R. Cífková

Hypertension is the most prevalent cardiovascular (CV) disorder, affecting 20–50% of the adult population in developed countries [1]. Prevalence of hypertension increases with age, rising steeply after the age of 50, and affecting more than 50% of this population.

Whenever comparing the prevalence of hypertension, one should be aware that this is heavily dependent on the definition of hypertension, population examined, number of blood pressure (BP) readings taken on each occasion and, finally, on the number of visits. A comparative analysis of hypertension prevalence and BP levels in six European countries, the US and Canada, based on the second BP reading, showed a 60% higher prevalence of hypertension in Europe compared with the US and Canada in population samples aged 35–64 years [2]. There were also differences in the prevalence of hypertension among European countries, with the highest rates in Germany (55%), followed by Finland (49%), Spain (47%), England (42%), Sweden (38%), and Italy (38%). Prevalences in the US and Canada were half the rates in Germany (28% and 27%, respectively).

Findings from the World Health Organization (WHO) MONItoring trends and determinants in CArdiovascular diseases (MONICA) project showed a remarkably higher prevalence of hypertension in Eastern Europe, and virtually no difference in the rates of controlled hypertension among Eastern and Western populations [3].

Global estimates of BP by age, sex, and sub-region show considerable variation in estimated levels (analyses based on data from about 230 surveys including 660 000 participants [4]). Age-specific mean systolic BP (SBP) values ranged from 114 to 164 mmHg for females, and from 117 to 153 mmHg for males. Females typically had lower SBP levels than males in the 30–44-year age groups but, in all sub-regions, SBP levels rose more steeply with age for females than males. Therefore, SBP levels in those aged ≥60 years tended to be higher in females. Sub-regions with consistently high mean SBP levels included parts of Eastern Europe and Africa. Mean SBP levels were lowest in Southeast Asia and parts of the Western Pacific.

The age-related rise in SBP is primarily responsible for an increase in both the incidence and prevalence of hypertension with increasing age [5]. The impressive increase in BP to hypertensive levels with age is also illustrated by Framingham data indicating that the 4-year rates of progression to hypertension are 50% for those 65 years and older with BP in the 130–139/85–89 mmHg range, and 26% for those with BP in the 120–129/80–84 mmHg range [6].

Renata Cífková, MD, PhD, FESC, Head, Department of Preventive Cardiology, Institute for Clinical and Experimental Medicine, Prague, Czech Republic

BLOOD PRESSURE AS A RISK FACTOR FOR CVD

Elevated BP as a risk factor for coronary heart disease (CHD), heart failure, cerebrovascular disease and renal failure in both men and women has been demonstrated in a large number of epidemiological studies [7–10]. Observational evidence is also available that BP levels correlate negatively with cognitive function and that hypertension is associated with an increased incidence of dementia [11]. Historically, more emphasis was placed on diastolic BP (DBP) than SBP as a predictor of cerebrovascular disease and CHD. This was reflected in the design of major randomized controlled trials of hypertension management, which used DBP as an inclusion criterion until the 1990s [12]. Individuals with isolated systolic hypertension were excluded by definition from such trials. Nevertheless, a large compilation of observational data before [7] and since the 1990s [13] confirms that both SBP and DBP show a continuous graded independent relationship with the risk of stroke and coronary events. Data from observational studies involving more than one million individuals have indicated that death from both CHD and stroke increases progressively and linearly from BP levels as low as 115 mmHg systolic and 75 mmHg diastolic upward [13]. The increased risks are present in all age groups ranging from 40 to 89 years old. For every 20 mmHg systolic or 10 mmHg diastolic increase in BP, there is a doubling of mortality from both CHD and stroke.

In addition, longitudinal data obtained from the Framingham Heart Study indicated that BP values in the 130–139/85–89 mmHg range are associated with a more than two-fold increase in relative risk from CVD compared with those with BP levels below 120/80 mmHg [14].

The apparently simple direct relationship between increasing SBP and DBP and CV risk is confounded by the fact that SBP rises throughout the adult years in the vast majority of populations, whereas DBP peaks at about age 60 in men and 70 in women, and falls gradually thereafter [15].

This observation helps to explain why a wide pulse pressure (SBP − DBP) has been shown in some observational studies to be a better predictor of adverse CV outcomes than either SBP or DBP individually [16] and to identify patients with systolic hypertension who are at specifically high risk [17]. However, the largest meta-analysis of observational data in almost one million patients in 61 studies (70% of which had been conducted in Europe) [13], showed both SBP and DBP were independently predictive of stroke and CHD mortality and more so than pulse pressure. This meta-analysis also confirmed the increasing contribution of pulse pressure after age 55.

It has been shown that, compared to normotensive individuals, those with an elevated BP more commonly have other risk factors for CV disease (CVD) (diabetes, insulin resistance, dyslipidaemia) [9, 18–20] and various types and degrees of target organ damage (TOD). Because risk factors may interact positively with each other, this also makes the overall CV risk of hypertensive patients not infrequently high when BP elevation is only mild or moderate [9, 14, 21].

The impact of hypertension on the incidence of CVD in the general population is best evaluated from the population-attributable risk or, more correctly, the population-attributable burden, which is the proportional reduction in average disease risk over a specified time interval that would be achieved by eliminating the exposure of interest from the population while the distribution of other risk factors remains unchanged [22]. For BP, attributable burden can therefore be defined as the proportion of disease that would not have occurred if BP levels had been at the same alternative distribution [23]. The statistics take into account both the prevalence of the risk factor (hypertension) and the strength of its impact (risk ratio) on CVD.

Because of the high prevalence of hypertension in the general population and its risk ratio, approximately 35% of atherosclerotic events are attributable to hypertension. The odds ratio or the relative risk to the individual increases with the severity of hypertension, but the attributable risk is greatest for mild hypertension because of its greater prevalence in the general population. Therefore, the burden of CVD arising from hypertension in the general population comes from those with relatively mild BP elevation [24]. About half of the CV events in the general population occur at BP levels below those recommended for treatment with antihypertensive medications. The burden of non-optimal BP is almost double that of the only previous global estimates [25]. Globally, approximately two-thirds of stroke, one-half of ischaemic heart disease, and approximately three-quarters of hypertensive disease were attributable to non-optimal BP in the year 2000. Worldwide, this equates to approximately 7.1 million deaths (12.8% of the total) and 64.3 million DALYs (1 DALY is one lost year of healthy life; 4.4% of the total). This indicates a need for vigorous non-pharmacological treatment of persons with high-normal BP and for initiating drug treatment in the vast majority of patients with mild hypertension based on their total CV risk.

CLASSIFICATION OF HYPERTENSION

There is a continuous relationship between the level of BP and CV risk. Any numerical definitions and classifications of hypertension are therefore arbitrary, and must be flexible, reflecting evidence of risk and availability of well-tolerated drugs.

The 2007 European Society of Hypertension–European Society of Cardiology (ESH-ESC) guidelines for the management of arterial hypertension [26] used the same BP classification introduced by JNC 6 [27] (Table 16.1), with the exception of the BP range of 130–139/85–89 mmHg referred to as 'borderline' hypertension by JNC 6 and 'high-normal' BP by the ESH-ESC guidelines. A new classification of BP was established by JNC 7 [28] coining the term 'prehypertension' for those with BPs ranging from 120 to 139 mmHg systolic and/or from 80 to 89 mmHg diastolic, reflecting new data on lifetime risk of hypertension, and the impressive increase in the risk of CV complications associated with the levels of BP previously considered to be normal [14].

Another difference between the European guidelines and JNC 7 is that the latter combines Grades 2 and 3 of hypertension into a single Stage 2 category (Table 16.1).

DIAGNOSTIC EVALUATION

Diagnostic procedures are aimed at:

1. Establishing BP levels.
2. Identifying secondary causes of hypertension.
3. Evaluating total CV risk by searching for other risk factors, TOD, and concomitant disease or established CV or renal disease.

Table 16.1 Blood pressure classifications

2007 ESH-ESC guidelines category	SBP/DBP (mmHg)	JNC 7 category
Optimal	<120/80	Normal
Normal	120–129/80–84	Prehypertension
High-normal	130–139/85–89	Prehypertension
Hypertension	≥140/90	Hypertension
Grade 1	140–159/90–99	Stage 1
Grade 2	160–179/100–109	Stage 2
Grade 3	≥180/110	Stage 2

DBP = diastolic blood pressure; SBP = systolic blood pressure.

The diagnostic procedures comprise:

1. Repeated BP measurements.
2. Medical history.
3. Physical examination.
4. Laboratory and instrumental investigations.

BP MEASUREMENT

BP is characterized by large variations both within and between days. Therefore, the diagnosis of hypertension should be based on multiple BP measurements taken on separate occasions. If BP is only slightly elevated, repeated measurements should be obtained over several months because there is often regression to normal levels. If a patient has a more marked BP elevation, evidence of hypertension-related organ damage or high or very high total CV risk, repeated measurements should be obtained over shorter periods of time such as weeks or days. BP can be measured by the doctor or the nurse in the office or the clinic (office or clinic BP), by the patient at home (home BP), or automatically over a 24-h period (ambulatory BP measurement).

Office or clinic BP measurement

The mercury sphygmomanometer has always been regarded as the gold standard for clinical measurement of BP, but this situation is likely to change in the near future. The potential of mercury spillage contaminating the environment has led to the decreased use or elimination of mercury in sphygmomanometers. Their use has been banned in some European countries. However, concerns regarding the accuracy of non-mercury sphygmomanometers have created new challenges for accurate BP determination. Other non-invasive devices (aneroid and auscultatory or oscillometric semi-automatic devices) can be used only if validated according to standardized protocols [29].

Ambulatory BP monitoring

Ambulatory BP monitoring (ABPM) provides information about BP during daily activities and sleep. BP has a reproducible circadian profile with higher values while awake and mentally and physically active, with much lower values during rest and sleep, and early morning increases for 3 or more hours during the transition from sleep to wakefulness. Several devices (mostly oscillometric) are available. However, only devices validated by international standardized protocols should be used. ABPM is usually several mmHg lower than office BP. In the population, office values of 140/90 mmHg correspond approximately to 24-h average values of 125–130/80 mmHg. Mean daytime and nighttime values are several mmHg higher and lower, respectively, than the 24-h means, but threshold values are more difficult to establish, as these are markedly influenced by behaviour during day or night (Table 16.2). Clinical decisions may be based on 24-h, day or night values but, preferably, on 24-h means. Virtually all national and international guidelines for the diagnosis and treatment of hypertension at least mention 24-h ABPM, noting its superiority over the office BP in diagnosing hypertension. Several studies in hypertensives have documented that 24-h ABPM was a better predictor of CV events than office BP [30–36]. There are only three studies in the general population showing the superiority of ABPM over office BP in predicting CV mortality [37–40]. The growing body of evidence may consequently include 24-h ABPM into the diagnostic algorithm of all national and international guidelines for hypertension management.

ABPM is currently used only in a minority of patients with hypertension but its use is gradually increasing. The monitors are reliable, reasonably convenient to wear, and generally

Table 16.2   Blood pressure thresholds (mmHg) for definition of hypertension with different types of measurements

Measurement	SBP	DBP
Office or clinic	140	90
24-h ambulatory	125–130	80
Home (self)	130–135	85

DBP = diastolic blood pressure; SBP = systolic blood pressure.

With permission [26].

accurate. Ambulatory monitoring can be regarded as the gold standard for the prediction of risk related to BP, since prognostic studies have been shown to predict clinical outcome better than conventional BP readings [41].

Home BP measurement

Self-measurements of BP at home cannot provide the extensive information on 24-h BP values provided by ABPM. However, it can provide values on different days in a setting close to daily life conditions. When averaged over a period of a few days, these values have been shown to share some of the advantages of ABPM, i.e. to have no white-coat effect and to be more reproducible and predictive of the presence and progression of organ damage than office values [42, 43]. Home BP measurements for suitable periods (e.g. a few weeks) before and during treatment can therefore be recommended because this relatively cheap procedure may improve patients' adherence to treatment regimens [44]. Home monitoring devices should be checked for accuracy every 1–2 years.

When advising self-measurement of BP at home, care [45] should be taken to:

▧ Advise only use of validated devices; none of the presently available wrist devices for measurement of BP is satisfactorily validated. Should any of these wrist devices become validated, the subject should be advised to keep the arm at heart level during measurement. The fact that a device has passed the validation criteria does not guarantee accuracy in the individual patient and it is essential that each device be checked for each patient before the readings are accepted as being valid.

▧ Choose semi-automatic devices rather than a mercury sphygmomanometer to avoid the difficulty posed by patients' instruction and errors originating from hearing problems in elderly individuals.

▧ Instruct the patient to make measurements in a sitting position after several minutes' rest. Inform him or her that values may differ between measurements because of spontaneous BP variability.

▧ Avoid asking for an excessive number of values to be measured and ensure that measurements include the period prior to drug intake in order to have information on the duration of the treatment effect.

▧ Remember that, as for ambulatory BP, normal values are lower for home than for office BP. Take 130–135/85 mmHg as the values of home BP corresponding to 140/90 mmHg measured in the office or clinic (Table 16.2).

▧ Give the patient clear instructions on the need to provide the doctor with proper documentation of the measured values and to avoid self-alterations of the treatment regimens.

▓ One factor delaying the wider use of home or self-monitoring in clinical practice was the lack of prognostic data. However, several prospective studies [46–49] have found that home BP predicts morbid events better than conventional clinical measurements. There is an increasing body of evidence that home BP may also predict TOD better than clinic BP.

The recent report from the Subcommittee of Professional and Public Education of the American Heart Association Council on High Blood Pressure Research [50] highlights the importance of using out-of-office BP measurements in making a diagnosis of hypertension.

Isolated office or white-coat hypertension

In some patients, office BP is persistently elevated while daytime or 24-h BP falls within their normality range. This condition is widely known as 'white-coat hypertension' [51], although the more descriptive and less mechanistic term 'isolated office (or clinic) hypertension' is preferable because the office ambulatory BP difference does not correlate with the office BP elevation induced by the alerting response to the doctor or the nurse, i.e. the true 'white-coat effect' [52]. Regardless of the terminology, evidence is now available that isolated office hypertension is not infrequent (about 10% in the general population [53]) and that it accounts for a noticeable fraction of individuals in whom hypertension is diagnosed. There is also evidence that, in individuals with isolated office hypertension, CV risk is less than in individuals with both office and ambulatory BP elevations [53]. Sustained hypertension may develop in some patients with white-coat hypertension, and the risk of stroke may increase after 6 years [54]. Several, although not all studies, however, have reported this condition to be associated with a prevalence of organ damage and metabolic abnormalities greater than that of normal subjects, which suggests that it may not be an entirely innocent phenomenon [55, 56].

Physicians should diagnose isolated office hypertension whenever office BP is ≥140/90 mmHg at several visits while 24-h and day ambulatory BP are <125–130/80 mmHg and <130–135/85 mmHg, respectively. Diagnosis can also be based on home BP values (average of several days' readings <135/85 mmHg). Identification should be followed by search for metabolic risk factors and TOD. Drug treatment should be instituted when there is evidence of organ damage or a high CV risk profile. Lifestyle changes and a close follow-up should, however, be implemented in all patients with isolated office hypertension for whom the doctor elects not to start pharmacological treatment.

Masked hypertension or isolated ambulatory hypertension or 'reversed white-coat' condition

Normal BP in the office and elevated BP elsewhere (e.g. at work or at home) is called masked hypertension or isolated ambulatory hypertension [49, 55, 57, 58]. These individuals have been shown to display a greater than normal prevalence of TOD [59] and may have a greater CV risk than truly normotensive individuals [49, 58]. Alcohol, tobacco, caffeine consumption and physical activity outside the office/clinic may contribute to this phenomenon. The prevalence of masked hypertension in treated hypertensives is about 10% [60] and is somewhat greater in the general population [61]. The clinic BP of patients with masked hypertension may underestimate the risk of CV events. A study of patients with treated hypertension showed that about one-third of those seen in a hypertension clinic had masked hypertension over a 5-year follow-up period; their relative risk of CV events was 2.28 as compared with patients whose BP was adequately controlled according to the criteria for both clinic BP and ambulatory BP [62]. Other studies have shown masked hypertension in patients with untreated hypertension and often in those with undiagnosed hypertension, where it is associated with an increased rate of TOD [59] and adverse prognosis [63]. Masked hypertension may be suspected on the basis of high BP readings taken at home, and one study has shown that masked hypertension diagnosed solely on the basis of home recordings is associated with increased mortality [49].

FAMILY AND PERSONAL HISTORY

A comprehensive family history should be obtained with particular attention to hypertension, diabetes, dyslipidaemia, premature CHD, stroke or renal disease.

A clinical history should include: (a) duration and previous levels of high BP; (b) symptoms suggestive of secondary causes of hypertension and intake of drugs or substances that can raise BP, such as liquorice, cocaine, amphetamines, oral contraceptives, steroids, nonsteroidal anti-inflammatory drugs, erythropoietin, cyclosporine; (c) lifestyle factors, such as dietary intake of fat (animal fat in particular), salt and alcohol, quantification of smoking and physical activity, weight gain since early adult life; (d) past history or current symptoms of coronary disease, heart failure, cerebrovascular or peripheral vascular disease, renal disease, diabetes mellitus, gout, dyslipidaemia, bronchospasm or any other significant illnesses, and drugs used to treat those conditions; (e) previous antihypertensive therapy, its results and adverse effects; and (f) personal, family and environmental factors that may influence BP, CV risk, as well as the course and outcome of therapy.

PHYSICAL EXAMINATION

In addition to BP measurement, physical examination should search for evidence of additional risk factors (in particular abdominal obesity), for signs suggesting secondary hypertension, and for evidence of organ damage.

LABORATORY INVESTIGATIONS

Laboratory investigations are also aimed at providing evidence of additional risk factors, at searching for hints for secondary hypertension, and at assessing absence or presence of TOD. The younger the patient, the higher the BP and the faster the development of hypertension, the more detailed the diagnostic work-up will be.

Routine tests

The latest ESH-ESC guidelines [26] recommend the following routine laboratory tests: fasting plasma glucose, total cholesterol, high-density lipoprotein (HDL) cholesterol, low-density lipoprotein (LDL) cholesterol, fasting triglycerides, serum potassium, serum uric acid, serum creatinine, estimated creatinine clearance (Cockroft-Gault formula) or glomerular filtration rate (MDRD formula), haemoglobin and haematocrit, urinalysis (complemented by microalbuminuria using dipstick test and microscopic examination); and an electrocardiogram (Table 16.3). The set of routine laboratory tests recommended by JNC 7 [28] is quite similar to the European ones, but does not include serum uric acid. On the other hand, it does contain calcium. Both the European guidelines and JNC 7 now put more emphasis on renal function by incorporating serum creatinine and/or estimated glomerular filtration rate (GFR). There is a strong relationship between decreases in GFR and increases in CV morbidity and mortality [64, 65]. Even small decreases in GFR increase CV risk. Serum creatinine may overestimate GFR. The optimal tests to determine GFR are debated but calculating GFR from the recent modifications of the Cockroft and Gault equation is useful [66].

A fasting glucose of 7.0 mmol/l (126 mg/dl) or a 2-h post-prandial glucose of 11 mmol/l (198 mg/dl) are now considered as threshold values for diabetes mellitus [67]. Impaired glucose tolerance (IGT) is defined as a 2-h post-load glucose of 7.8–11.1 mmol/l (140–199 mg/dl). The category of impaired fasting glucose (IFG) was introduced to designate

Table 16.3 Laboratory tests as recommended by the 2007 ESH-ESC guidelines and JNC 7

2007 ESH-ESC guidelines	JNC 7
Routine tests	
Fasting plasma glucose	Plasma glucose
Serum total cholesterol	Serum total cholesterol
Serum LDL cholesterol	
Serum HDL cholesterol	Serum HDL cholesterol
Fasting serum triglycerides	Fasting serum triglycerides
Serum uric acid	
	Calcium
Serum creatinine	Serum creatinine or estimated GFR
Estimated creatinine clearance or GFR	
Serum potassium	Serum potassium
Haemoglobin and haematocrit	Haematocrit
Urinalysis (complemented by	Urinalysis
microalbuminuria using dipstick	
and urinary sediment examination)	
Electrocardiogram	Electrocardiogram
Recommended tests	*Optional tests*
Echocardiogram	
Carotid ultrasound	
	hs-CRP
	Urinary albumin excretion or albumin/creatinine ratio
Quantitative proteinuria	
(if dipstick test positive)	
Funduscopy (in severe hypertension)	
Ankle-brachial index	
Glucose tolerance test (if fasting plasma	
glucose 5.6 mmol/l [100 mg/dl])	
Home and 24-h ABPM	
Pulse-wave velocity	
Extended evaluation (domain of the specialist)	
Complicated hypertension: tests of	
cerebral, cardiac and renal function	
Search for secondary hypertension:	Screening tests for identifiable hypertension:
measurement of renin, aldosterone,	estimated GFR, CT angiography, dexamethasone
corticosteroids, catecholamines;	suppression test, drug screening,
arteriography; renal and adrenal	24-h urinary metanephrine and nor-metanephrine,
ultrasound; computer-assisted tomography;	24-h urinary aldosterone or other
brain magnetic resonance imaging	mineralocorticoids, Doppler renal artery flow
	study, MR renal angiography, sleep study
	with O_2 saturation, TSH, serum PTH

ABPM = ambulatory blood pressure monitoring; CRP = C-reactive protein; CT = computed tomography; GFR = glomerular filtration rate; HDL = high-density lipoprotein; hs-CRP = high-sensitivity CRP; LDL = low-density lipoprotein; MR = magnetic resonance; PTH = parathyroid hormone; TSH = thyroid stimulating hormone.

the zone between the upper limit of normal fasting plasma glucose and the lower limit of diabetic plasma fasting glucose, much as IGT designates the zone between the upper limit of normal 2-h plasma glucose and the lower limit of diabetic 2-h plasma glucose. The Expert Committee [68] defined normal fasting plasma glucose as lower than 5.6 mmol/l

(100 mg/dl). Patients with IFG and/or IGT are now referred to as having 'pre-diabetes', indicating the relatively high risk for development of diabetes in these patients [69].

There is ongoing debate on which test is superior. Fasting plasma glucose remains the test of choice in clinical practice where costs, convenience and reproducibility are important considerations. For research studies, or in clinical situations in which it is important, to the extent possible, to rule in or out every case of diabetes, or every case of IFG/IGT, fasting plasma glucose and 2-h plasma glucose should be performed. Confirmatory testing is recommended to diagnose diabetes by fasting plasma glucose tests (on separate days).

Optional tests

Urinary albumin excretion evaluation is recommended by JNC 7 except for those with diabetes or kidney disease, for whom annual measurements should be made. The presence of albuminuria, even in the setting of normal GFR, is also associated with an increase in CV risk [70–72]. Urinary albumin excretion should be monitored on an annual basis in high-risk groups such as those with diabetes or renal disease [28].

The list of optional or recommended tests is much shorter in JNC 7. The European guidelines make every effort to search for TOD. Echocardiography is undoubtedly much more sensitive than electrocardiography in diagnosing left ventricular hypertrophy [73] and predicting CV risk [74]. An echocardiographic examination may help in more precisely classifying the overall risk of the hypertensive patient and in directing therapy.

Ultrasound examination of the carotid arteries with measurement of the intima–media complex thickness, and detection of plaques [75], has repeatedly been shown to predict occurrence of both stroke and myocardial infarction. It can usefully complement echocardiography in making risk stratification of hypertensive patients more precise. The relation between carotid artery intima–media thickness and CV events is continuous, but a threshold ≥0.9 mm can be taken as a conservative estimate of significant alteration.

In contrast to the 1930s, when Keith et al.'s [76] classification of hypertensive retinal changes in four grades was formulated, nowadays most hypertensive patients present early, and haemorrhages and exudates (grade 3), and papilloedema (grade 4) are very rarely observed. An evaluation of 800 hypertensive patients attending a hypertension out-patient clinic [77] showed that the prevalence of grades 1 and 2 retinal changes was as high as 78% (in contrast to 43% for carotid plaques, 22% for left ventricular hypertrophy, and 14% for microalbuminuria). It is, therefore, doubtful whether grades 1 and 2 retinal changes can be used as a sign of TOD to stratify global CV risk, whereas grades 3 and 4 are certainly markers of severe hypertensive complications.

The increasing interest in SBP and pulse pressure as predictors of CV events [78], stimulated by trial evidence of the beneficial effects of lowering BP in the elderly and in isolated systolic hypertension, has encouraged the development of techniques for measuring large artery compliance. A large body of important pathophysiological, pharmacological and therapeutic information has accumulated [79–81]. Two of these techniques have further been developed for possible use as diagnostic procedures, namely pulse wave velocity (PWV) measurement [82] and the augmentation index measurement (Sphygmocor device) [83, 84]. Aortic stiffness, measured through carotid–femoral PWV, has an independent predictive value for all-cause and CV mortality, fatal and non-fatal coronary events, and fatal strokes not only in patients with uncomplicated essential hypertension [81, 85, 86], but also in patients with type 2 diabetes [87], end-stage renal disease (ESRD) [88, 89], elderly subjects [90–92], and the general population [93, 94]. The relation between aortic stiffness and CV events is continuous, but a threshold >12 m/s can be taken as a conservative estimate of significant alteration in middle-aged hypertensives.

The carotid augmentation index and pulse pressure are both independent predictors of CV events in the hypertensive patients of the Conduit Artery Function Evaluation (CAFE) study [95], an ancillary study of the Anglo-Scandinavian Cardiac Outcomes Trial (ASCOT) trial [96], and predict all-cause mortality in ESRD patients [97, 98]. However, data concerning the predictive values of both these parameters in other patient groups and in the general population are scarce. Further longitudinal studies should, therefore, be performed to ascertain the predictive value of central pulse pressure and augmentation index.

Additionally, three emerging risk factors – (1) high-sensitivity C-reactive protein (hs-CRP), a marker of inflammation; (2) homocysteine; and (3) elevated heart rate – have been proposed by JNC 7.

(1) Although hs-CRP has been reported to predict the incidence of CV events in several clinical settings [99], its added value in determining total CV risk is uncertain [100] except in patients with the metabolic syndrome in whom hs-CRP values have been reported to be associated with a further marked increase in risk [101]. Several studies, including the Framingham Heart Study, have demonstrated that individuals with LDL cholesterol within the normal range and elevated hs-CRP had a higher CV event rate as compared with those with low CRP and high LDL cholesterol [102]. Other studies have shown that elevated CRP is associated with higher CV event rates, particularly in women [103].

(2) Epidemiological studies conducted over the past 25 years have provided ample support for the association of mild hyperhomocysteinaemia with an elevated risk of atherothrombosis [104]. Several large, prospective trials have been initiated over the past 5 years to study the consequences on CV events of lowering serum homocysteine concentrations with the use of folic acid, vitamin B12 and vitamin B6. The ease of administration of these inexpensive, naturally occurring co-factors, has offered a straightforward approach to test the homocysteine hypothesis. Recently, three interventional studies in individuals with overt CVD have been completed [105–107]. The data are quite consistent that there is no clinical benefit in the use of folic acid and vitamin B12 (with or without the addition of vitamin B6) in patients with established vascular disease. The three completed clinical trials do not provide evidence to support the preventive use of B-vitamin supplements. Ongoing large clinical trials and the planned meta-analysis of all trials [108] will answer the remaining relevant clinical questions.

(3) Although the association between elevated resting heart rate and CV morbidity and mortality has been demonstrated in a large number of epidemiological studies, elevated heart rate is not yet considered to be a risk factor for CHD. This is mainly due to the lack of studies demonstrating that reduction of a high heart rate in non-cardiac patients can improve prognosis. An elevated heart rate appeared to be a weak predictor of death from CHD in females. All data on the possible importance of heart rate lowering are retrospective and a demonstration of the benefits of reducing heart rate pharmacologically is limited to patients with myocardial infarction or heart failure. Not a single prospective trial has been designed to specifically evaluate whether therapeutic lowering of heart rate in cardiac patients and, particularly, in hypertensives, might beneficially modify CV outcomes [109].

Extended evaluation

Both JNC 7 and the European guidelines list a battery of additional diagnostic procedures indicated to identify secondary forms of hypertension, which may account for 5–10% of adult patients with hypertension. Simple screening for secondary forms of hypertension can be obtained from clinical history, physical examination, and routine laboratory tests. Furthermore, a secondary form of hypertension is suggested by a severe BP elevation, sudden onset of hypertension, and BP responding poorly to drug therapy. In these cases, specific diagnostic procedures may become necessary, as outlined in Table 16.3.

TOTAL CARDIOVASCULAR RISK

Historically, therapeutic intervention thresholds for the treatment of CV risk factors such as BP, blood cholesterol, and blood sugar, had been based on various arbitrary cut-points for the individual risk factors. Because risk factors cluster [110] and there is a graded association between each risk factor and overall CV risk [111], the contemporary approach to treatment is to determine the threshold, at least for cholesterol and BP reduction, based on the calculation of estimated coronary [112, 113] or CV (coronary + stroke) [114, 115] risk over a defined, relatively short-term (e.g. 5–10-year) period.

The methods used to assess total CV risk vary among the different guidelines. JNC 7 estimates the 10-year risk for both fatal and non-fatal CHD by SBP and presence of other risk factors. The easy and rapid calculation of a Framingham risk score using published tables (National Cholesterol Education Program [NCEP]) [116] may assist the physician and patient in demonstrating the benefits of treatment.

Most risk estimation systems are based on the Framingham Study [21]. While this database has been shown to be reasonably applicable to some European populations [117], estimates require recalibration in other populations [118] due to important differences in the incidence of coronary and stroke events. The main disadvantage associated with an intervention threshold based on relatively short-term absolute risk is that younger adults (particularly women), despite having more than one major risk factor, are unlikely to reach treatment thresholds despite being at high risk relative to their peers. By contrast, most elderly men (e.g. >70 years) will often reach treatment thresholds whilst being at very little increased risk relative to their peers. This situation results in most resources being concentrated on the oldest subjects, whose potential lifespan, despite intervention, is relatively limited, while young subjects at high relative risk remain untreated despite, in the absence of intervention, a predicted significant shortening of their otherwise much longer potential lifespan [119, 120].

On the basis of these considerations, total CV risk classification may be stratified as suggested in Table 16.4. The terms *low*, *moderate*, *high* and *very high added risk* are calibrated to indicate, approximately, an absolute 10-year risk of CHD of <15%, 15–20%, 20–30% and >30%, respectively, according to Framingham criteria [18], or an approximate absolute risk of fatal CHD <4%, 4–5%, 5–8%, and >8% according to the Systemic Coronary Risk Evaluation (SCORE) chart [115].

Table 16.5 indicates the most common risk factors, TOD, diabetes and established CV or renal disease, to be used to stratify risk. The following is a summary of major changes in the 2003 and 2007 ESH-ESC guidelines [121, 26].

(1) Obesity is indicated as 'abdominal obesity', in order to give specific attention to an important sign of the metabolic syndrome [122]; (2) diabetes is listed as a separate criterion in order to underline its importance as a risk factor, at least twice as large as in the absence of diabetes [123]; (3) microalbuminuria is indicated as a sign of subclinical organ damage/TOD, but proteinuria as a sign of renal disease; (4) a slight elevation of serum creatinine concentration is taken as a sign of TOD and concentrations of 115–133 μmol/l (1.3–1.5 mg/dl) in men and 107–124 μmol/l (1.2–1.4 mg/dl) in women, and concentrations >133 μmol/l (>1.5 mg/dl) in men and >124 μmol/l (>1.4 mg/dl) in women as renal disease [124, 125]; (5) the list of renal markers of organ damage has been expanded to include estimates of creatinine clearance by the Cockcroft-Gault formula or of GFR by the MDRD formula [66], because of the evidence that these estimated values are a more precise index of the CV risk accompanying renal dysfunction; (6) generalized or focal narrowing of the retinal arteries is omitted among signs of TOD as too frequently seen in subjects aged 50 years or older [77], but retinal haemorrhages and exudates as well as papilloedema are listed as established CV disease; (7) carotid femoral PWV >12 m/s (reflecting aortic stiffness) has been added to the list of subclinical organ damage. (8) A low ankle-brachial

Table 16.4 Stratification of risk to quantify prognosis

Other risk factors and disease history	Blood pressure (mmHg)				
	Normal SBP 120–129 or DBP 80–84	High-normal SBP 130–139 or DBP 85–89	Grade 1 SBP 140–159 or DBP 90–99	Grade 2 SBP 160–179 or DBP 100–109	Grade 3 SBP ≥180 or DBP ≥110
No other risk factors	Average risk	Average risk	Low-added risk	Moderate-added risk	High-added risk
1–2 risk factors	Low-added risk	Low-added risk	Moderate-added risk	Moderate-added risk	Very high-added risk
3 or more risk factors, MS or TOD or diabetes	Moderate-added risk	High-added risk	High-added risk	High-added risk	Very high-added risk
Established CV or renal disease	Very high-added risk	Very high-added risk	Very high-added risk	Very high-added risk	Very high-added risk

DBP = diastolic blood pressure; MS = metabolic syndrome; SBP = systolic blood pressure; TOD = target organ damage.

With permission [26].

Table 16.5 Factors influencing prognosis

Risk factors for cardiovascular disease used for stratification	Subclinical organ damage	Diabetes mellitus	Established CV or renal disease

• Levels of systolic and diastolic BP
• Levels of pulse pressure (in the elderly)
• Age (M >55 years; W >65 years)
• Smoking
• Dyslipidaemia
  –TC >5.0 mmol/l (100 mg/dl) or;
  –LDL-c >3.0 mmol/l (115 mg/dl) or;
  –HDL-c: M <1.0 mmol/l (40 mg/dl), W <1.2 mmol/l (46 mg/dl)
  –TG >1.7 mmol/l (150 mg/dl)
• Fasting plasma glucose 5.6–6.0 mmol/l (102–125 mg/dl)
• Abnormal glucose tolerance test
• Abdominal obesity (waist circumference M >102 cm, W >88 cm)
• Family history of premature cardiovascular disease (at age <55 years M, <65 years W)
	• Left ventricular hypertrophy (electrocardiogram: Sokolow-Lyon >38 mm; Cornell >2440 mm × ms; echocardiogram: LVMI M ≥125; W ≥110 g/m²)
	• Ultrasound evidence of arterial wall thickening (carotid IMT ≥0.9 mm) or atherosclerotic plaque
	• Carotid-femoral pulse wave velocity >12 m/s
	• Ankle-brachial index <0.9
	• Slight increase in serum creatinine M: 115–133 μmol/l (M 1.3–1.5 mg/dl) W: 107–124 μmol/l (W 1.2–1.4 mg/dl)
	• Low estimated GFR (<60 ml/min/1.73 m²) or creatinine clearance (<60 ml/min)
	• Microalbuminuria 30–300 mg/24 h or albumin-creatinine ratio: M ≥22, W ≥31 mg/g creatinine
		• Fasting plasma glucose ≥7.0 mmol/l (126 mg/dl)
		• Post-prandial plasma glucose >11.0 mmol/l (198 mg/dl)
			• Cerebrovascular disease: ischaemic stroke; cerebral haemorrhage; transient ischaemic attack
			• Heart disease: myocardial infarction; angina; coronary revascularization; heart failure
			• Renal disease: diabetic nephropathy; renal impairment (serum creatinine M >133 μmol/l or >1.5 mg/dl; W >124 μmol/l or >1.4 mg/dl); proteinuria (>300 mg/24 h)
			• Peripheral artery disease
			• Advanced retinopathy: haemorrhages or exudates; papilloedema

GFR = glomerular filtration rate; HDL = high-density lipoprotein; IMT = intima-media thickness; LDL = low-density lipoprotein; LVMI = left ventricular mass index; M = men; TC = total cholesterol; TG = total triglycerides; W = women.

index (ABI < 0.9) is listed as a relatively easy-to-obtain marker of artherosclerotic disease and increased total CV risk.

Both 2003 and 2007 ESH-ESC guidelines emphasize that, in addition to CV risk factors, the presence of subclinical organ damage (TOD) confers an increased total CV risk.

TREATMENT OF HYPERTENSION

HYPERTENSION CONTROL

Hypertension is poorly controlled worldwide, with <25% controlled in developed countries, and <10% in developing countries [1]. Hypertension control rates also vary within countries by age, gender, race/ethnicity, socioeconomic status, education, and quality of healthcare [126]. Awareness of hypertension has improved in the US and other Western countries over the past decade, but remains inadequate as only a proportion of those who are aware of their diagnosis are treated, and an even smaller number of those receiving treatment are treated adequately. Sadly, however, the most important parameter likely to have an impact on public health is neither the number of those who are aware of their hypertension nor the number taking steps to improve it but, rather, the percentage whose BP is under control [127].

GOALS OF TREATMENT

The primary goal of treatment of the patient with high BP is to achieve maximum reduction in the long-term total risk of CV morbidity and mortality. This requires treatment of all the reversible risk factors identified, including smoking, dyslipidaemia, or diabetes and established CV or renal disease, as well as treatment of the raised BP *per se*.

As to the BP goal to be achieved, randomized trials comparing less with more intensive treatment [128–131] have shown that, in diabetic patients, more intensive BP lowering is more protective [128, 130, 132, 133]. This is not yet conclusively established in non-diabetic subjects; however, because the only trial not exclusively involving diabetics is the Hypertension Optimal Treatment (HOT) study [132], which, because of the small DBP differences achieved (2 mmHg) between the groups randomized to ≤90, 85 or 80 mmHg, was unable to detect significant differences in the risk of CV events (except for myocardial infarction) between adjacent target groups.

However, the results of the HOT study have confirmed that there is no increase in CV risk in the patients randomized to the lowest target group, which is relevant to clinical practice because setting lower BP goals allows a greater number of subjects at least to meet the traditional ones. Furthermore, a subgroup analysis of the HOT study [134] suggests that, except for smokers, a reduction of DBP to an average of 82 rather than 85 mmHg significantly reduces major CV events in non-diabetic patients at high/very high risk (50% of HOT study patients), as well as in patients with previous ischaemic heart disease, in patients older than 65 years, and in women.

Finally, in patients with a history of stroke or transient ischaemic attack, the Perindopril Protection against Recurrent Stroke Study (PROGRESS) [135] showed lower CV mortality and morbidity by reducing DBP to 79 mmHg (active treatment group) rather than 83 mmHg (placebo group). Similar observations have been made in patients with coronary disease although the role of BP reduction in this trial has been debated [136].

As far as SBP is concerned, evidence of a greater benefit by a more aggressive reduction is limited to the United Kingdom Prospective Diabetes Study (UKPDS), which has shown, through retrospective analysis of the data, fewer CV morbid events at values below 120–130 as compared with 140 mmHg. However, most trials have been unable to reduce SBP below 140 mmHg and, in no trials on diabetic and non-diabetic patients, have values below 130 mmHg been achieved [136].

A *post hoc* analysis of the INternational VErapamil SR and Trandolapril STudy (INVEST) trial showed that, in hypertensive patients with CHD who were treated with sustained-release verapamil or atenolol to lower BP, increased risk for all-cause death and myocardial infarction was associated with DBP below 70–80 mmHg [137].

As for patients with non-diabetic renal disease, data about the effects of more or less intensive BP lowering on CV events are scanty: the HOT study was unable to find any significant reduction in CV events in the subset of patients with plasma creatinine >115 μmol/l (>1.3 mg/dl) [134] or >133 μmol/l (>1.5 mg/dl) [138] when subjected to more vs. less intensive BP lowering (139/82 vs. 143/85 mmHg). However, none of these trials suggests an increased CV risk at the lowest BP achieved.

In conclusion, on the basis of current evidence from trials, it can be recommended that BP, both systolic and diastolic, be intensively lowered to at least below 140/90 mmHg and to definitely lower values if tolerated, in all hypertensive patients, and below 130/80 mmHg in diabetics and in high or very high risk patients, such as those with established CV or renal disease (stroke, myocardial infarction, renal dysfunction, proteinuria). The achievable goal may depend on the pre-existing BP level and systolic values below 140 mmHg may be difficult to achieve, particularly in the elderly.

LIFESTYLE CHANGES

Lifestyle measures should be instituted in all patients including individuals with high-normal BP and patients who require drug treatment. The purpose is to lower BP and to control other risk factors and clinical conditions. A substantial body of evidence strongly supports the concept that multiple dietary factors affect BP [139]. Well-established dietary modifications that lower BP are reduced salt intake, weight loss, and moderation of alcohol consumption (among those who drink). Over the past decade, increased potassium intake and consumption of dietary patterns based on the Dietary Approaches to Stop Hypertension (DASH) diet (a diet rich in fruit, vegetables, and low-fat dairy products, with a reduced content of dietary cholesterol as well as saturated and total fat), [140] have emerged as effective strategies that also lower BP. The effects of sodium reduction on BP tend to be greater in blacks, middle-aged, and older persons and in individuals with hypertension, diabetes, or chronic kidney disease. These groups tend to have a less responsive renin–angiotensin–aldosterone system [141]. The recommended adequate sodium intake has been recently reduced from 2.4 to 1.5 g/day (65 mmol/day) [142].

A substantial and largely consistent body of evidence from observational studies and clinical trials documents that weight is directly associated with BP. In one meta-analysis, mean SBP and DBP reductions associated with an average weight loss of 5.1 kg were 4.4 and 3.6 mmHg, respectively [143].

Everyone who is able should engage in regular aerobic physical activity such as brisk walking, at least 30 min/day, most days of the week [144, 145]. Combinations of two or more lifestyle modifications can achieve better results [146]. For overall CV risk reduction, patients should be strongly counselled to quit smoking.

DRUG TREATMENT

The main benefit of antihypertensive treatment is due to BP lowering *per se*. A head-to-head comparison of major classes of antihypertensive drugs did not find any significant differences in major CV outcomes or CV mortality [147]. Similar conclusions were reached in another meta-analysis on behalf of the National Institute for Health and Clinical Excellence (NICE) in the United Kingdom [148] and a quantitative overview of recent clinical trials [149]. However, specific drug classes may differ in some effects or in special patient groups. Antihypertensive drugs are not equal in terms of adverse events in individual patients.

Benefits of antihypertensive treatment have been shown in large controlled trials using the following classes of antihypertensive drugs: diuretics, β-blockers, calcium channel blockers, angiotensin-converting enzyme (ACE) inhibitors, and angiotensin-receptor antagonists. JNC 7 strongly recommends thiazide-type diuretics as the preferred initial agents [150], underlining their tolerability and low cost.

On the contrary, the European guidelines [26] are much more liberal in selecting the initial antihypertensive agent, taking into account the fact that the majority of patients will need a combination of at least two drugs to achieve BP control.

Within the array of available agents, the choice of drugs will be influenced by many factors including:

(1) The previous, favourable or unfavourable experience of the individual patient with a given class of compounds.
(2) The cost of drugs, either to the individual patient or to the health provider, although cost considerations should not predominate over efficacy and tolerability in any individual patient.
(3) The CV risk profile of the individual patient.
(4) The presence of TOD or established CV or renal disease and diabetes.
(5) The presence of other coexisting disorders that may either favour or limit the use of particular classes of antihypertensive drugs.
(6) The possibility of interactions with drugs used for other conditions present in the patient.

The physician should tailor the choice of drugs to the individual patient, after taking all these factors, together with patient preference, into account. Indications and contraindications of specific drug classes are listed in Table 16.6.

A revolutionary approach in drug treatment of hypertension is highlighted by the updated recommendations for management of hypertension issued by NICE in the UK, developed by the National Collaborating Centre for Chronic Conditions and the British Hypertension Society (BHS) [151]. These new guidelines formally acknowledge that the evidence base for treating hypertension was focused mainly on patients over 55 years of age with overt vascular disease and that there is an alarming absence of data in younger (<55 years) individuals.

In the elderly, the BP-lowering effect is pre-eminent in deriving treatment benefit, and calcium channel blockers or thiazide-type diuretics are the two most clinically effective and cost-effective drug classes for initiating antihypertensive therapy in this age group. As they often need combination therapy, addition of an ACE inhibitor (or an angiotensin-receptor blocker, if an ACE inhibitor is not tolerated) is recommended as step 2. As step 3, the combination of an ACE inhibitor + calcium channel blocker + thiazide-type diuretic is recommended. For individuals younger than 55 years, the initiation of antihypertensive therapy is recommended with an ACE inhibitor rather than with a calcium channel blocker or a thiazide-type diuretic.

The position of β-blockers has been challenged; they are no longer preferred as routine initial therapy in hypertension without CHD. In head-to-head comparative trials, β-blockers were usually less effective in reducing major CV events, particularly stroke [152, 153]. They are more likely to induce diabetes [154] and have an unfavourable effect on the metabolic profile, particularly in combination with diuretics [155].

On the other hand, β-blockers should not be withdrawn in CHD patients; they should still be considered for patients with increased sympathetic nervous activity, women of child-bearing potential (as they should not be given ACE inhibitors or angiotensin II-receptor antagonists), and in patients with intolerance of or contraindications to ACE inhibitors and

Table 16.6 Indications and contraindications for the major classes of antihypertensive drugs

Class	Conditions favouring the use	Contraindications Compelling	Contraindications Possible
Diuretics (thiazides)	Isolated systolic hypertension (elderly) Heart failure Hypertension in blacks	Gout	Metabolic syndrome Glucose intolerance Pregnancy
Diuretics (loop)	End-stage renal disease Heart failure		
Diuretics (anti-aldosterone)	Heart failure Post-myocardial infarction	Renal failure Hyperkalaemia	
β-blockers	Angina pectoris Post-myocardial infarction Heart failure (up-titration) Glaucoma Pregnancy Tachyarrhythmias	Asthma A-V block (grade 2 or 3)	Peripheral artery disease Metabolic syndrome Glucose intolerance Athletes and physically active patients Chronic obstructive pulmonary disease
Calcium antagonists (dihydropyridines)	Isolated systolic hypertension (elderly) Angina pectoris LV hypertrophy Carotid/coronary atherosclerosis Pregnancy Hypertension in blacks		Tachyarrhythmias Heart failure
Calcium antagonists (verapamil, diltiazem)	Angina pectoris Carotid atherosclerosis Supraventricular tachycardia	A-V block (grade 2 or 3) Heart failure	

Table 16.6 (*continued*)

Class	Conditions favouring the use	Contraindications	
		Compelling	Possible
ACE inhibitors	Heart failure LV dysfunction Post-myocardial infarction Diabetic nephropathy Non-diabetic nephropathy LV hypertrophy Carotid atherosclerosis Proteinuria/microalbuminuria Atrial fibrillation Metabolic syndrome	Pregnancy Angioneurotic oedema Hyperkalaemia Bilateral renal artery stenosis	
Angiotensin-receptor antagonists (AT$_1$-blockers)	Heart failure Post-myocardial infarction Diabetic nephropathy Proteinuria/microalbuminuria LV hypertrophy Atrial fibrillation Metabolic syndrome ACE inhibitor-induced cough	Pregnancy Hyperkalaemia Bilateral renal artery stenosis	
α-blockers	Prostatic hyperplasia (BPH) Hyperlipidaemia	Orthostatic hypotension	Heart failure

ACE = angiotensin-converting enzyme; A-V = atrio-ventricular; LV = left ventricular.
With permission [26].

angiotensin II-receptor antagonists. A recent meta-analysis re-examining the efficacy of β-blockers in the treatment of hypertension showed that β-blockers reduced major CV outcomes in younger patients in placebo-controlled trials. In active comparator trials, β-blockers demonstrated an efficacy similar to that of other antihypertensive agents in younger, but not in older, patients with the excess being particularly high for stroke [156].

By contrast, without hard clinical endpoint data for younger people, the NICE/BHS guidelines recommend ACE inhibitors (or an angiotensin II-receptor antagonist if the ACE inhibitor is not tolerated) for initiating therapy in hypertensives younger than 55 years.

ANTIPLATELET THERAPY

Antiplatelet therapy, in particular low-dose aspirin, has been shown to reduce the risk of stroke and myocardial infarction in patients with unstable angina, acute myocardial infarction, stroke, transient ischaemic attack, or other clinical evidence of vascular disease [157]. The HOT study [129] showed a significant 15% reduction in major CV events and a 36% reduction in acute myocardial infarction, with no effect on stroke (but no increase in risk of intracerebral haemorrhage) in relatively well-treated hypertensives receiving, on top of their antihypertensive medication, 75 mg of acetylsalicylic acid (ASA) or placebo. However, these benefits were associated with a 65% increase in risk of major haemorrhagic events (mostly gastrointestinal bleeding). Patients with serum creatinine >115 μmol/l (>1.3 mg/dl), with higher total CV risk at baseline, or higher baseline SBP or DBP, had a favourable balance between benefits and harm of aspirin [158]. The 2007 ESC-ESH guidelines recommend antiplatelet therapy, in particular low-dose aspirin in hypertensive patients with previous CV events, provided there is no excessive risk of bleeding. Low-dose aspirin should also be considered in hypertensive patients without a history of CVD, aged over 50 years, with a moderate increase in serum creatinine, or with a high total CV risk. Lowering BP to values lower than 140/90 mmHg (or close to that value) should precede the initiation of ASA treatment.

LIPID-LOWERING THERAPY

Two trials – Antihypertensive and Lipid-Lowering Treatment to Prevent Heart Attack Trial (ALLHAT) [159] and ASCOT [160] – have evaluated the benefits associated with the use of statins, specifically in patients with hypertension. ALLHAT compared the effect of 40 mg/day pravastatin with usual care in over 10 000 patients, 14% of whom had established vascular disease. The differential effect of pravastatin on total and LDL cholesterol (11% and 17%, respectively) was smaller than expected due to extensive statin use in the usual care group and was associated with a modest, non-significant 9% reduction in fatal CHD and non-fatal myocardial infarction, and a 9% reduction in fatal and non-fatal stroke. There was no impact on all-cause mortality, which was the primary endpoint of the trial. By contrast, the results of ASCOT, which also included over 10 000 hypertensive patients, showed a 36% reduction in the primary endpoint of total CHD and non-fatal myocardial infarction, and a 27% reduction in fatal and non-fatal stroke associated with the use of atorvastatin 10 mg/day compared with placebo in patients with total cholesterol <6.5 mmol/l (250 mg/dl) [160].

There is no doubt that lipid-lowering therapy, and statins in particular, should be part of comprehensive treatment of hypertension reducing total CV risk. JNC 7 [28] refers to NCEP, Adult Treatment Panel (ATP) III [95] whereas the 2007 ESH-ESC guidelines recommend considering statins in hypertensive patients up to the age of 80 with overt CHD, peripheral artery disease, stroke, and long-standing type 2 diabetes with the goal of achieving total cholesterol <4.5 mmol/l (175 mg/dl) and LDL cholesterol <2.5 mmol/l (100 mg/dl) and lower, if possible. Lower goals, i.e., 4 and 2 mmol/l (155 and 80 mg/dl), respectively, may also be considered [26]. Patients without overt CVD or with high CV risk should also be considered for statin treatment if their baseline total and LDL cholesterol levels are not elevated.

As there is compelling evidence from recent clinical trials favouring aggressive lipid-lowering therapy, the 2006 Update of the American Heart Association/American College of Cardiology (AHA/ACC) guidelines for secondary prevention for patients with coronary and other atherosclerotic vascular disease further reduces the goals for LDL cholesterol to 2.0 mmol/l (<70 mg/dl) [161].

ACKNOWLEDGEMENTS

Supported by grant No. MZO 00023001 awarded by the Ministry of Health of the Czech Republic.

REFERENCES

1. Kearney PM, Whelton M, Reynolds K, Whelton PK, He J. Worldwide prevalence of hypertension: a systematic review. *J Hypertens* 2004; 22:11–19.
2. Wolf-Maier K, Cooper RS, Banegas JR *et al*. Hypertension prevalence and blood pressure levels in 6 European countries, Canada and the United States. *JAMA* 2003; 289:2363–2369.
3. Strasser T. Hypertension: the East European experience. *Am J Hypertens* 1998; 11:756–758.
4. Lawes CMM, Vander Hoorn S, Law MR, Elliott P, MacMahon S, Rodgers A. Blood pressure and the global burden of disease 2000. Part I: Estimates of blood pressure levels. *J Hypertens* 2006; 24:413–422.
5. Franklin SS, Gustin W, Wong ND *et al*. Hemodynamic patterns of age-related changes in blood pressure. The Framingham Heart Study. *Circulation* 1997; 96:308–315.
6. Vasan RS, Larson MG, Leip EP, Kannel WB, Levy D. Assessment of frequency of progression to hypertension in nonhypertensive participants in the Framingham Heart Study. A cohort study. *Lancet* 2001; 358:1682–1686.
7. MacMahon S, Peto R, Cutler J *et al*. Blood pressure, stroke, and coronary heart disease. Part 1. Prolonged differences in blood pressure: prospective observational studies corrected for the regression dilution bias. *Lancet* 1990; 335:765–774.
8. Kannel WB. Blood pressure as a cardiovascular risk factor: prevention and treatment. *JAMA* 1996; 275:1571–1576.
9. Assmann G, Schulte H. The Prospective Cardiovascular Münster (PROCAM) study: prevalence of hyperlipidemia in persons with hypertension and/or diabetes mellitus and the relationship to coronary heart disease. *Am Heart J* 1988; 116(pt 2):1713–1724.
10. Walker WG, Neaton JD, Cutler JA, Neuwirth R, Cohen JD. Renal function change in hypertensive members of the Multiple Risk Factor Intervention Trial. Racial and treatment effects. The MRFIT Research Group. *JAMA* 1992; 268:3085–3091.
11. Skoog I, Lernfelt B, Landahl S *et al*. 15-year longitudinal study of blood pressure and dementia. *Lancet* 1996; 347:1141–1145.
12. Collins R, Peto R, MacMahon S *et al*. Blood pressure, stroke, and coronary heart disease. Part 2. Short-term reductions in blood pressure: overview of randomised drug trials in their epidemiological context. *Lancet* 1990; 335:827–839.
13. Lewington S, Clarke R, Qizilbash N, Peto R, Collins R. Age-specific relevance of usual blood pressure to vascular mortality: A meta-analysis of individual data for one million adults in 61 prospective studies. Prospective Studies Collaboration. *Lancet* 2002; 360:1903–1913.
14. Vasan RS, Larson MG, Leip EP *et al*. Impact of high-normal blood pressure on the risk of cardiovascular disease. *N Engl J Med* 2001; 345:1291–1297.
15. Primatesta P, Brookes M, Poulter NR. Improved hypertension management and control. Results from the Health Survey for England 1998. *Hypertension* 2001; 38:827–832.
16. Franklin SS, Larson MG, Khan SA *et al*. Does the relation of blood pressure to coronary heart disease risk change with aging? The Framingham Heart Study. *Circulation* 2001; 103:1245–1249.
17. Benetos A, Zureik M, Morcet J *et al*. A decrease in diastolic blood pressure combined with an increase in systolic blood pressure is associated with a higher cardiovascular mortality in men. *J Am Coll Cardiol* 2000; 35:673–680.

18. Cardiovascular disease risk factors: new areas for research. *Report of a WHO Scientific Group. WHO Technical Report Series 841.* World Health Organization, Geneva, 1994.

19. Isomaa B, Almgren P, Tuomi T *et al.* Cardiovascular morbidity and mortality associated with the metabolic syndrome. *Diabetes Care* 2001; 24:683–689.

20. Cuspidi C, Ambrosioni E, Mancia G, Pessina AC, Trimarco B, Zanchetti A. Role of echocardiography and carotid ultrasonography in stratifying risk in patients with essential hypertension: the Assessment of Prognostic Risk Observational Survey. *J Hypertens* 2002; 20:1307–1314.

21. Anderson KM, Wilson PW, Odell PM, Kannel WB. An updated coronary risk profile. A statement for health professionals. *Circulation* 1991; 83:356–362.

22. Rockhill B, Newman B, Weinberg C. Use and misuse of population attributable fractions. *Am J Public Health* 1998; 88:15–19.

23. Murray CJ, Lopez AD. On the comparable quantification of health risks; lessons from the Global Burden of Disease Study. *Epidemiology* 1999; 10:594–605.

24. Kannel WB. Update on hypertension as a cardiovascular risk factor. In: Mancia G (ed.). *Manual of Hypertension.* Churchill Livingstone, London, 2002, pp 4–19.

25. Lawes CMM, Vander Hoorn S, Law MR, Elliott P, MacMahon S, Rodgers A. Blood pressure and the global burden of disease 2000. Part II: Estimates of attributable burden. *J Hypertens* 2006; 24:423–430.

26. Mancia G, De Backer G, Dominiczak A *et al.* 2007 Guidelines for the management of arterial hypertension. *J Hypertens* 2007; 25:1105–1187.

27. National High Blood Pressure Education Program. The sixth report of the Joint National Committee on Prevention, Detection, Evaluation, and Treatment of High Blood Pressure: The JNC 7 Report. *Arch Intern Med* 1997; 157:2413–2446.

28. Chobanian AV, Bakris GL, Black HR *et al.* The seventh report of the Joint National Committee on Prevention, Detection, Evaluation and Treatment of High Blood Pressure: the JNC 6 Report. *JAMA* 2003; 289:2560–2572.

29. O'Brien E, Waeber B, Parati G, Staessen J, Myers MG. Blood pressure measuring devices: recommendations of the European Society of Hypertension. *BMJ* 2001; 322:531–536.

30. Verdechia P, Porcellati C, Schillaci G *et al.* Ambulatory blood pressure – an independent predictor of prognosis in essential hypertension. *Hypertension* 1994; 24:793–801.

31. Redon J, Campos C, Narciso ML, Rodicio JL, Pascal JM, Ruilope LM. Prognostic value of ambulatory blood pressure monitoring in refractory hypertension – a prospective study. *Hypertension* 1998; 31:712–718.

32. Staessen JA, Thijs L, Fagard R *et al.*, for the Systolic Hypertension in Europe Trial Investigators. Predicting cardiovascular risk using conventional vs ambulatory blood pressure in older patients with systolic hypertension. *JAMA* 1999; 282:539–546.

33. Khattar RS, Swales JD, Banfield A, Dore C, Senior R, Lahiri A. Prediction of coronary and cerebrovascular morbidity and mortality by direct continuous ambulatory blood pressure monitoring in essential hypertension. *Circulation* 1999; 100:1071–1076.

34. Kario K, Shimada K, Schwarz JE, Matsuo T, Hoshide S, Pickering TG. Silent and clinically overt stroke in older Japanese subjects with white-coat and sustained hypertension. *J Am Coll Cardiol* 2001; 38:238–245.

35. Clement DL, De Buyzere ML, De Bacquer DA *et al.*; for the Office Ambulatory Blood Monitoring Study Investigators. Prognostic value of ambulatory blood pressure recordings in patients with treated hypertension. *N Engl J Med* 2003; 348:2407–2415.

36. Pierdomenico SD, Lapenna D, Bucci A *et al.* Cardiovascular and renal events in uncomplicated mild hypertensive patients with sustained and white-coat hypertension. *Am J Hypertens* 2004; 17:876–881.

37. Ohkubo T, Imai Y, Tsuhi I *et al.* Prediction of mortality by ambulatory blood pressure monitoring versus screening blood pressure measurements. A pilot study in Ohasama. *J Hypertens* 1997; 15:357–364.

38. Ohkubo T, Hozawa A, Nagai K *et al.* Prediction of stroke by ambulatory blood pressure monitoring versus screening blood pressure measurements in a general population: the Ohasama study. *J Hypertens* 2000; 18:847–854.

39. Björklund K, Lind L, Zethelius B, Andrén B, Lithell H. Isolated ambulatory hypertension predicts cardiovascular morbidity in elderly men. *Circulation* 2003; 107:1297–1303.

40. Hansen TW, Jeppesen J, Rasmussen S, Ibsen H, Torp-Pedersen C. Ambulatory blood pressure and mortality: a population based study. *Hypertension* 2005; 45:499–504.

41. Pickering TG, Shimbo D, Haas D. Ambulatory blood pressure monitoring. *N Engl J Med* 2006; 354:2368–2374.

42. Mancia G, Zanchetti A, Agabiti-Rosei E *et al*. Ambulatory blood pressure is superior to clinic blood pressure in predicting treatment induced regression of left ventricular hypertrophy. *Circulation* 1997; 95:1464–1470.

43. Sakuma M, Imai Y, Nagai K *et al*. Reproducibility of home blood pressure measurements over a 1-year period. *Am J Hypertens* 1997; 10:798–803.

44. Zarnke KB, Feagan BG, Mahon JL, Feldman RD. A randomized study comparing a patient-directed hypertension management strategy with usual office-based care. *Am J Hypertens* 1997; 10:58–67.

45. O'Brien E, Asmar R, Beilin L *et al.*, on behalf of the European Society of Hypertension Working Group on Blood Pressure Monitoring. European Society of Hypertension Recommendations for Conventional, Ambulatory and Home Blood Pressure Measurement. *J Hypertens* 2003; 21:821–848.

46. Tsuji I, Imai Y, Nagai K *et al*. Proposal of reference values for home blood pressure measurement: prognostic criteria based on a prospective observation of the general population in Ohasama, Japan. *Am J Hypertens* 1997; 10(pt 1):409–418.

47. Imai Y, Ohkubo T, Tsuji I *et al*. Prognostic value of ambulatory and home blood pressure measurements in comparison to screening blood pressure measurements: a pilot study in Ohasama. *Blood Press Monit* 1996; 1(suppl 2):S51–S58.

48. Ohkubo T, Imai Y, Tsuji I *et al*. Reference values for 24-hour ambulatory blood pressure monitoring based on a prognostic criterion: the Ohasama Study. *Hypertension* 1998; 32:255–259.

49. Bobrie G, Chatellier G, Genes N *et al*. Cardiovascular prognosis of 'masked hypertension' detected by blood pressure self-measurement in elderly treated hypertensive patients. *JAMA* 2004; 291:1342–1349.

50. Pickering TG, Hall JE, Appel LJ *et al*. Recommendations for blood pressure measurement in humans and experimental animals. Part I: Blood pressure measurement in humans; a statement for professionals from the subcommittee of Professional and Public Education of the Am Heart Association Council on High Blood Pressure Research. *Hypertension* 2005; 45:142–161.

51. Pickering T, James GD, Boddie C, Hrashfield GA, Blank S, Laragh JH. How common is white coat hypertension? *JAMA* 1988; 259:225–228.

52. Parati G, Ulian L, Santucci C, Omboni S, Mancia G. Difference between clinic and daytime blood pressure is not a measure of the white coat effect. *Hypertension* 1998; 31:1185–1189.

53. Pickering TG, Coats A, Mallion JM, Mancia G, Verdecchia P. Task Force V. White-coat hypertension. *Blood Press Monit* 1999; 4:333–341.

54. Verdecchia P, Reboldi GP, Angeli F *et al*. Short- and long-term incidence of stroke in white-coat hypertension. *Hypertension* 2005; 45:203–208.

55. Sega R, Trocino G, Lanzarotti A *et al*. Alterations of cardiac structure in patients with isolated office, ambulatory or home hypertension. Data from the general PAMELA population. *Circulation* 2001; 104:1385–1392.

56. Mancia G, Facchetti R, Bombelli M, Grossi G, Sega R. Long-term risk of mortality associated with selective and combined elevation in office, home, and ambulatory blood pressure. *Hypertension* 2006; 47:846–853.

57. Wing LMH, Brown MA, Beilin LJ, Ryan P, Reid C. Reverse white coat hypertension in older hypertensives. *J Hypertens* 2002; 20:639–644.

58. Björklund K, Lind L, Zethelius B, Andren B, Lithell H. Isolated ambulatory hypertension predicts cardiovascular morbidity in elderly men. *Circulation* 2003; 107:1297–1302.

59. Liu JE, Roman MJ, Pini R, Schwartz JE, Pickering TG, Devereux RB. Cardiac and arterial target organ damage in adults with elevated ambulatory and normal office blood pressure. *Ann Intern Med* 1999; 131:564–572.

60. Mallion JM, Genés N, Vaur L *et al*. Detection of masked hypertension by home blood pressure: is the number of measurements an important issue? *Blood Press Monitoring* 2004; 9:301–305.

61. Bombelli M, Sega R, Facchetti R *et al*. Prevalence and clinical significance of a greater ambulatory versus office blood pressure ('reversed white coat' condition) in a general population. *J Hypertens* 2005; 23:513–520.

62. Pierdomenico SD, Lapenna D, Bucci A *et al*. Cardiovascular outcome in treated hypertensive patients with responder, masked, false resistant, and true resistant hypertension. *Am J Hypertens* 2005; 18:1422–1428.

63. Bjorklund K, Lind L, Zethelius B, Berglund L, Lithell H. Prognostic significance of 24-h ambulatory blood pressure characteristics for cardiovascular morbidity in a population of elderly men. *J Hypertens* 2004; 22:1691–1697.

64. Mann JF, Gerstein HC, Pogue J, Bosch J, Yusuf S. Renal insufficiency as a predictor of cardiovascular outcomes and the impact of ramipril: the HOPE randomized trial. *Ann Intern Med* 2001; 134:629–636.

65. Beddhu S, Allen-Brady K, Cheung AK *et al*. Impact of renal failure on the risk of myocardial infarction and death. *Kidney Int* 2002; 62:1776–1783.

66. Levey AS, Bosch JP, Lewis JB, Greene T, Rogers N, Roth D. A more accurate method to estimate glomerular filtration rate from serum creatinine: a new prediction equation. Modification of Diet in Renal Disease Study Group. *Ann Intern Med* 1999; 130:461–470.

67. The Expert Committee on the Diagnosis and Classification of Diabetes Mellitus. Report of the Expert Committee on the diagnosis and classification of diabetes mellitus. *Diabetes Care* 1997; 20:1183–1197.

68. The Expert Committee on the Diagnosis and Classification of Diabetes Mellitus: Follow-up report on the diagnosis of diabetes mellitus. *Diabetes Care* 2003; 26:3160–3167.

69. Diagnosis and classification of diabetes mellitus. *Diabetes Care* 2004; 27:S5–S10.

70. Jensen JS, Feldt-Rasmussen B, Strandgaard S, Schroll M, Borch-Johnsen K. Arterial hypertension, microalbuminuria, and risk of ischemic heart disease. *Hypertension* 2000; 35:898–903.

71. Gerstein HC, Mann JF, Yi Q *et al*. Albuminuria and risk of cardiovascular events, death, and heart failure in diabetic and nondiabetic individuals. *JAMA* 2001; 286:421–426.

72. Garg JP, Bakris GL. Microalbuminuria: marker of vascular dysfunction, risk factor for cardiovascular disease. *Vasc Med* 2002; 7:35–43.

73. Reichek N, Devereux RB. Left ventricular hypertrophy: relationship of anatomic, echocardiographic and electrocardiographic findings. *Circulation* 1981; 63:1391–1398.

74. Levy D, Garrison RJ, Savage DD, Kannel WB, Castelli WP. Prognostic implications of echocardiographically determined left ventricular mass in the Framingham Heart Study. *N Engl J Med* 1990; 322:1561–1566.

75. Simon A, Gariepy J, Chironi G, Megnien J-L, Levenson J. Intima–media thickness: a new tool for diagnosis and treatment of cardiovascular risk. *J Hypertens* 2002; 20:159–169.

76. Keith NH, Wagener HP, Barker MW. Some different types of essential hypertension: their course and prognosis. *Am J Med Sci* 1939; 197:332–343.

77. Cuspidi C, Macca G, Salerno M *et al*. Evaluation of target organ damage in arterial hypertension: which role for qualitative funduscopic examination? *Ital Heart J* 2001; 2:702–706.

78. Benetos A, Safar M, Rudnich A *et al*. Pulse pressure: a predictor of long-term cardiovascular mortality in a French male population. *Hypertension* 1997; 30:1410–1415.

79. Safar ME, Frohlich ED. The arterial system in hypertension: a prospective view. *Hypertension* 1995; 26:10–14.

80. Giannattasio C, Mancia G. Arterial distensibility in humans. Modulating mechanisms, alterations in diseases and effects of treatment. *J Hypertens* 2002; 20:1889–1900.

81. Laurent S, Cockcroft J, van Bortel L *et al.*, on behalf of the European Network for Non Invasive Investigation of Large Arteries. Expert consensus document on arterial stiffness: methodological issues and clinical applications. *Eur Heart J* 2006; 27:2588–2605.

82. Laurent S, Boutouyrie P, Asmar R *et al*. Aortic stiffness is an independent predictor of all-cause and cardiovascular mortality in hypertensive patients. *Hypertension* 2001; 37:1236–1241.

83. O'Rourke MF. From theory into practice. Arterial hemodynamics in clinical hypertension. *J Hypertens* 2002; 20:1901–1915.

84. Pauca AL, O'Rourke MF, Kon ND. Prospective evaluation of a method for estimating ascending aortic pressure from the radial artery pressure waveform. *Hypertension* 2001; 38:932–937.

85. Boutouyrie P, Tropeano AI, Asmar R *et al*. Aortic stiffness is an independent predictor of primary coronary events in hypertensive patients: a longitudinal study. *Hypertension* 2002; 39:10–15.

86. Laurent S, Katsahian S, Fassot C, Tropeano AI, Laloux B, Boutouyrie P. Aortic stiffness is an independent predictor of fatal stroke in essential hypertension. *Stroke* 2003; 34:1203–1206.

87. Cruickshank K, Riste L, Anderson SG, Wright JS, Dunn G, Gosling RG. Aortic pulse-wave velocity and its relationship to mortality in diabetes and glucose intolerance: an integrated index of vascular function? *Circulation* 2002; 106:2085–2090.

88. Blacher J, Guerin AP, Pannier B, Marchais SJ, Safar ME, London GM. Impact of aortic stiffness on survival in end-stage renal disease. *Circulation* 1999; 99:2434–2439.

89. Shoji T, Emoto M, Shinohara K *et al*. Diabetes mellitus, aortic stiffness, and cardiovascular mortality in end-stage renal disease. *J Am Soc Nephrol* 2001; 12:2117–2124.

90. Meaume S, Benetos A, Henry OF *et al*. Aortic pulse wave velocity predicts cardiovascular mortality in subjects >70 years of age. *Arterioscler Thromb Vasc Biol* 2001; 21:2046–2050.

91. Sutton-Tyrrell K, Najjar SS, Boudreau RM *et al.*, Health ABC Study. Elevated aortic pulse wave velocity, a marker of arterial stiffness, predicts cardiovascular events in well-functioning older adults. *Circulation* 2005; 111:3384–3390.

92. Mattace-Raso FU, van der Cammen TJ, Hofman A *et al.* Arterial stiffness and risk of coronary heart disease and stroke: the Rotterdam Study. *Circulation* 2006; 113:657–663.

93. Shokawa T, Imazu M, Yamamoto H *et al.* Pulse wave velocity predicts cardiovascular mortality: findings from the Hawaii-Los Angeles-Hiroshima study. *Circ J* 2005; 69:259–264.

94. Willum-Hansen T, Staessen JA, Torp-Pedersen C *et al.* Prognostic value of aortic pulse wave velocity as index of arterial stiffness in the general population. *Circulation* 2006; 113:664–670.

95. Williams B, Lacy PS, Thom SM *et al.*, CAFE Investigators; Anglo-Scandinavian Cardiac Outcomes Trial Investigators; CAFE Steering Committee and Writing Committee. Differential impact of blood pressure-lowering drugs on central aortic pressure and clinical outcomes: principal results of the Conduit Artery Function Evaluation (CAFE) study. *Circulation* 2006; 113:1213–1225.

96. Dahlof B, Sever PS, Poulter NR *et al.*, ASCOT Investigators. Prevention of cardiovascular events with an antihypertensive regimen of amlodipine adding perindopril as required versus atenolol adding bendroflumethiazide as required, in the Anglo-Scandinavian Cardiac Outcomes Trial-Blood Pressure Lowering Arm (ASCOT-BPLA): a multicentre randomised controlled trial. *Lancet* 2005; 366:895–906.

97. Safar ME, Blacher J, Pannier B *et al.* Central pulse pressure and mortality in end-stage renal disease. *Hypertension* 2002; 39:735–738.

98. London GM, Blacher J, Pannier B, Guerin AP, Marchais SJ, Safar ME. Arterial wave reflections and survival in end-stage renal failure. *Hypertension* 2001; 38:434–438.

99. Ridker PM. Clinical application of C-reactive protein for cardiovascular disease detection and prevention. *Circulation* 2003; 107:363–369.

100. Wang TJ, Gona P, Larson MG *et al.* Multiple biomarkers for the prediction of first major cardiovascular events and death. *N Engl J Med* 2006; 355:2631–2639.

101. Ridker PM, Buring JE, Cook NR, Rifai N. C-reactive protein, the metabolic syndrome, and risk of incident cardiovascular events: an 8-year follow-up of 14 719 initially healthy American women. *Circulation* 2003; 107:391–397.

102. Ridker PM, Rifai N, Rose L, Buring JE, Cook NR. Comparison of C-reactive protein and low-density lipoprotein cholesterol levels in the prediction of first cardiovascular events. *N Engl J Med* 2002; 347:1557–1565.

103. Ridker PM, Hennekens CH, Buring JE, Rifai N. C-reactive protein and other markers of inflammation in the prediction of cardiovascular disease in women. *N Engl J Med* 2000; 342:836–843.

104. Homocysteine Studies Collaboration. Homocysteine and risk of ischemic heart disease and stroke: a meta-analysis. *JAMA* 2002; 288:562–573.

105. Toole JF, Malinow MR, Chambless LE *et al.* Lowering homocysteine in patients with ischemic stroke to prevent recurrent stroke, myocardial infarction, and death: the Vitamin Intervention for Stroke Prevention (VISP) randomized controlled trial. *JAMA* 2004; 291:565–575.

106. Bønaa KH, Njølstad I, Ueland PM *et al.* Homocysteine lowering and cardiovascular events after acute myocardial infarction. *N Engl J Med* 2006; 354:1578–1588.

107. The Heart Outcomes Prevention Evaluation (HOPE) 2 Investigators. Homocysteine lowering with folic acid and B vitamins in vascular disease. *N Engl J Med* 2006; 354:1567–1577.

108. B-Vitamin Treatment Trialists' Collaboration. Homocysteine-lowering trials for prevention of cardiovascular events: a review of the design and power of the large randomized trials. *Am Heart J* 2006; 151:282–287.

109. Palatini P, Benetos A, Grassi G *et al.* Identification and management of the hypertensive patient with elevated heart rate: statement of the European Society of Hypertension Consensus Meeting. *J Hypertens* 2006; 24:603–610.

110. Zanchetti A. The hypertensive patient with multiple risk factors: is treatment really so difficult? *Am J Hypertens* 1997; 10:223S–229S.

111. Stamler J, Wentworth D, Neaton JD. Is relationship between serum cholesterol and risk of premature death from coronary heart disease continuous and graded? Findings in 356,222 primary screenees of the Multiple Risk Factor Intervention Trial (MRFIT). *JAMA* 1986; 256:2823–2828.

112. Pyörälä K, De Backer G, Graham I, Poole-Wilson P, Wood D. Prevention of coronary heart disease in clinical practice. Recommendations of the Task Force of the European Society of Cardiology, European Atherosclerosis Society and European Society of Hypertension. *Eur Heart J* 1994; 15:1300–1331.

113. Wood D, De Backer G, Faergeman O, Graham I, Mancia G, Pyörälä K. Prevention of coronary heart disease in clinical practice. Recommendations of the Second Joint Task Force of European and other Societies on Coronary Prevention. *Eur Heart J* 1998; 19:1434–1503.

114. Jackson R. Updated New Zealand cardiovascular disease risk–benefit prediction guide. *BMJ* 2000; 320:709–710.

115. Conroy RM, Pyörälä K, Fitzgerald AP *et al*. Estimation of ten-year risk of fatal cardiovascular disease in Europe: the SCORE Project. *Eur Heart J* 2003; 11:987–1003.

116. Third Report of the National Cholesterol Education Program (NCEP). Expert Panel on Detection, Evaluation, and Treatment of High Blood Cholesterol in Adults (Adult Treatment Panel III). NIH Publication 02-5215. *Circulation* 2002; 106:3143–3420.

117. Haq IU, Ramsay LE, Yeo WW, Jackson PR, Wallis EJ. Is the Framingham risk function valid for northern European populations? A comparison of methods for estimating absolute coronary risk in high risk men. *Heart* 1999; 81:40–46.

118. Menotti A, Puddu PE, Lanti M. Comparison of the Framingham risk function-based coronary chart with risk function from an Italian population study. *Eur Heart J* 2000; 21:365–370.

119. Simpson FO. Guidelines for antihypertensive therapy: problems with a strategy based on absolute cardiovascular risk. *J Hypertens* 1996; 14:683–689.

120. Zanchetti A. Antihypertensive therapy. How to evaluate the benefits. *Am J Cardiol* 1997; 79:3–8.

121. 2003 European Society of Hypertension-European Society of Cardiology guidelines for the management of arterial hypertension. Guidelines Committee. *J Hypertens* 2003; 21:1011–1053.

122. Reaven G. Metabolic syndrome: pathophysiology and implications for management of cardiovascular disease. *Circulation* 2002; 106:286–288.

123. Zanchetti A, Ruilope LM. Antihypertensive treatment in patients with type-2 diabetes mellitus: what guidance from recent controlled randomized trials? *J Hypertens* 2002; 20:2099–2110.

124. Zanchetti A, Hansson L, Dahlof B *et al*. Effects of individual risk factors on the incidence of cardiovascular events in the treated hypertensive patients of the Hypertension Optimal Treatment Study. HOT Study Group. *J Hypertens* 2001; 19:1149–1159.

125. Ruilope LM, Salvetti A, Jamerson K *et al*. Renal function and intensive lowering of blood pressure in hypertensive participants of the hypertension optimal treatment (HOT) study. *J Am Soc Nephrol* 2001; 12:218–225.

126. He J, Muntner P, Chen J, Roccella EJ. Factors associated with hypertension control in the general population of the United States. *Arch Intern Med* 2002; 162:1051–1058.

127. Elliott WJ. In: Kaplan NM (ed.). *The Current Inadequate Control of Hypertension: How Can We Do Better? Hypertension Therapy Annual*. Martin Dunitz, London, 2000, pp 1–25.

128. Schrier RW, Estacio RO, Esler A, Mehler P. Effects of aggressive blood pressure control in normotensive type 2 diabetic patients on albuminuria, retinopathy and stroke. *Kidney Int* 2002; 61:1086–1097.

129. Hansson L, Zanchetti A, Carruthers SG *et al*. Effects of intensive blood-pressure lowering and low-dose aspirin in patients with hypertension: principal results of the Hypertension Optimal Treatment (HOT) randomised trial. *Lancet* 1998; 351:1755–1762.

130. UK Prospective Diabetes Study Group. Tight blood pressure control and risk of macrovascular and microvascular complications in Type 2 diabetes. UKPDS38. *Br Med J* 1998; 317:703–713.

131. Estacio RO, Jeffers BW, Hiatt WR, Biggerstaff SL, Gifford N, Schrier RW. The effect of nisoldipine as compared with enalapril on cardiovascular outcomes in patients with non-insulin independent diabetes and hypertension. *N Engl J Med* 1998; 338:645–652.

132. Zanchetti A, Hansson L, Ménard J *et al*. Risk assessment and treatment benefit in intensively treated hypertensive patients of the Hypertension Optimal Treatment (HOT) study for the HOT Study Group. *J Hypertens* 2001; 19:819–825.

133. Blood Pressure Lowering Treatment Trialists' Collaboration. Effects of ACE inhibitors, calcium antagonists, and other blood-pressure-lowering drugs: results of prospectively designed overviews of randomised trials. *Lancet* 2000; 356:1955–1964.

134. Zanchetti A, Hansson L, Clement D *et al.*, on behalf of the HOT Study Group. Benefits and risks of more intensive blood pressure lowering in hypertensive patients of the HOT Study with different risk profiles: does a J-shaped curve exist in smokers? *J Hypertens* 2003; 21:797–804.

135. PROGRESS Collaborative Study Group. Randomised trial of perindopril based blood pressure-lowering regimen among 6108 individuals with previous stroke or transient ischaemic attack. *Lancet* 2001; 358:1033–1041.

136. Mancia G, Grassi G. Systolic and diastolic blood pressure control in antihypertensive drug trials. *J Hypertens* 2002; 20:1461–1464.
137. Messerli FM, Mancia G, Conti CR *et al.* Dogma disputed: can aggressively lowering blood pressure in hypertensive patients with coronary artery disease be dangerous? *Ann Int Med* 2006; 144:884–893.
138. Ruilope LM, Salvetti A, Jamerson K *et al.* Renal function and intensive lowering of blood pressure in hypertensive participants of the hypertension optimal treatment (HOT) study. *J Am Soc Nephrol* 2001; 12:218–225.
139. Appel LJ, Brands MW, Daniels SR, Karanja N, Elmer PJ, Sacks FM. Dietary approaches to prevent and treat hypertension. A scientific statement from the American Heart Association. *Hypertension* 2006; 47:296–308.
140. Sacks FM, Svetkey LP, Vollmer WM *et al.* Effects on blood pressure of reduced dietary sodium and the Dietary Approaches to Stop Hypertension (DASH) diet. DASH-Sodium Collaborative Research Group. *N Engl J Med* 2001; 344:3–10.
141. He FJ, Makandu ND, MacGregor GA. Importance of the renin system for determining blood pressure fall with acute salt restriction in hypertensive and normotensive whites. *Hypertension* 2001; 38:321–325.
142. Institute of Medicine. *Dietary Reference Intakes: Water, Potassium, Sodium Chloride, and Sulfate,* 1st edition. National Academy Press, Washington, DC, 2004.
143. Neter JE, Stam BE, Kok FJ, Grobbee DE, Gelejinse JM. Influence of weight reduction on blood pressure: a meta-analysis of randomized controlled trials. *Hypertension* 2003; 42:878–884.
144. Kelley GA, Kelley KS. Progressive resistance exercise and resting blood pressure: a meta-analysis of randomized controlled trials. *Hypertension* 2000; 35:838–843.
145. Whelton SP, Chin A, Xin X, He J. Effect of aerobic exercise on blood pressure: a meta-analysis of randomized, controlled trials. *Ann Intern Med* 2002; 136:493–503.
146. Appel LJ, Champagne CM, Harsha DW *et al.* Effects of comprehensive lifestyle modification on blood pressure control. Main results of the PREMIER clinical trial. Writing Group of the PREMIER Collaborative Research Group. *JAMA* 2003; 289:2083–2093.
147. Blood Pressure Lowering Treatment Trialists Collaboration. Effects of different blood-pressure-lowering regimens on major cardiovascular events: results of prospectively-designed overview of randomized trials. *Lancet* 2003; 362:1527–1545.
148. National Institute of Clinical Excellence (NICE) Clinical Guideline 18 – management of hypertension in adults in primary care, 2004. Available at: www.nice.org.uk/ CG18NICEguideline. Accessed 12 October 2004.
149. Staessen JA, Wang JG, Thijs L *et al.* Cardiovascular prevention and blood pressure reduction: a quantitative overview updated until 1st March 2003. *J Hypertens* 2003; 21:1055–1076.
150. The ALLHAT Officers and Coordinators for the ALLHAT Collaborative Research Group. Major outcomes in high-risk hypertensive patients randomized to angiotensin-converting enzyme inhibitor or calcium channel blocker vs diuretic: the Antihypertensive and Lipid-Lowering Treatment to Prevent Heart Attack Trial (ALLHAT). *JAMA* 2002; 288:2981–2997.
151. NICE/BHS. Clinical guideline 34: hypertension: management of hypertension in adults in primary care: http:www.niveco.org.uk/G034guidance (accessed 28 June 2006).
152. Dahlöf B, Devereux RB, Kjeldsen SE; for the LIFE Study Group. Cardiovascular morbidity in the Losartan Intervention for Endpoint reduction in hypertension study (LIFE): a randomized trial against atenolol. *Lancet* 2002; 359:995–1003.
153. Dahlöf B, Sever PAS, Poulter NP, for the ASCOT Investigators. Prevention of cardiovascular events with an antihypertensive regimen of amlodipine adding perindopril as required versus adding dendrofluomethiazide as required, in the Anglo-Scandinavian Cardiac Outcomes Trials–Blood Pressure Lowering Arm (ASCOT-BPLA): a multicenter randomized controlled trial. *Lancet* 2005; 366:895–906.
154. Mancia G, Grassi G, Zanchetti A. New-onset diabetes and antihypertensive drugs. *J Hypertens* 2006; 24:3–10.
155. Mason JM, Dickinson HO, Nicolson DJ, Campbell F, Ford GA, Williams B. The diabetogenic potential of thiazide-type diuretic and beta-blocker combinations in patients with hypertension. *J Hypertens* 2005; 3:1777–1781.
156. Khan N, McAlister FA. Re-examining the efficacy of beta-blockers for the treatment of hypertension: a meta-analysis. *CMAJ* 2006; 174:1737–1742.
157. Antithrombotic Trialists' Collaboration. Collaborative meta-analysis of randomized trials of antiplatelet therapy for prevention of death, myocardial infarction, and stroke in high risk patients. *BMJ* 2002; 324:71–86.

158. Zanchetti A, Hansson L, Dahlöf B *et al.* Benefit and harm of low-dose aspirin in well-treated hypertensives at different baseline cardiovascular risk. *J Hypertens* 2002; 20:2301–2307.

159. The ALLHAT Officers and Coordinators for the ALLHAT Collaborative Research group. Major outcomes in moderately hypercholesterolemic, hypertensive patients randomized to pravastatin vs usual care. The Antihypertensive and Lipid-Lowering Treatment to Prevent Heart Attack Trial (ALLHAT-LLT). *JAMA* 2002; 288:2998–3007.

160. Sever PS, Dahlöf B, Poulter NR *et al.*, for the ASCOT Investigators. Prevention of coronary and stroke events with atorvastatin in hypertensive patients who have average or lower-than-average cholesterol concentrations in the Anglo-Scandinavian Cardiac Outcomes Trials–Lipid Lowering Arm (ASCOT-LLA): a multicentre randomized controlled trial. *Lancet* 2003; 361:1149–1158.

161. Smith SC, Allen J, Blair SN *et al.* AHA/ACC Guidelines for Secondary Prevention for Patients With Coronary and Other Atherosclerotic Vascular Disease: 2006 Update. Endorsed by the National Heart, Lung and Blood Institute. *Circulation* 2006; 113:2363–2372.

17

Heart rate as a risk factor

M. T. Cooney, A. L. Dudina, D. Ward, I. M. Graham

INTRODUCTION

Resting heart rate is one of the most easily obtained measures of cardiovascular health. Increased resting heart rate is associated with increased total and cardiovascular mortality in general as well as coronary artery disease (CAD) and hypertensive populations. Although resting pulse rate can be quickly and reliably assessed, it is often overlooked as an index of cardiovascular risk. In this chapter, we address:

- The evidence for an association between cardiovascular mortality and increased resting heart rate and its utility as a variable for the estimation of cardiovascular risk.
- The possible mechanisms for the association between heart rate and mortality.
- Whether the association is likely to be causal.
- The likelihood of benefit from reducing heart rate.

ANIMAL STUDIES

Smaller mammals tend to have higher heart rates and shorter life spans than larger ones. There is a semi-logarithmic, inverse relationship between heart rate and life expectancy; as the heart rate of different mammalian species increases, the life expectancy decreases. Humans are the only exception [1]. This relationship has been graphically illustrated by Levine, as shown in Figure 17.1. One explanation for the association between body size and heart rate is that smaller body sizes require higher metabolic rates and consequent elevated heart rates.

The number of heart beats in a lifetime is constant amongst the various species of mammal within one order of magnitude (mean $= 7.4 \pm 5.6 \times 10^8$), despite a 40-fold difference in life expectancy. The number of heart beats per lifetime in each of the species of mammal is plotted against life expectancy in Figure 17.2.

If inter-species differences in heart rate determine longevity, the next question is whether heart rate also determines disease and life expectancy *within* a species. Kaplan *et al.* [2] studied the effect of propranolol on coronary artery atherosclerosis (CAA) in monkeys. Fifteen monkeys were given propranolol mixed with an atherogenic diet and 15 controls were

Marie Therese Cooney, MB BCh, BAO, MRCPI, Research Fellow in Cardiology, Department of Cardiology, The Adelaide and Meath Hospital, Tallaght, Dublin, Ireland

Alexandra L. Dudina, MB, Research Fellow in Cardiology, Department of Cardiology, The Adelaide and Meath Hospital, Tallaght, Dublin, Ireland

Deirdre Ward, MRCPI, Consultant Cardiologist, Department of Cardiology, The Adelaide and Meath Hospital, Tallaght, Dublin, Ireland

Ian M. Graham, FRCPI, FESC, Consultant Cardiologist; Professor of Cardiovascular Medicine, Trinity College, Dublin; Professor of Preventive Cardiology, Royal College of Surgeons in Ireland

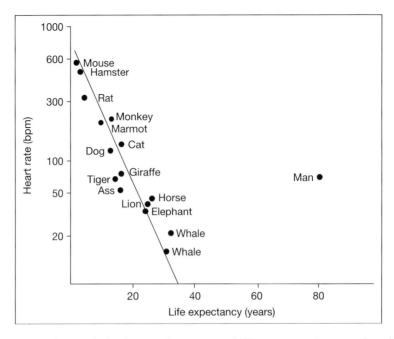

Figure 17.1   Inverse linear relation between heart rate and life expectancy in mammals and humans.

given only an atherogenic diet. All of the monkeys were examined for CAA after 26 months. Previous studies had shown socially dominant monkeys to be predisposed to the development of atherosclerosis when fed an atherogenic diet. Here, the dominant monkeys in the control group exhibited significantly exacerbated CAA. However, treated dominant monkeys did not develop exacerbated CAA (mean atherosclerosis = 0.71 mm² in dominant untreated and 0.23 mm² in dominant treated [0.43 and 0.30 in treated and untreated subordinates respectively]). These effects were independent of blood lipids, blood pressure and resting heart rate. The authors conclude that propranolol reduces the development of atherosclerosis in behaviourally predisposed monkeys.

A similar study has been performed by Beere *et al.* [3]. The effect of lowered heart rate achieved by means of sinoatrial node ablation on monkeys fed an atherogenic diet was assessed. The extent of coronary atherosclerosis after 6 months was compared to that seen in control monkeys who underwent a sham operation. The monkeys with sinoatrial ablation had significantly lower heart rates, as seen on telemetry, and significantly less atherosclerosis formation. The average lesion area in the low heart rate group was only one-third of that seen in the high heart rate group, despite no difference in blood lipids, blood pressure or body weight.

Further evidence that an elevated heart rate has a direct effect on atherogenesis in humans as well as animals was provided by Perski *et al.* [4]. Progression of atherosclerosis and its relationship to heart rate was studied in 56 men who had survived a first myocardial infarction (MI) which occurred before the age of 45 [4]. All of the participants had two angiograms with an interval of 4–7 years between them. 24-hour heart rate monitoring was undertaken at the time of the re-angiography. High minimum heart rate on 24-hour monitoring was associated with progression of both diffuse lesions and distinct stenoses. An increase in minimum heart rate of 5 beats per minute (bpm) corresponded to an increase in stenosis progression score of 0.27 (95% confidence interval [CI] 0.24–0.31). Although it is difficult to be certain that the increase in heart rate was an effect of more rapidly developing disease rather than a cause, the effect of increased minimum heart rate was independent of other

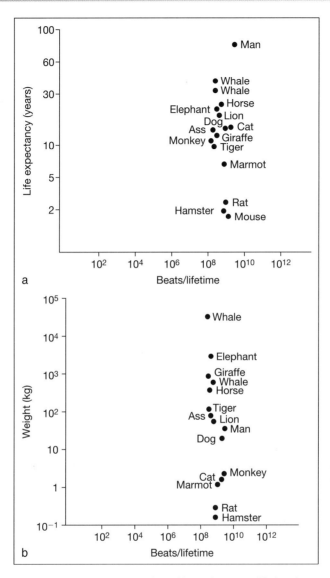

Figure 17.2 Relation between life expectancy and total heart beats per lifetime in mammals and humans.

factors including age, low-density lipoprotein cholesterol (LDL-c)/high-density lipoprotein cholesterol (HDL-c) ratio, lipoprotein (a), fibrinogen, hypertension, smoking and the presence of β-blocker therapy.

EPIDEMIOLOGICAL STUDIES

Several longitudinal studies have examined the effect of increasing heart rate on coronary heart disease (CHD) and cardiovascular disease (CVD) in the general population as well as subgroups of people including those with CAD, the elderly, hypertensives and diabetics. Table 17.1 represents a summary of each of the main studies that have examined the effect of heart rate on cardiovascular endpoints in the general population.

Table 17.1 Epidemiological studies in the general population

References	Study population	Number and gender	Follow-up (years)	Age group	Endpoints	Effect of elevated heart rate	Qualification of effect (CVD mortality) (multivariate)	Covariates included/others
Filipovsky et al. [7]	Paris Prospective Study	4907 men	17	Middle-aged	Total mortality / CV mortality	Potential independent RF / Not significant		Sports activity and BMI included
Jouven et al. [45]	Paris Prospective Study	7746 men	22	43–52	Fatal MI / Sudden death	Independent RF / Independent RF	1.22 (1.12–1.49) for each increase of 10.2 bpm	No exercise covariate
Benetos et al. [11]	French IPC	12 123 men 7263 women	17	40–69	Total mortality / CV mortality	Predictor in both genders / Independent RF in men only	61–80: 1.35 (1.01–1.80) 81–100: 1.44 (1.04–2) >100: 2.18 (1.37–3.47) Compared to <60 men only	Physical activity included; Subgroup analyses – effect persisted in: HTN and non-HTN, >65 and <65
Kristal-Boneh et al. [46]	CORDIS	3527 men	8	mean 48 years	CV mortality	Independent RF	1.95 (1.1–3.8) >70 compared to <70	Sports activity included. Many haematological factors included
Seccareccia et al. [47]	MATISS	2533 men	9.7	40–69	CV mortality	Independent RF	2.54 (1.25–5.16) >70 compared to <70	Arm circumference and adjusted FEV_1 considered surrogates for exercise
Shaper et al. [10]	Brit Reg Heart Study	7735 men	8	40–59	CHD mortality / Sudden death	Independent RF / Independent RF	3.3 (1.4–7.8) / 5.2 (1.4–18.7) >90 compared to <60	Physical activity included; Persisted in subgroup HTN vs. non-HTN

Study	Cohort	Sample	Years	Age	Outcome	Result	Effect size	Comments
Kannel et al. [14]	Framingham	5070 men and women	30	35–64 and 65–94	CV mortality (2-year incidence)	Independent in men not women. Related univariate in women also (gradients steeper in men)	Standardized regression coefficients for effect of heart rate on 2-year CVD mortality: men (35–64) 0.288 ($P < 0.001$) men (65–94) 0.147 ($P < 0.05$)	No exercise/fitness covariate. Effect persisted in men after exclusion of those with interim CAD development
Gillum et al. [9]	NHANES	5136 white men and women	9.9	45–74	CV mortality (whites)	RF in both – univariate Multivariate men only	White men: 1.44 (1.08–1.92)	Authors report that inclusion of BMI and physical activity did not change results, figures not given
		859 black men and women	10.3	45–74	CV mortality (blacks)	RF in both – univariate Multivariate black women only	Black women: 3.03 (1.46–6.28) >84 compared to <74	
Reunanen et al. [8]		5598 men 5119 women	23	30–59	Total mortality CV mortality	Univariate associated Univariate associated but not significant after addition of SBP to model		
Dyer et al. [6]	3 Chicago Industry Studies	1233 men 1899 men 5784 men	15 17 5	40–59 40–55 45–64	CHD Sudden death	Not significant on multivariate analysis Independent RF in 2 of 3 studies		No exercise covariate

Table 17.1 (continued)

References	Study population	Number and gender	Follow-up (years)	Age group	Endpoints	Effect of elevated heart rate	Qualification of effect (CVD mortality) (multivariate)	Covariates included/others
Greenland et al. [5]	Chicago Heart Association Detection Project in Industry	18 787 men 14 994 women	22	18–74 – divided into 3 age groups	CHD mortality	Increased HR significantly associated with CHD mortality in men 18–39 and 40–59, women 40–59. Only remained after addition of SBP to model in women 40–59 and men 18–39	RR per each increase of 12 bpm (1 standard deviation) Men 18–39: 1.20 (1.02–1.42) Women 40–59: 1.13 (1.01–1.28)	No exercise covariate
Okamura et al. [51]		3856 men	16.5	30–59	CV mortality	Independent RF men 30–59	Men: 2.55 (95%CI 1.22–5.31) comparing >74 bpm to <60 bpm	Albumin included No exercise covariate
		4944 women		Over 60		Independent RF women 30–59	Women: 3.61 (95% CI 1.34–9.72) comparing 70–77 bpm to <60 bpm	

BMI = body mass index; CAD = coronary artery disease; CHD = coronary heart disease; CV = cardiovascular; FEV_1 = forced expiratory volume in 1 second; HTN = hypertensive; MI = myocardial infarction; RF = risk factor; SBP = systolic blood pressure.

Many factors may potentially confound the relationship between cardiovascular risk and heart rate. Hypertension and heart rate are intrinsically linked, so it is important to include this as a covariate in the multivariate analysis. Another possible confounder is exercise, as this may contribute some of its beneficial effect on cardiovascular risk through heart rate reduction, but also has many other proven beneficial effects independent of heart rate, such as elevation of HDL-c. A specific note has been made in Table 17.1 to indicate which of the studies have exercise/physical activity included as a covariate. In addition, the odds ratio or relative risk has only been reported if it continued to be significant after multivariate analysis, which includes systolic blood pressure (SBP), unless otherwise stated.

THE EFFECT OF INCREASING HEART RATE ON CARDIOVASCULAR MORTALITY IN MEN FROM THE GENERAL POPULATION

Heart rate has been demonstrated to be an independent risk factor for the development of CVD in men in the majority of the studies listed in Table 17.1. In a minority of the studies, the effect was no longer significant after multivariate adjustment. This was the case in the Chicago Heart Association Detection in Industry study by Greenland *et al.* [5] (except for the male subgroup aged 18–39), the three Chicago Industry studies by Dyer *et al.* [6], the first of the Paris Prospective studies by Filipovsky *et al.* [7] and the study in the Finnish population by Reunanen *et al.* [8]. In the latter study, the authors pointed out that the association lost statistical significance after the addition of SBP; this effect was also seen in the study by Greenland *et al.* In the National Health and Nutrition Examination Study (NHANES) study, the effect of elevated heart rate on CVD mortality was significant on multivariate analysis in white, but not black men [9].

The finding of the association becoming non-significant with the addition of SBP into the model has prompted some to postulate that the effect of heart rate on CVD mortality may be mediated through hypertension. Two sources of evidence would dispute this. The first is the evidence from the other studies, in which heart rate continued to have an effect when SBP was included as a covariate. There are eight of these listed in Table 17.1. The second piece of evidence comes from subgroup analyses. These were done in two of the studies, Shaper *et al.* [10] and Benetos *et al.* [11]. These studies examined the effect of heart rate in both the hypertensive and non-hypertensive groups and concluded that heart rate remained an independent risk factor in both (see also Figure 17.4). Gillman *et al.* [12] demonstrated that increased heart rate continued to be an independent risk factor for cardiovascular mortality in hypertensive men, with an odds ratio of 1.48 (95% CI 1.05–2.09 per 40 bpm increase in heart rate). A large study by Thomas *et al.* [13] of 60 343 hypertensive men, showed the relative risk associated with a heart rate >80 bpm vs. a heart rate <80 bpm to be 1.48 (95% CI 1.22–1.78) in men under 65 and 1.32 (95% CI 1.11–1.56) in men over 65.

Of the eight studies in which heart rate is shown to be an independent risk factor, five contain physical activity (or surrogate markers for this) as a covariate in the multivariate analysis. This suggests that the effect of elevated heart rate on cardiovascular risk is not merely as a result of elevated heart rate acting as a proxy for a sedentary lifestyle. In an attempt to rule out the possibility of undiagnosed CHD and consequent elevated heart rate confounding the relationship, the authors of the Framingham study re-analysed the relationship after exclusion of those who developed CHD in the interim [14]. The effect remained significant in this re-analysis.

The odds ratios and relative risks shown in Table 17.1 associated with increasing heart rate suggest that the risk of CVD mortality associated with increasing heart rate is both strong and graded. This is illustrated in Figure 17.3, which shows the adjusted relative risks of ischaemic heart disease (IHD) and sudden death associated with various categories of heart rate, as demonstrated in the study by Shaper *et al.* [10]. The authors of the Framingham study commented that there were no indications of any critical or threshold values which could be labelled as safe or hazardous.

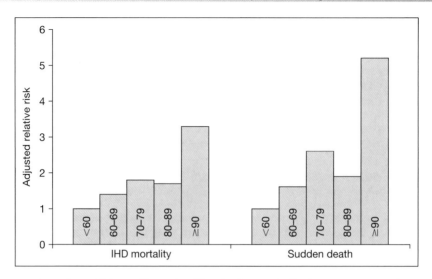

Figure 17.3   Age-adjusted CV mortality and sudden death rates in five heart rate groups in men in the British Regional Heart Study. With permission [10].

THE EFFECT OF ELEVATED HEART RATE ON CARDIOVASCULAR MORTALITY IN WOMEN IN THE GENERAL POPULATION

In women, the relationship between heart rate and cardiovascular risk is less clear. In general, it is more difficult to demonstrate the association of risk factors to cardiovascular events and mortality in women. This may be in part because women develop CVD on average 10 years later than men. This means that, at any given age, a longer follow-up time will be required for sufficient events to occur to demonstrate a significant relationship. Also, many of the older studies, especially those based on cohorts derived from industry, did not include women. Of the studies listed in Table 17.1, only the Framingham study, the French IPC study, the NHANES study, the Chicago Heart Association Detection Project in Industry, the Japanese study by Okamura *et al.* and the study by Reunanen *et al.* included women. The Framingham study showed that total and cardiovascular death were, in general, related to increasing heart rate at all ages. The risk gradient associated with increasing heart rate was steeper in men than in women for both total and cardiovascular mortality. After adjustment for other cardiovascular risk factors, the relationship to total, but not cardiovascular, mortality remained independent in women. Of the studies listed in Table 17.1, only the NHANES study (in black women only), the Japanese study and the Chicago study (in women aged 40–59), actually demonstrated an independent effect in women.

A study by Perk *et al.* [15] is interesting in this regard because it included women who were over the age of 70 at study entry and followed them for 6 years. Four hundred and twenty-two people were included. Only total mortality was analysed. The relative odds ratio comparing heart rate >77 bpm to less than this was 3.37 (95% CI 0.96–11.8) for total mortality, adjusted for previous CVD, hypertension, anaemia, congestive heart failure (CHF), smoking and level of exercise. This was statistically significant when those on β-blockers were removed from the analysis (rollover risk [ROR] = 8.5 [95% CI 1.19–60.1]). The association was not significant in men.

Chang *et al.* [16] studied the effect of increasing heart rate on mortality in a group of disabled (mobility or self-care difficulty with mini-mental test score >18, older [>65] women).

The women were from the Women's Health and Aging Study 1 (WHAS1). The hazard ratio for total mortality comparing a heart rate >90 bpm to 60–89 bpm was 2.0 (95% CI 1.2–3.3). This was adjusted for age, disease status, cardiovascular risk factors, physical activity, and physical and pulmonary function. The same analysis was repeated in the subgroup with no previous clinical or electrocardiographic evidence of ischaemic heart disease. The hazard ratio was 2.3 (95% CI 0.98–5.3), but it did not reach statistical significance. The authors suggested that subclinical heart failure could be causing some of the effects and that controlling for ejection fraction would have been useful.

Gillman et al. [12] studied the association between increased heart rate and cardiovascular mortality in a group of 2037 men and 2493 women from the Framingham study who had hypertension. On univariate analysis, increased heart rate was associated with increased risk of cardiovascular and all-cause mortality over the follow-up period of 34 years. However, after adjustment for age, SBP, cholesterol, cigarette smoking, glucose intolerance and left ventricular hypertrophy, increased heart rate was significantly associated with all-cause mortality in men and women, but with cardiovascular mortality in men only.

PREDICTIVE ABILITY OF ELEVATED HEART RATE IN THE ELDERLY

Cardiovascular risk factors such as cholesterol and smoking tend to lose their predictive power for morbidity and mortality in older age. The Cardiovascular Study in the Elderly (CASTEL, [15]) evaluated the effect of increasing heart rate on cardiovascular mortality in 763 men and 1175 women over the age of 65, followed up for 12 years. An elevated heart rate was found to be an independent predictor of cardiovascular mortality in older men but not in older women. The relative risk of cardiovascular mortality in men associated with the fifth quintile of heart rate compared to the three intermediate quintiles was 1.38 (95% CI 0.94–2.03; $P = 0.005$). This was adjusted for age, body mass index (BMI), total cholesterol (TC), HDL-c, triglycerides, glucose, uric acid, creatinine, forced expiratory volume in 1 second (FEV_1), CHD, CHF, diabetes, hypertension, intermittent claudication, history of cerebrovascular accident (CVA), sedentariness, alcohol intake, smoking and regular medication.

Palatini et al. [17] have added to this work by addressing the question of whether this association held in hypertensive elderly patients. In a group of elderly people (1557 men, 3138 women) with untreated systolic hypertension, elevated heart rate was associated with both total and cardiovascular mortality. Univariate analysis of the effect of increasing heart rate on cardiovascular and total mortality was similar in men and women, so multivariate analysis was done on men and women together. Comparing those with heart rates >79 bpm to those with rates less than this, the hazard ratio for total mortality was 1.88 (95% CI 1.33–2.67; $P < 0.01$) and 1.60 (95% CI 0.99–2.58; $P = 0.05$) for cardiovascular mortality. These figures were adjusted for sex, age, smoking, drinking status, SBP, previous CVD, diabetes, haemoglobin. Further adjustment for other lipid and haematological parameters and BMI did not change the results. Interestingly, ambulatory heart rate measurement did not add prognostic information to that provided by clinic heart rate.

The Chicago Heart Association Study listed in Table 17.1 included a group of men and women aged 60–74 years [5]. Elevated heart rate was not an independent risk factor in this age group. The Framingham study also analysed the effect by age groups (34–64 and 65–94) and the independent association seen held in men in both groups. Also described above are studies by Chang et al. and Perk et al., which demonstrate a significant independent association in older women.

As demonstrated above, the results of studies investigating the effect in women and in the elderly are not in complete agreement with each other. Differences in study populations, lengths of follow-up and methodologies may be responsible for the different results and conclusions regarding similar issues.

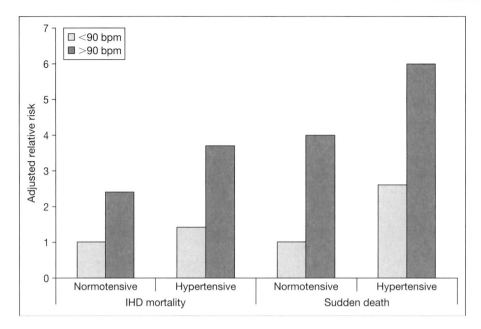

Figure 17.4   Adjusted relative risk of CHD mortality and sudden death associated with heart rate >90 bpm or <90 bpm in hypertensive and normotensive men in the British Regional Heart Study. With permission [10].

THE EFFECT OF ELEVATED HEART RATE ON RISK OF SUDDEN DEATH IN THE GENERAL POPULATION

Some of the studies in Table 17.1 have looked at sudden death specifically and the increased risk of sudden death associated with elevated heart rate. The mechanisms by which elevated heart rate predisposes to sudden death are unclear. An obvious explanation would be that an elevated heart rate is associated with other risk factors including physical inactivity, lipoprotein abnormalities and previous cardiovascular health. However, in the case of the study by Shaper *et al.* [10], all of these were included in the multivariate analysis. Here an adjusted relative risk for sudden death of 5.2 (95% CI 1.4–18.7) comparing those with heart rate <90 bpm to heart rate >90 bpm was demonstrated. A subgroup analysis in those with and without hypertension was also performed: elevated heart rate was associated with an increased risk of sudden death in both groups, as shown in Figure 17.4. The combination of elevated heart rate and hypertension led to a relative risk of 6.0 (95% CI 2.4–15.2). The effect of elevating heart rate on increasing risk of sudden death was also demonstrated in men in the CASTEL study and in men in the Framingham study, as described above.

EPIDEMIOLOGICAL STUDIES INVESTIGATING THE EFFECT OF ELEVATED HEART RATE IN CAD PATIENTS

Table 17.2 describes the studies that have examined the effect of elevated heart rate in people who have evidence of previous CAD. These studies show considerable heterogeneity, with some looking at the effect of 30-day or in-hospital mortality in patients directly after acute MI and others looking at long-term prognosis in those with stable CHD.

Table 17.2 Epidemiological studies in the population with previous coronary heart disease

References	Study group	Number	Follow-up	Endpoint	When heart rate taken	Odds ratio/ relative risk	Covariates	Subgroup analyses/ others
Hathaway et al. [48]	GUSTO-I trial	1081 patients with acute STEMI	30 days	30-day mortality	Admission heart rate – independent RF, U-shaped relationship	1.49 (1.41–1.59) 84 bpm compared to 60 bpm	Ejection fraction or infarct size are not included in multivariate analysis, Killip class is included	Includes a nomogram for predicting outcome, heart rate is a variable
Copie et al. [49]		579 with acute MI	2 years	Sudden death Non-sudden CV death	Mean pre-discharge heart rate on 24-h monitor	HR superior to LVF in predicting sudden death, HR var superior for sens >40%, same for sens <40% Non-sudden death, all three predict equally		
Disegni et al. [19]	SPRINT	1044 patients with MI	1 year	In-hospital mortality 1-year mortality	Admission heart rate independent RF for both	In-hospital mortality: 1.36 (1.08–1.72) 1-year mortality 1.45 (1.15–1.84) per 15 bpm increase	Severity of heart failure, cardiomegaly on chest X-ray, 4× normal limit of CK and LDH included as covariates	Subgroups: association significant only in mild CHF. Excess 1-year mortality in HR >90, identical in men and women

Table 17.2 (continued)

References	Study group	Number	Follow-up	Endpoint	When heart rate taken	Odds ratio/ relative risk	Covariates	Subgroup analyses/ others
Diaz et al. [20]	CASS	24 913 stable CHD (proven or suspect) men and women analysed together	14.7 years	CV mortality	Baseline HR	1.31 (1.15–1.48) >83 compared to <62	Recreational activity Diuretics β-blockers Antiplatelet meds Lipid-lowering meds No. diseased coronary vessels Ejection fraction	Extensive subgroup analysis for total mortality: association held in all groups: men vs. women, <65 vs. >65, HTN vs. non-HTN, DM vs. non-DM, BMI >27 vs. BMI <27, EF <50% vs. >50%, β-blockers vs. non-β-blockers
Wong et al. [18]	Framingham	464 male and 233 female patients post-MI	9.7 years	Re-infarction CHD mortality	Heart rate approximately 1-year after MI	Elevated HR significantly increased risk of coronary death, not re-infarction on univariate but not multivariate analysis		

Hjalmarson et al. [50]	1807 patients less than 12 h post-MI	At least 3 months (1410 – 1 year)	All-cause mortality	Admission HR	Independent RF – no RR P = 0.004	Degree of heart failure, Age, Max CK, Max urea, Prev AMI, Prev CHF

AMI = acute myocardial infarction; bpm = beat per minute; BMI = body mass index; CHD = coronary heart disease; CHF = congestive heart failure; CK = creatinine kinase; CV = cardiovascular; DM = diabetes mellitus; EF = ejection fraction; HR = heart rate; HTN = hypertension; LDH = lactute dehydrogenase; LVF = left ventricular failure; MI = myocardial infarction; RF = risk factor; RR = relative risk; STEMI = ST-elevation myocardial infarction.

One important factor in assessing the relationship in this population is the fact that larger infarcts with consequent reduction in left ventricular function will be associated with increased heart rate. Therefore, any relationship between elevated heart rate and poorer outcome could be confounded by this: elevated heart rate could be acting as a proxy for reduced left ventricular function. The correlation between worsening degrees of heart failure and increasing heart rate is well established [18]. Some of the studies include ejection fraction as a covariate in the multivariate analysis; note has been made of this in the table.

Firstly, we will consider the studies looking at heart rate in acute MI patients. Disegni et al. [19] assessed the effect of admission heart rate in 1044 acute MI patients. Admission heart rate was shown to be an independent risk factor for in-hospital and 1-year mortality. An increase of 15 bpm in admission heart rate was associated with a hazard ratio of 1.36 (95% CI 1.08–1.72). This was independent of factors including previous MI, diabetes, SBP, anterior MI, severity of CHF, cardiomegaly on chest X-ray, creatinine kinase (CK) elevation (4× upper limit) and lactate dehydrogenase (LDH) elevation (4× upper limit). While clinical markers of severity of heart failure were included, ejection fraction was not. Interestingly, in subgroup analyses of none, mild, moderate and severe CHF, elevated heart rate was only significantly associated with increased mortality in mild CHF. Hathaway et al. studied admission heart rate in a similar number of acute MI patients. Again, elevated heart rate was an independent risk factor for 30-day mortality. However, only a clinical marker of heart failure (Killip class) was used as a covariate in the multivariate analysis. In summary, elevated admission heart rate is clearly related to increased short- and intermediate-term outcome in acute MI patients, but whether the association could be due to confounding is uncertain.

A study by Diaz et al. [20] of a large number of stable patients with proven or suspected coronary heart disease is noteworthy for several reasons. Twenty-four thousand, nine hundred and thirteen subjects were followed for a median of 14.7 years. Several factors were included as covariates including ejection fraction as a continuous variable, number of vessels affected and several medical treatments as detailed in the table. The hazard ratio for heart rate >83 bpm compared to <62 bpm was 1.31 (99% CI 1.15–1.48), indicating that elevated heart rate is an independent risk factor for cardiovascular death in the long term in this population. Extensive subgroup analysis was done on the relationship between total mortality and elevated heart rate. The association held in each, including those with ejection fraction greater and less than 50%. In a previous smaller study, Wong et al. [18] demonstrated that elevated heart rate was associated with increased risk of CHD mortality but not non-fatal re-infarction in the long term. This relationship was not statistically significant in multivariate analysis.

POSSIBLE MECHANISMS FOR THE ASSOCIATION OF ELEVATED HEART RATE AND INCREASED RISK OF CARDIOVASCULAR MORTALITY

It has been suggested that the association between elevated heart rate and both vascular and non-vascular mortality may be explained by lack of physical fitness and poor general health. However, many of the studies quoted above that have shown an effect have adjusted for these possible confounders in their analyses. This, coupled with the fact that numerous trials have shown a benefit from heart rate reduction in those with CAD, suggest a need to look for mechanisms whereby heart rate may relate to the development of disease and hence prognosis directly.

The mechanism by which heart rate reduction protects the myocardium is not yet fully elucidated. However, it has been postulated that a low heart rate may be exerting its effect in a number of ways including protecting from ischaemia and arrhythmias as well as protecting from atherogenesis and plaque rupture.

Heart rate is a critical determinant of myocardial oxygen consumption in patients with CAD. Other factors are contractility and end systolic stress. β-blockers reduce the mechanical work and oxygen demand secondary to their negative inotropic and chronotropic effects. The reduction of myocardial oxygen consumption and prolongation of diastole and myocardial perfusion are thought to be two of the main mechanisms responsible for the improvement in outcome due to heart rate reduction in the treatment of CAD patients.

It has been demonstrated that the autonomic nervous system plays a critical role in the genesis of sudden cardiac death. Sympathetic activation is known to promote the occurrence of life-threatening ventricular arrhythmias, whereas increased vagal tone exerts a protective and anti-fibrillatory effect [21, 22]. This is likely to be one explanatory factor in the particularly strong association between increasing heart rate and sudden death.

Elevated heart rates have been shown to increase the progression of atherosclerosis in both humans and animals, as described above. A mechanism for this may be the haemodynamic effects of increased heart rate. It is known that heart rate, along with systemic blood pressure, modulates flow velocity and shear stress oscillation. Alterations in both of these haemodynamic forces may predispose to the development of coronary atherosclerosis.

It has been suggested that elevated heart rate may be involved in coronary plaque disruption, the central pathophysiological mechanism underlying acute coronary syndromes and the progression of coronary atherosclerosis. Heidland and Strauer [23] retrospectively analysed 106 patients who underwent coronary angiography twice within 6 months. Fifty-three patients had initially smooth stenosis and developed plaque disruption by the time of the second angiogram. These were matched with 53 individuals with initially smooth stenoses who did not have evidence of coronary plaque disruption on the second examination. Logistic regression identified positive associations between plaque disruption and elevated heart rate (as measured on 24-hour monitoring at first angiogram), left ventricular mass above 270 g and a negative association with the use of β-blockers. It should be noted that other cardiovascular risk factors were not included in the multivariate model. The authors pointed out that blood pressure was similar in both groups initially, but higher in the disruption group at the time of the second angiogram.

One of the Chicago studies showed a U-shaped relationship between heart rate and sudden death, indicating that bradycardia is also associated with sudden death: this is probably as a result of conduction abnormalities. Baseline electrocardiograph (ECG) conduction abnormalities were excluded from the analysis in many of the other studies including CASTEL and, presumably for this reason, did not show this association with bradycardia.

ASSOCIATIONS OF ELEVATED HEART RATE INCLUDING THE METABOLIC SYNDROME

Singh [24] and Martin et al. [25] have studied the relationship between other cardiovascular risk factors and elevated resting heart rate. Singh found that both genetic and environmental factors (including BMI, SBP and diastolic blood pressure (DBP), smoking and alcohol consumption) are associated with elevated resting heart rate. Martin et al. estimated the heritability of resting heart rate to be 26%, and obtained significant evidence of linkage for resting heart rate on chromosome 4q. These authors also demonstrated that those with elevated resting heart rate, especially females, tended to have higher glucose and insulin levels. Their mean values for waist circumference, triglycerides, BMI, SBP and DBP also tended to be higher, combined with lower HDL-c levels. This complex is easily recognized as the metabolic syndrome, prompting the question – *is elevated heart rate part of this syndrome?*

A recent review by Cook et al. [26] has suggested the possibility that reduced bioavailability of nitric oxide may be involved in the pathogenesis of elevated resting heart rate. Much evidence exists which describes the role of nitric oxide as a mediator of cardiac autonomic control. For example, it has been demonstrated in both animals and humans that nitric oxide augments vagal tone and has an inhibitory effect on the sympathetic nervous system [27–29]. Given that it has been demonstrated that elevated heart rates are associated with sympathetic overactivity [30], the possibility of decreased bioavailability of nitric oxide as an aetiological factor in the pathogenesis of elevated heart rates seems reasonable. Furthermore, a substantial body of evidence links sympathetic overactivity to insulin resistance and the metabolic syndrome [31], which adds weight to the speculation that elevated heart rate is another component of the syndrome.

DOES HEART RATE REDUCTION RESULT IN CLINICAL BENEFIT?

We have reviewed the increasing evidence that a fast resting heart rate is associated with an increased risk of ischaemic events and sudden death, particularly in those with established CAD. The relationship will be more likely to be one of cause and effect if it can be shown that reducing heart rate improves outcome. β-adrenergic blocking drugs are now established therapy in both stable CHD and heart failure, and also reduce heart rate. We now examine some of the evidence for the benefit of β-blockers in ischaemic heart disease and in cardiac failure. Subsequently, we will review the key question as to whether heart rate reduction is one of the mechanisms by which β-blockers exert their beneficial effect in these conditions, and whether clinical benefit is likely with newer drugs such as ivabradine, which have a selective effect on heart rate.

β-BLOCKADE IN CORONARY ARTERY DISEASE PATIENTS – GUIDELINES

The recently published European Guidelines on the treatment of stable angina stress the importance of β-blocker therapy for patients post-MI [32]. Their use in post-MI and heart failure patients is recommended as a class 1 recommendation with a level of evidence of A. A recent meta-regression analysis of the effects of different β-blockers on mortality found non-significant benefits of acute treatment, but a significant 24% relative risk reduction in mortality with long-term secondary preventive treatment (see Table 17.3) [33]. The guidelines of the American Heart Association and the American College of Cardiology state that it is usual to titrate the dose of β-blocker to achieve a resting heart rate of 55–60 bpm, in the treatment of stable angina, or <50 bpm in severe angina provided there are no contraindications [34].

β-BLOCKADE BENEFIT IN HEART FAILURE TRIALS

A meta-analysis of the effect of β-blocker therapy in stable heart failure (mainly New York Heart Association [NYHA] class II or III) was undertaken by Brophy et al. [35]. Twenty-two randomized placebo-controlled trials were identified, all of which had mortality as an outcome and a follow-up period of greater than 3 months. Trials using β-blockers with intrinsic sympathomimetic activity were excluded. Most of the trials used metoprolol, bisoprolol or carvedilol. Total mortality and rates of hospitalization were significantly reduced in the group receiving β-blocker therapy (Table 17.3).

EVIDENCE THAT HEART RATE REDUCTION IS A MECHANISM OF BENEFIT IN β-BLOCKADE

The beneficial effects of β-blocker therapy both in post-MI and heart failure patients have been discussed. We will now consider further the issue of whether this benefit can be attributed to the heart rate-lowering properties of β-blockers.

A study by Thackray et al. [36] published in 2006 is particularly interesting as the objective of the study was to determine whether the beneficial effect of β-blockers on ventricular function in patients with cardiac failure is mediated through reduction of heart rate.

Table 17.3 Relative and absolute benefits of β-blockade in the post-MI and congestive cardiac failure populations, from meta-analyses

Outcome measure	Post-MI [33]	Congestive cardiac failure [35]
Odds ratio for total mortality	0.76 (95% CI 0.70–0.83)	0.65 (95% CI 0.53–0.80)
Lives saved per 100 treated for 1 year	1.3 (95% CI 0.7–1.8)	3.8 (95% CI 2.1–5.3)

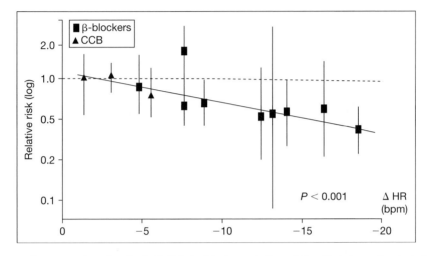

Figure 17.5 Meta-regression of randomized clinical trials demonstrating relationship between heart rate lowering and benefits on cardiac and sudden death observed with β-blockers in post-MI patients. CCB = calcium channel blocker. With permission [37].

A group of 49 pacemaker-dependent patients, with symptomatic left ventricular (LV) dysfunction (ejection fraction [EF] 26 ± 9% at baseline) were randomized to either lower rate (60 ppm) pacing or higher rate (80 ppm) pacing. All of the patients were receiving β-blocking treatment. Mean LV end-diastolic and systolic volumes increased with higher rate vs. lower rate pacing, whereas LV ejection fraction declined. All of these results were statistically significant. The authors concluded that reversal of β-blocker-induced bradycardia has deleterious effects on ventricular function, suggesting that heart rate reduction is an important mediator of its effects. It should be noted that the numbers completing the study protocol were small, 12 in the higher rate group and 13 in the lower rate group.

A recently presented meta-regression by Cucherat [37] has investigated the effect of reducing heart rate in patients post-MI on the risk of cardiac death, sudden death and re-infarction. Of 24 randomized controlled trials evaluating the effect of long-term β-blocker or calcium channel blocker treatment in patients post-MI, 14 gave information on both heart rate reduction and mortality. The association between log odds ratio for cardiovascular events and heart rate reduction was investigated. A statistically significant relationship was found between heart rate reduction and log odds ratio for cardiac death, sudden death and re-infarction as shown in Figure 17.5. Each 10 bpm reduction in the heart rate is estimated to reduce the odds ratio of cardiac death by about 26%.

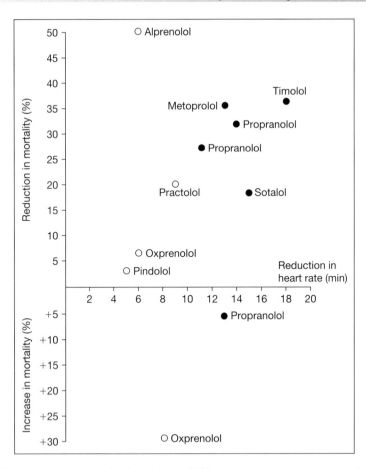

Figure 17.6   Relation between reduction in heart rate (difference between treatment groups) and percentage of reduction in mortality in large, prospective, double-blind trials with β-blockers. Open circles = β-blockers with intrinsic sympathomimetic activity; $r = 0.6$; $P < 0.05$. With permission [38].

Kjekshus [38] reviewed the subject in 1986 by examining β-blocker trials. These included both β-blockade as acute and long-term treatment of post-MI. Eight early intervention trials were analysed. In each, patients were given intravenous β-blocker within 12 h of the onset of pain. There was a wide difference in the heart rate reduction seen with different β-blockers (10.5–22.8%). There was an almost linear relationship relating the heart rate reduction to reduction in size of the infarct ($r = 0.97$; $P < 0.001$). The average reduction of infarct size with acute administration of β-blocker therapy was 24.4%.

The effect of β-blockade on long-term outcome in survivors of MI was also assessed. Data from 11 randomized, placebo-controlled trials were analysed. All but one of the trials had follow-up periods of 1 year or greater. As shown in Figure 17.6, there is an association between the degree of reduction in heart rate and mortality, apart from the smaller trials; with greater heart rate reduction causing greater decreases in mortality. A similar relationship is seen between heart rate reduction and reduction in non-fatal re-infarction, however the results were not significant in all of these. β-blockers with intrinsic sympathomimetic activity, including practolol, oxprenolol and pindolol caused lesser reductions in heart rate and caused less benefit in terms of mortality and morbidity. The exception to this is alprenolol, however the number of patients included here was low. The study concludes that heart rate is an important mechanism by which β-blockers improve mortality post-MI but not necessarily the only mechanism of benefit.

It has been suggested by Kjekshus in his review on β-blockers and their mechanism of benefit, that non-β1 selective β-blockers, which block β2 receptors, may also have an additional benefit. A possible mechanism is blockage of the transient hypokalaemia caused by activation of β2 adrenoceptors, thereby reducing the possibility of ventricular fibrillation.

HEART RATE REDUCTION AND ITS EFFECT ON PROGNOSIS IN CARDIAC FAILURE

The COMET (Carvedilol Or Metoprolol European Trial) trial compared the effect of carvedilol and metoprolol on subsequent death and events in a population with cardiac failure. They showed that carvedilol was superior to metoprolol in improving left ventricular function in this group. The influence of heart rate reduction in patients with heart failure has been studied in the COMET population by Metra *et al.* [39]. They found that, after adjustment for conventional cardiovascular risk factors, subsequent outcome over a 4.8 year follow-up period was independently related to resting heart rate at 4 months post study enrolment, but not significantly related to baseline resting heart rate or change in heart rate over the 4 months since starting on β-blocker.

EFFECT OF PURE HEART RATE REDUCTION BY IVABRADINE – A NEW SELECTIVE I_f INHIBITOR

I_f, a mixed Na^+ and K^+ inward current activated by hyperpolarization and modulated by the autonomic nervous system, is one of the most important ionic currents for regulating pacemaker activity in the sinoatrial node. Ivabradine is a novel specific heart rate-lowering agent that acts in sinoatrial node cells by selectively inhibiting the pacemaker I_f current in a dose-dependent manner. It is unique in that it appears to be a pure heart rate-lowering medication without other effects. The effect of ivabradine (5, 7.5 and 10 mg) in stable angina patients compared to atenolol 100 mg has been evaluated in a randomized trial [40]. Nine hundred and thirty-nine stable angina patients were randomized to receive either atenolol or ivabradine. The effect was assessed at 4 and 16 weeks of therapy by means of an exercise stress test. The differences in total exercise duration were measured in both the ivabradine and atenolol groups. There was no significant difference between the improvements in the total exercise time achieved in the two treatment groups. The number of anginal attacks per week also decreased in both groups. This is interesting as it shows that a medication that purely lowers heart rate is similar to a β-blocker in terms of exercise tolerance and anginal symptoms in stable angina patients. There are to date no published data on the effect of ivabradine on hard endpoints such as MI and mortality. This is being addressed in studies of the effect of ivabradine in subjects with stable CAD and impaired left ventricular function [41] and systolic heart failure [42].

IS THE RELATIONSHIP BETWEEN HEART RATE AND CVD AND TOTAL MORTALITY ONE OF CAUSE AND EFFECT?

To examine whether the relationship between heart rate and CVD is causal we will assess whether the relationship satisfies the causal criteria. This has been summarized in Table 17.4. Here, we have given each of the criteria a score (0 – minimum, 3 – maximum) to indicate the weight of evidence supporting fulfilment of that criterion. This is based on the evidence

Table 17.4 Summary of the weight of evidence supporting fulfilment of causal criteria for heart rate and cholesterol

	Heart rate	Total cholesterol
Biologically plausible	2	3
Strong	3	3
Temporal sequence	2	3
Graded	3	3
Consistent	1–2	3
Agreement between disciplines	2	3
Treatable	3	3
Benefit results	1	3

presented above. For comparison, total cholesterol – a well-established cardiovascular risk factor, is assessed in the same way.

SHOULD ASYMPTOMATIC OR ASYMPTOMATIC HYPERTENSIVE PATIENTS, FREE OF CARDIOVASCULAR DISEASE WITH ELEVATED HEART RATES BE TREATED WITH RATE-LOWERING MEDICATION?

If resting heart rate has been shown to be an independent risk factor for the development of CVD in the general population, then the question arises – *should we promote heart rate reduction in healthy, asymptomatic patients as a means of further improving primary prevention*? The primary consideration in management of the patient with elevated heart rate should be a careful investigation to rule out the many possible conditions that manifest themselves as a result of an elevated heart rate. Amongst the many possible secondary causes of elevated heart rate are lack of physical fitness, hypoxaemia, anaemia, alcoholism, chronic anxiety, hyperthyroidism and iatrogenic tachycardia through medications. Treating secondary causes and lifestyle measures, including increasing exercise, preventing anxiety and avoidance of toxins including caffeine, should be the first recommendations.

No trials have yet been done to evaluate the benefit of heart rate reduction in the general population by pharmacological means. A recent statement from the European Society of Hypertension consensus meeting suggests that a trial of heart rate lowering in asymptomatic hypertensive patients is required as the first step in answering this question [43]. They suggest that the best approach would be to treat all of the hypertensive patients with the same antihypertensive drug, with neutral heart rate activity and then randomize the patients to a bradycardic agent with neutral effects on blood pressure or placebo. Ivabradine may be appropriate here. They have suggested that the trial would need to contain 3800 participants.

SHOULD RESTING HEART RATE BE INCLUDED IN RISK ESTIMATION SYSTEMS?

Currently, total risk estimation systems are used widely in clinical practice in guiding primary prevention measures, for example the Systemic Coronary Risk Evaluation (SCORE) and HeartScore risk estimation systems [44]. Given that resting heart rate has been shown to be an independent risk factor for CVD in the general population, should resting heart rate be included in these risk estimation systems? The major components of risk estimation – smoking, blood cholesterol and blood pressure – are not only modifiable but are associated with proven benefit from reduction. However, since the benefits of heart rate reduction in healthy people are unproven, the answer at present is a qualified 'yes'. This subject is currently being pursued by the SCORE investigators.

REFERENCES

1. Levine H. Rest heart rate and life expectancy. *J Am Coll Cardiol* 1997; 30:1104–1106.
2. Kaplan JR, Manuck SB, Adams MR, Weingand KW, Clarkson TB. Inhibition of coronary atherosclerosis by propranolol in behaviorally predisposed monkeys fed an atherogenic diet. *Circulation* 1987; 76:1364–1372.
3. Beere P, Glagov S, Zarins C. Retarding effect of lowered heart rate on coronary atherosclerosis. *Science* 1984; 226:180–182.
4. Perski A, Olsson G, Landou C, de Faire U, Theorell T, Hamsten A. Minimum heart rate and coronary atherosclerosis: independent relations to global severity and rate of progression of angiographic lesions in men with myocardial infarction at a young age. *Am Heart J* 1991; 123:609–616.
5. Greenland P, Daviglus M, Dyer A. Resting heart rate is a risk factor for Cardiovascular and Noncardiovascular Mortality: The Chicago Heart Association Detection Project in Industry. *Am J Epidemiol* 1999; 149:853–862.
6. Dyer AR, Persky V, Stamler J *et al*. Heart rate as a prognostic factor for coronary heart disease and mortality: findings in three Chicago epidemiologic studies. *Am J Epidemiol* 1980; 112:736–749.
7. Filipovsky J, Ducimetiere P, Safar M. Prognostic significance of exercise heart rate and blood pressure in middle-aged men. *Hypertension* 1992; 20:333–339.
8. Reunanen A, Karjalainen J, Ristola P, Heliovaara M, Knekt P, Aromaa A. Heart rate and mortality. *J Intern Med* 2000; 247:231–239.
9. Gillum R, Makuc D, Feldman J. Pulse rate, coronary heart disease, and death: the NHANES I Epidemiologic Follow-up Study. *Am Heart J* 1991; 121:172–177.
10. Shaper AG, Wannamethee G, Macfarlane PW, Walker M. Heart rate, ischaemic heart disease and sudden death in middle-aged British men. *Br Heart J* 1993; 70:49–55.
11. Benetos A, Rudnichi A, Thomas F, Safar M, Guize L. Influence of heart rate on mortality in a French population: role of age, gender, and blood pressure. *Hypertension* 1999; 33:44–52.
12. Gillman MW, Kannel WB, Belanger A, D'Agostino RB. Influence of heart rate on mortality among persons with hypertension: The Framingham Study. *Am Heart J* 1993; 125:1148–1154.
13. Thomas F, Rudnichi A, Bacri A-M, Bean K, Guize L, Benetos A. Cardiovascular mortality in hypertensive men according to presence of associated risk factors. *Hypertension* 2001; 37:1256–1261.
14. Kannel WB, Kannel C, Paffenbarger RS, Cupples LA. Heart rate and cardiovascular mortality: The Framingham Study. *Am Heart J* 1987; 113:1489–1494.
15. Perk G, Stessman J, Ginsberg G, Bursztyn M. Sex differences in the effect of heart rate on mortality in the elderly. *J Am Geriatr Soc* 2003; 51:1260–1264.
16. Chang M, Havlik RJ, Corti MC, Chaves PH, Fried LP, Guralnik JM. Relation of heart rate at rest and mortality in the women's health and aging study. *Am J Cardiol* 2003; 92:1294–1299.
17. Palatini P, Thijs L, Staessen JA *et al*. Predictive value of clinic and ambulatory heart rate for mortality in elderly subjects with systolic hypertension. *Arch Intern Med* 2002; 162:2313–2321.
18. Wong ND, Cupples LA, Ostfeld AM, Levy D, Kannel WB. Risk factors for long-term coronary prognosis after initial myocardial infarction: The Framingham Study. *Am J Epidemiol* 1989; 130:469–480.
19. Disegni E, Goldbourt U, Reicher-Reiss H *et al*. The predictive value of admission heart rate in patients with suspected or proven coronary artery disease. *Eur Heart J* 1995; 48:1197–1205.
20. Diaz A, Bourassa MG, Guertin MC, Tardif JC. Long-term prognostic value of resting heart rate in patients with suspected or proven coronary artery disease. *Eur Heart J* 2005; 26:967–974.
21. Myers R, Pearlman A, Hyman R *et al*. Beneficial effect of vagal stimulation and bradycardia during experimental acute myocardial ischaemia. *Circulation* 1974; 49:943–947.
22. James R, Arnold J, Allen J *et al*. The effects of heart rate, myocardial ischaemia and vagal stimulation on the threshold for ventricular fibrillation. *Circulation* 1977; 55:311–317.
23. Heidland U, Strauer B. Left ventricular muscle mass and elevated heart rate are associated with coronary plaque disruption. *Circulation* 2001; 104:1477–1482.
24. Singh B. Increased heart rate as a risk factor for cardiovascular disease. *Eur Heart J Suppl* 2003; 5:G3–G9.
25. Martin LJ, Comuzzie AG, Sonnenberg GE *et al*. Major qualitative trait locus for resting heart rate maps to a region on chromosome 4. *Hypertension* 2004; 43:1146–1151.
26. Cook S, Togni M, Schaub MC, Wenaweser P, Hess OM. High heart rate: a cardiovascular risk factor? *Eur Heart J* 2006; 27:2387–2393.
27. Chowdhary S, Vaile JC, Fletcher J, Ross HF, Coote JH, Townend JN. Nitric oxide and cardiac autonomic control in humans. *Hypertension* 2000; 36:264–269.

28. Conlon K, Collins T, Kidd C. The role of nitric oxide in the control by the vagal nerves of the heart of the ferret. *Exp Physiol* 1998; 83:469–480.

29. Sartori C, Lepori M, Scherrer U. Interaction between nitric oxide and the cholinergic and sympathetic nervous system in cardiovascular control in humans. *Pharmacol Ther* 2005; 106:209–220.

30. Grassi G, Vailati S, Bertinieri G *et al*. Heart rate as a marker of sympathetic activity. *J Hypertens* 1998; 16:1635–1639.

31. Egan B. Insulin resistance and the sympathetic nervous system. *Curr Hypertens Rep* 2003; 5:247–254.

32. Yusuf S, Wittes J, Friedman L. Overview of results of randomised clinical trials in heart disease. 1. Treatments following myocardial infarction. *JAMA* 1988; 260:2088–2093.

33. Freemantle N, Urdahl H, Eastaugh J, Hobbs FD. What is the place of beta-blockade in patients who have experienced a myocardial infarction with preserved left ventricular function? Evidence and (mis)interpretation. *Prog Cardiovasc Dis* 2002; 44:243–250.

34. Gibbons R, Abrams J, Chatterjee K *et al*. ACC/AHA 2002 guideline for the management of patients with chronic stable angina. *Circulation* 2003; 107:149–158.

35. Brophy J, Joseph L, Rouleau J. β-blockers in congestive heart failure: a Bayesian meta-analysis. *Ann Intern Med* 2001; 134:550–560.

36. Thackray S, Ghosh JM, Wright GA *et al*. The effect of altering heart rate on ventricular function in patients with heart failure treated with β-blockers. *Am Heart J* 2006; 152:713.

37. Cucherat M. Relationship between heart rate lowering and benefits on cardiac and sudden death observed with β-blockers in post MI patients. A meta-regression of randomised clinical trials. *Eur Heart J* 2006; 27(Abstract suppl):590.

38. Kjekshus J. Importance of heart rate in determining beta-blocker efficacy in acute and long-term acute myocardial infarction intervention trials. *Am J Cardiol* 1986; 57:43F–49F.

39. Metra M, Torp-Pedersen C, Swedberg K *et al*. Influence of heart rate, blood pressure, and beta-blocker dose on outcome and the differences in outcome between carvedilol and metoprolol tartrate inpatients with chronic heart failure: results from the COMET trial. *Eur Heart J* 2005; 26:2259–2268.

40. Tardif J, Ford I, Tendera M, Bourassa MG, Fox K, for the INITIATIVE Investigators. Efficacy of ivabradine, a new slective I_f inhibitor, compared with atenolol in patients with chronic stable angina. *Eur Heart J* 2005; 26:2529–2536.

41. Fox K, Ferrari R, Tendera M, Steg PG, Ford I, on behalf of the BEAUTIFUL Steering Committee. Rationale and design of a randomized, double-blind, placebo-controlled trial of ivabradine in patients with stable coronary artery disease and left ventricular systolic dysfunction: the morBidity–mortality EvAlUaTion of the I_f inhibitor ivabradine in patients with coronary disease and left ventricULar dysfunction (BEAUTIFUL) Study. *Am Heart J* 2006; 152:860–866.

42. http://www.controlled-trials.com/

43. Palatini P, Benetos A, Grassi G *et al*. Identification and management of the hypertensive patient with elevated heart rate: Statement of a European Society of Hypertension Consensus Meeting. *J Hypertens* 2006; 24:603–610.

44. Conroy R, Pyörälä K, Fitzgerald A *et al*. Estimation of ten-year risk of fatal cardiovascular disease in Europe: the SCORE project. *Eur Heart J* 2003; 24:987–1003.

45. Jouven X, Desnos M, Guerot C. Predicting sudden death in the population: The Paris Prospective Study. *Circulation* 1996; 99:1978–1983.

46. Kristal-Boneh E, Silber H, Harari G, Froom P. The association of resting heart rate with cardiovascular, cancer and all-cause mortality. Eight year follow-up of 3527 male Israeli employees (the CORDIS Study). *Eur Heart J* 2000; 21:116–124.

47. Seccareccia F, Pannozzo F, Dima F *et al*. Heart rate as a predictor of mortality: the MATISS project. *Am J Pubic Health* 2001; 91:1258–1263.

48. Hathaway WR, Peterson ED, Wagner GS *et al*. Prognostic significance of admission electrocardiogram in acute myocardial infarction. GUSTO-I investigators. Global utilization of streptokinase and t-PA for occluded coronary arteries. *JAMA* 1998; 279:387–391.

49. Copie X, Hnatkova K, Staunton A, Fei L, Camm AJ, Malik M. Predictive power of increased heart rate versus depressed left ventricular ejection fraction and heart rate variability for risk stratification after myocardial infarction. Results of a two-year follow-up study. *J Am Coll Cardiol* 1996; 27:270–276.

50. Hjalmarson A, Gilpin EA, Kjekshus J *et al*. Influence of heart rate on mortality after acute myocardial infarction. *Am J Cardiol* 1990; 65:547–553.

51. Okamura T, Hayakawa T, Kadowaki T *et al*. Resting heart rate and cause-specific death in a 16.5-year cohort study of the Japanese general population. *Am Heart J* 2004; 147:1024–1032.

18

Cardiovascular risk estimation and management – concluding remarks

R. B. D'Agostino, Sr, I. M. Graham

Geoffrey Rose's classic monograph, *The Strategy of Preventive Medicine*, contains several remarks that are as pertinent now as they were 25 years ago:

'It is better to be healthy than ill or dead. That is the beginning and the end of the only real argument for preventive medicine. It is sufficient'.

'The primary determinants of disease are mainly economic and social, and therefore its remedies must also be economic and social. Medicine and politics cannot and should not be kept apart'.

'Small but widespread risks – a public health disaster?'

Bearing these in mind, we now summarise a few key messages from the individual chapters of this book. We have allowed ourselves the editorial privilege of some additional comments based on our own research and experience

CHAPTER 1 – CARDIOVASCULAR EPIDEMIOLOGY: BACKGROUND AND PRINCIPLES OF CARDIOVASCULAR DISEASE PREVENTION

A *risk factor* may be defined as a characteristic of an individual that is associated with an increased risk of the development of a specific disease such as cardiovascular disease (CVD). By 1965, the criteria to establish whether or not a risk factor is likely to be directly causal had been defined by Austin Bradford Hill. Cigarette smoking, raised blood cholesterol and high blood pressure are now accepted as causal risk factors for atherosclerotic cardiovascular disease. While multiple other social, environmental, behavioural and genetic factors may modify these primary causes, or have additional effects, they remain dominant. Cardiovascular risk is strongly associated with increasing age, but age should be regarded more as exposure time than as a causal factor.

All recent guidelines on cardiovascular disease prevention stress the fact that atherosclerosis is usually the product of multiple interacting risk factors. For this reason, epidemiological studies such as Framingham and SCORE and all recent guidelines on cardiovascular disease prevention have tried to develop simple tools to allow the busy clinician to estimate the simultaneous impact of several factors on CVD risk.

Ralph B. D'Agostino, Sr, PhD, Professor of Mathematics/Statistics and Public Health, Director of Data Management and Statistical Analysis of Framingham Study, Mathematics and Statistics Department, Framingham Study, Boston University, Boston, Massachusetts, USA

Ian M. Graham, FRCPI, FESC, Consultant Cardiologist; Professor of Cardiovascular Medicine, Trinity College, Dublin; Professor of Preventive Cardiology, Royal College of Surgeons in Ireland

Preventive strategies include both the population and the high-risk approach. It is now clear that both are necessary. While high risk people gain most from preventive advice, most deaths in a population come from people at only slightly increased risk, merely because they are more numerous – Rose's *'public health disaster'*.

Risk estimation at the extremes of age poses challenges. All elderly people are at high risk, and the age at which risk factor modification ceases to be beneficial requires further study. Young people may be at low risk or low absolute risk of cardiovascular disease, and yet they may be exposed to very high relative risks.

There is a seeming paradox in that women are generally stated to be at lower risk of cardiovascular disease than men and yet ultimately more women than men die of CVD. This is because they do so at a later age, so that mortality rates in young and middle aged persons are indeed higher in men. Women are often offered less intensive risk evaluation and management.

CHAPTER 2 – FROM EPIDEMIOLOGICAL RISK TO CLINICAL PRACTICE BY WAY OF STATISTICS – A PERSONAL VIEW

For nearly half a century, cardiovascular epidemiologists have been aware that multiple factors impact on the risk of cardiovascular disease. Early attempts to model risk estimation used discriminate function analysis because of the computer time required to undertake logistic regression analysis. Most recent risk estimation systems utilise Cox or Weibull techniques. Most progress in this field has come from the Framingham investigators. Others, such as Jackson in New Zealand and the early European Joint Task Force recommendations attempted to simplify the presentation of Framingham-based data. The SCORE project, used in more recent European recommendations, used a similar format, but based on data on 205 000 subjects from 12 European studies. An interactive, electronic risk estimation system was developed by the Danish PRECARD investigators, and lessons from PRECARD were used to develop the electronic version of SCORE, HeartScore.

Estimation of risk will always be just that – an estimate. It will never achieve as high a predictive value as a test that reliably diagnoses a disease as opposed to estimating the likelihood of its development. However, the current risk estimation systems are becoming robust enough to usefully guide clinical decision-making with regard to risk management.

CHAPTER 3 – ENDPOINTS, MORTALITY AND MORBIDITY

An 'endpoint' is the occurrence of a specific disease event. It may be 'hard' and unequivocal, such as death, 'soft' and subjective such as chest pain, or intermediate such as an acute coronary syndrome.

Although an increased risk of cardiovascular death automatically implies an additional risk of a non-fatal event such as a non-fatal acute coronary syndrome or stroke, clinicians intuitively wish for risk estimation systems that evaluate the risk of both fatal and non-fatal events. While there could be no disagreement about total deaths, and categories of cardiovascular deaths are reasonably well standardised through the International Classification of Diseases, definitions of non-fatal events pose a number of problems. In particular, definitions of CVD events and diagnostic criteria have changed substantially over the past quarter of a century. Ascertainment rates vary between different studies. Therapeutic advances will reduce event rates.

Risk estimation is only valuable if the advice that results will benefit the person being assessed. This requires reasonably accurate risk estimation, and an estimation of likely benefit from intervention on the basis of randomized control trials. Early trials, such as those of statins for cholesterol lowering, concentrated on reductions in cardiovascular and total mortality. Newer therapies are unlikely to produce major additional changes in mortality – the law of diminishing returns. Thus, recent trials focus on 'total cardiovascular endpoints', a heterogeneous composite that is not always reproducible.

Challenges for the future of cardiovascular risk estimation include the development of universally agreed definitions of both fatal and non-fatal endpoints, quantification of the incremental effect on risk estimation of adding other risk markers, and further studies to ascertain whether the use of total risk estimation results in unequivocal patient benefit.

CHAPTER 4 – GENETICS, FAMILY HISTORY AND RISK ESTIMATION IN THE YOUNG

Autopsy studies from the 1950s indicated that atherosclerosis is already frequently evident in young adults, and it is now clear that the process may start in childhood and possibly *in utero*. Although absolute CVD risks over the next decade may be low in young persons, this may conceal a high relative risk, and a high absolute risk in middle age. This issue is addressed in chapter 11.

The simplest and most useful way to assess long-term risk of CVD in young persons remains the estimation of the long-term consequences of maintaining current patterns of high risk behaviour such as smoking, unhealthy nutrition and inactivity, and the consequences of failing to correct hypertension, dyslipidaemia, hyperglycaemia and other modifiable physiological and biochemical characteristics.

Inherited susceptibility to CVD can be assessed by taking a family history and, in the rare cases of monogenic disorders, by the cautious use of molecular genetic analysis. The vision of a 'portfolio' of polymorphisms that would determine an individual's risk of disease and indeed his or her likely reaction to lifestyle and environmental factors remains unfulfilled.

CHAPTER 5 – MANAGEMENT OF CARDIOVASCULAR RISK IN THE OLDER PERSON

The next 50 years will see a huge increase in both the number and proportion of elderly people, especially women. Increasing longevity means longer exposure to risk factors. While CVD mortality in younger persons may be declining in developed societies, much of this decline reflects a shifting of the burden to older people. The global burden of CVD is rising, especially in developing nations such as China and India, which already experience more CVD than all of the developed countries combined.

Older persons are more likely to have additional manifestations of CVD, including left ventricular hypertrophy, diastolic dysfunction, conduction system disease, heart failure and aortic stenosis.

The prevalence of hypertension increases with age. It remains a risk factor in the elderly, and treatment is probably indicated at all ages, although benefits may reduce and side effects increase. Hypotension may reflect underlying disease and may also be associated with increased mortality.

Blood cholesterol levels tend to fall in old people, perhaps because those with very high levels have died, and because of wasting diseases such as cancer. Both low and high cholesterol levels may be associated with increased mortality in the old. Statin therapy appears to reduce vascular disease risk. The rise in all-cause mortality with increasing age would suggest that subjects in their mid 80s may not live long enough to benefit from statin therapy.

Smoking cessation appears to be associated with benefit at all ages. However, advice to quit should be tempered with humanity in those fortunate enough to survive to old age – the 'privileged survivors'.

Future research will explore the relevance of conventional risk factors, from episodic hypotension to cognitive decline. Further randomized controlled trials of risk factor management in the elderly are needed, especially in view of the predicted substantial increase in the elderly population.

CHAPTER 6 – OVERWEIGHT, PHYSICAL INACTIVITY, INSULIN RESISTANCE, IMPAIRED GLUCOSE TOLERANCE, DIABETES, THE METABOLIC SYNDROME AND CARDIOVASCULAR RISK

Increasing body weight is associated with an increased likelihood of high blood pressure, increased blood triglyceride and LDL cholesterol with reduced HDL cholesterol levels, impaired glucose tolerance, diabetes and consequent premature CVD. The clustering of central obesity with these factors has become known as the metabolic syndrome. These are now major and increasing public health problems in both developed and developing societies.

Regular moderate-intensity physical activity coupled with a healthy diet and avoidance of weight gain is highly effective in avoiding the progression from impaired glucose tolerance and the metabolic syndrome to diabetes. These measures also reduce the risks of both the occurrence and recurrence of CVD.

These observations raise questions of fundamental importance to the health of future generations. Should the emphasis be on the promotion of healthy lifestyles, or on salvage with drug treatments? What would we wish for our children? While both will be necessary, the balance of the investment of resources deserves detailed debate.

CHAPTER 7 – ESTIMATION OF CARDIOVASCULAR RISK: CLOSE ENOUGH IS NOT GOOD ENOUGH

Current risk management guidelines acknowledge 60 years of epidemiological and clinical trial research based on total and calculated LDL cholesterol measures in establishing therapeutic targets and levels of risk that trigger interventions. Current risk estimation systems also include age, gender, blood pressure and smoking, whereas most therapeutic trials have examined the effects of treating single risk factors, usually blood pressure or total or LDL cholesterol.

If one uses receiver operator curves (ROC) to evaluate how much conventional lipid measures and blood pressure add to the information derived from age and sex alone with regard to risk estimation, the increase in the area under the ROC is quite modest, from about 0.73 to 0.796 (chance alone would produce a figure of 0.5; 1.0 is perfection; 0.7–0.8 is regarded as acceptable and >0.8 as very good).

Smaller LDL particles are more atherogenic than large ones. Since each particle of LDL contains one apoB molecule, a high apoB level at any given LDL level would imply more small LDL particles and increased atherogenicity. ApoB cholesterol would therefore be expected to be a better risk estimator than LDL cholesterol. It is also a measurement, not a calculation, with automated, standardised methodology. Indeed, it may well be a better estimator of CVD risk than total or LDL cholesterol although differences to date have been modest.

Those developing guidelines for clinicians are constrained by the need to find the evidence that changes in recommendations are likely to result in measurable patient benefit. Clinical trials based on apoB rather than on total or LDL cholesterol would make it easier for them to seem less conservative in their recommendations. There is another possibility – that risk stratification based on apoB would identify individuals who are at *less* than expected risk for their level of LDL cholesterol.

CHAPTER 8 – NEW BIOMARKERS OF CARDIOVASCULAR DISEASE

In the context of CVD risk estimation, a biomarker may be defined as a measurable and quantifiable biological variable that serves as an index of disease risk. It may be a blood, urine or tissue test; a recording such as blood pressure or an electrocardiogram; or an image such as carotid–intimal thickness, echocardiogram or CT coronary angiogram. Thus biomarkers may be *serological* (blood tests), *structural* (imaging modalities such as ultrasound or CT), or *functional* (such as blood pressure or ankle-brachial index). In addition, they may be *antecedent* (identifying risk), *screening tests* for subclinical disease, *diagnostic tests* for the presence of overt disease, or *prognostic markers* to aid estimation the likelihood of disease recurrence or complications.

An ideal biomarker would result in a measurable improvement in patient management. It should be accurate, reproducible, acceptable to the patient, easy to interpret and affordable. It should have been evaluated on a wide variety of subjects and its performance in terms of sensitivity, specificity and positive and negative predictive value known. It should explain a useful proportion of the outcome in question, such as the occurrence of CVD.

This chapter tabulates the performance of serological, structural and functional biomarkers, based particularly on data from the Framingham heart study. Of nearly 40 biomarkers, the ones linked most strongly to future disease are abnormal lipids, apoB, Lp(a), high sensitivity CRP, homocysteine, natriuretic peptide and blood pressure, although few except apoB add usefully to the powerful effect of lipids and blood pressure in the Framingham Heart Study risk score. None except lipids and blood pressure track with disease treatment. This may reflect a lack of effective therapies and of trial data, or simply that the marker has no clinical utility.

The effect of biomarkers on myocardial vulnerability is also assessed and tabulated, and the relevance of different markers at different stages in the ischaemic cascade is illustrated.

CHAPTER 9 – RISK IN THOSE WITH ESTABLISHED DISEASE

There is no logical reason that the same risk factors that caused a myocardial infarction (MI) in the first place should not also determine the likelihood of further atherosclerotic events. In general this is so. They include hyperlipidaemia, hypertension, smoking, disturbed glucose metabolism, elevated CRP, disturbed endothelial function, homocysteine and psychosocial factors such as depression and social isolation. Other factors also operate, especially in the early stages. These include the size of the index MI, the number and severity of the coronary occlusions, the number of previous MIs and the presence of ventricular dysrhythmias. The biggest single factor improving long term prognosis is probably smoking cessation, which is associated with a halving of long term mortality. This is greater than any known drug effect.

Similar factors seem to determine prognosis in angina, atypical angina and after coronary artery bypass surgery and percutaneous interventions.

Prognostic factors after a stroke or transient cerebral ischaemic event include the factors associated with the index event, atrial fibrillation, coronary artery disease, hypertension, diabetes, inflammatory markers, high homocysteine levels, smoking and hormone replacement therapy.

CHAPTER 10 – SOCIOECONOMIC ASPECTS OF RISK ESTIMATION

Socioeconomic aspects at population level

There are marked *regional differences* in CVD mortality – even within Europe, CHD mortality is four to five times higher in the East than it is in the South-West. The main risk factors (smoking, blood cholesterol, blood pressure and body mass index) explain about 30% percent of these differences in men and 45% in women. It is likely that both between and within countries socioeconomic factors are major determinants of differences in CHD mortality, including poverty, stress, unemployment and consequent adverse health behaviours. Conventional, dietary and psychosocial factors are all determined by social conditions that should be highly relevant to health policy makers.

Socioeconomic factors at individual level

Social class is a powerful determinant of both cardiovascular mortality and morbidity; it is indeed true that *'the poor die young'*. Key factors are low socioeconomic status, lack of social support, social isolation, stress at work and outside work and negative emotions including depression and hostility.

Neither Framingham not the SCORE risk estimation systems include social class, although socioeconomic factors are dealt with in detail in the current European guidelines on prevention. Does this matter, since the impact of social factors is mediated in part at least through adverse effects on conventional risk factors? Also, what is the practicing clinician to do about a person's socioeconomic state? Perhaps the key message is that the socially deprived are likely to be at increased risk, and may be less well equipped to deal with their increased risk. They may need extra time and help with appropriate and comprehensible methods of communication to facilitate lifestyle change, and a healthcare system that allows access to advice, counselling, investigations and appropriate interventions and medication. Whether the simple expedient of giving money to the deprived would increase health is not known.

CHAPTER 11 – RISK ESTIMATION SYSTEMS IN CLINICAL USE: SCORE, HEARTSCORE AND THE FRAMINGHAM SYSTEM

Risk estimation poses several challenges for the busy health professional – to identify those at risk quickly and easily; to assess the individual components of total risk; to decide who needs lifestyle intervention or medication and to avoid over-treating low risk persons.

Certain persons declare themselves to be at high risk. These are individuals who have already had a vascular event, those with very high levels of blood pressure or cholesterol and those with diabetes mellitus. For others, risk is usually the product of a number of interacting factors, and here risk estimation systems may help identify those who need risk management advice and those who do not. For example, a 60-year-old woman with a blood cholesterol of 8 mmol/l (310 mg/dl) but no other risk factors has a 2% chance of a fatal CVD event over the next 10 years. In contrast, a man of the same age with a cholesterol level of only 5 mmol/l (190 mg/dl) may be at 10 times *higher* risk if he is a hypertensive smoker.

Both the Framingham and SCORE investigators have developed risk estimation systems that attempt to make risk estimation easier for the busy clinician. These are presented and illustrated in this chapter. Both use rather simple but well validated measures of risk. Framingham is derived from a homogeneous and meticulously documented population. SCORE is derived from a much larger data set, but one that is more heterogeneous. Many new risk markers are not included but can be if evidence that they usefully improve risk estimation is forthcoming.

It is likely that the contribution of newer markers will be modest. Many other risk estimation systems are available; within Scotland and the United Kingdom, ASSIGN and QRISK have attempted to include social class/social deprivation into risk estimation.

All risk estimation systems share common problems. If they are to be applied to different cultures, they may require recalibration to adjust for different mortality rates and risk factor distributions. They will overestimate risk in populations with a falling CVD mortality, and underestimate it if mortality is rising; again, recalibration to allow for such time trends may be helpful. The low absolute risk observed in younger persons may conceal a very substantial relative risk; for this reason, the SCORE investigators have prepared a relative risk chart to assist in counselling younger persons who may need intensive lifestyle advice.

CHAPTER 12 – EPIDEMIOLOGICAL RESEARCH AND PREVENTIVE CARDIOLOGY: LESSONS FROM FRAMINGHAM

For six decades, the Framingham investigators have reported on the prevalence, incidence, clinical manifestations, lifetime risk, prognosis, time trends and predisposing factors for atherosclerotic CVD. They coined the term 'risk factor', recognized the multifactorial nature of CVD in most cases, and devised multivariable CVD risk profiles that have made risk assessment accessible to clinicians as well as providing guidance to other leaders in preventive cardiology.

Some of the key associations between risk factors and CVD found in the Framingham study were summarised in chapter one; the list is expanded somewhat here:

- Coronary heart disease
  - Smoking
  - Cholesterol
  - Blood pressure
  - ECG abnormalities
  - Diabetes
  - Menopause
  - Triglycerides
  - Psychosocial factors
  - Type A behaviour
  - Isolated systolic hypertension

- Stroke
  - Blood pressure
  - Atrial fibrillation
  - Smoking
  - Left ventricular enlargement

- New risk factors for coronary heart disease
  - Fibrinogen
  - Homocysteine
  - Lipoprotein (a)
  - Apolipoprotein E
  - Proteinuria and microalbuminuria
  - C-reactive protein

The frequency and lethality of CVD was defined, as was the high likelihood of sudden death and the fact that the disease may be clinically silent even when advanced. It was recognized that the apparent 'protection' enjoyed by women merely reflects a time delay of about 10 years. The huge economic burden imposed by CVD, still the largest single killer of Americans, was stressed.

Several clinical misconceptions were corrected. There is no such entity as 'benign' hypertension, even if some individuals escape the effects of the risk associated with raised blood pressure. If anything, systolic blood pressure is a better measure of risk than diastolic.

Left ventricular hypertrophy is an ominous indicator of an adverse prognosis, and not merely a compensatory mechanism. The risk associated with atrial fibrillation does not just depend on the presence of co-existent CHD. It is a powerful risk factor for stroke, especially in the elderly. After decades of debate, the strong, graded and causal relationship between blood cholesterol and CVD risk was accepted, as was the inverse relationship with HDL cholesterol level. The increased risk associated with central obesity, impaired glucose intolerance, the 'metabolic syndrome' and type II diabetes was defined. The causal role of smoking in CVD as well as cancer was stressed, as was the benefit of even moderate exercise.

These findings are generalisable far beyond the town of Framingham and, in general, seem to apply to all countries and to all cultures. Thus, the Framingham study has informed preventive cardiology and health policy worldwide.

CHAPTER 13 – ELECTRONIC AND INTERACTIVE RISK ESTIMATION

Paper-based risk charts are limited in several ways: they are limited in the number of variables that can be accommodated, are cumbersome to update and do not interact with management guidelines.

Early attempts at electronic risk estimation were limited by the data and techniques available, were mostly developed by private industry and were not linked to management guidelines. Not surprisingly, they were not received with enthusiasm by either clinicians or scientific bodies.

With the advent of Windows™ based programming and the vision of the Danish PRE-CARD investigators, the possibility of an interactive method of total risk estimation linked to practical management advice became a reality. This facilitated a collaboration with the SCORE investigators to utilise the large SCORE data set to develop a web-based interactive risk estimation system that was integrated with the current European risk guidelines called HeartScore, available through *www.heartscore.org*. Because not all clinicians are online in their day-to-day practice, a stand-alone version has been developed and is currently undergoing testing.

CHAPTER 14 – MANAGEMENT OF SPECIFIC BEHAVIOURAL RISK FACTORS-EXERCISE, OBESITY AND SMOKING

Health professionals generally recognize that inactivity and obesity are both direct and indirect risk factors in that they affect both blood pressure and blood lipid levels as well as impacting directly on risk. They are often aware that smoking cessation is more effective in reducing risk than any current drug therapy. Yet helping patients to change behaviour is difficult, time consuming and requires more skill and training than simply writing a prescription that may often be the line of least resistance.

Lifestyle change is more difficult for those who are socially deprived through low income, poor education or social isolation; those under stress at work or at home; those experiencing depression, anxiety or hostile emotions; and if the advice given is complex or confusing.

Practical tips to help behaviour change include:

- Developing a sympathetic alliance with the patient
- Explaining carefully the relationship between lifestyle and disease
- Using this to gain commitment to attempt lifestyle change
- Involving the patient in identifying the risk factors to change
- Exploring barriers to change
- Helping to design a lifestyle change plan
- Realistic encouragement: "*any increase in exercise is good*"
- Reinforcing efforts to change
- Regular follow-up
- Using the help of all other healthcare staff who may be available

CHAPTER 15 – MANAGEMENT OF SPECIFIC RISK FACTORS – LIPIDS

It was pointed out in chapter 11 that a person with hyperlipidaemia as their only risk factor may be at far lower risk than a person with a much lower, 'average' western level of cholesterol (e.g. 5mmol/l; 190mg/dl) if the latter has multiple other risk factors. For this reason, total risk estimation may help to avoid both over- and under-treatment of hyperlipidaemia. This is the basis for recommending total risk estimation before making management decisions.

In evaluating a person with hyperlipidaemia, three initial steps are suggested:

1. Is hyperlipidaemia really present? Laboratory error is not unknown. Regression-dilution bias means that random extreme levels may be lower when repeated. A repeat fasting lipid estimation is the first step.
2. Could the hyperlipidaemia be secondary to another condition such as hypothyroidism, diabetes, renal failure, alcoholism, obesity, cholestasis or drugs such as steroids? It is embarrassing to give a statin to a person when treatment of their hypothyroidism turns out to be all that is required. Some individuals with hypertriglyceridaemia respond dramatically to calorie and/or alcohol restriction.
3. If hyperlipidaemia is confirmed and is not secondary, total risk estimation will guide management decisions.

Very high lipid levels, hyperlipidaemia in the context of a high total risk, and failure to respond to dietary advice and alcohol restriction will often indicate a need for drug treatment. Statins are the most effective therapy for hypercholesterolaemia, aided if necessary by ezetemibe and, occasionally, by ion exchange resins, fibrates or nicotinic acid. The latter two increase the likelihood of liver dysfunction and myopathy modestly.

Calorie and alcohol control are the initial measures in managing hypertriglyceridaemia. The response to statins is variable and unpredictable. Fibrates are generally more effective, although proof of clinical benefit is weak. Nicotinic acid is effective and also increases HDL cholesterol and modestly reduces LDL cholesterol. Omega-3 fatty acids reduce triglycerides and may improve prognosis after an acute coronary syndrome.

Overall, multiple randomized control trials indicate unequivocally that reduction of raised blood cholesterol levels in high risk subjects reduces both total and cardiovascular mortality. There is now considerable agreement with regard to target levels between American and European guidelines.

CHAPTER 16 – MANAGEMENT OF SPECIFIC RISK FACTORS – HYPERTENSION

Hypertension is an extremely prevalent risk factor, especially in the elderly. It is a risk factor for CHD, heart failure, stroke, renal failure and probably dementia in both men and women. Risk rises progressively from levels below 120/80mmHg. Other risk factors tend to accompany raised blood pressure, the presence of which should trigger a search for such factors. The presence of end-organ damage indicates increased risk.

Blood pressure varies both within and between days; serial measurements as well as evaluation of total risk should be performed before management decisions are made except in extreme cases. Not surprisingly, there is a growing body of evidence that 24-hour ambulatory BP is a better predictor of CVD risk that office BP measurement. Office levels of 140/90mmHg equate crudely to average 24-hour figures of 125/80mmHg.

Most guidelines recommend a target blood pressure of <140/90mmHg, and <130/80mmHg in high-risk persons such as those with established CVD or diabetes. Effective blood pressure control is more important than the choice of any particular agent or agents.

CHAPTER 17 – HEART RATE AS A RISK FACTOR

Increased heart rate is a fascinating risk associate in that it relates to reduced life expectancy both between and within animal species, and in both healthy humans and in those with CVD. Heart rate reduction by means of physical training is probably of benefit in high risk but otherwise healthy persons, but there is no evidence to date to support drug treatment in such persons.

Beta-blockade reduces mortality in subjects after myocardial infarction and in those with heart failure. It is likely that this relates to heart rate reduction. Whether selective, non β-blocker-related heart rate reduction is beneficial is a key question that has yet to be answered. To date, heart rate fulfils many but not all of the criteria required to establish it as a causal risk factor for CVD.

Abbreviations

4S	Scandinavian Simvastatin Survival Study
ABI	ankle–brachial index
ABPM	ambulatory blood pressure monitoring
ACC	American College of Cardiology
ACE	angiotensin-converting enzyme
ACS	acute coronary syndrome
AD	Alzheimer's disease
ADA	American Diabetes Association
ADMA	asymmetrical dimethylarginine
AF	atrial fibrillation
AFCAPS/TexCAPS	Air Force/Texas Coronary Atherosclerosis Prevention Study
AHA/ACC	American Heart Association/American College of Cardiology
ALLHAT	Antihypertensive and Lipid-Lowering Treatment to Prevent Heart Attack Trial
AP	angina pectoris
apo	apolipoprotein
ARIC	Atherosclerosis Risk in Communities
ASA	acetylsalicylic acid
ASCOT	Anglo-Scandinavian Cardiac Outcomes Trial
ATP III	Third Report of the Adult Treatment Panel
AV	atrioventricular
BHS	British Hypertension Society
BMI	body mass index
BNP	B-type natriuretic peptide or brain natriuretic peptide (*check context*)
BP	blood pressure
bpm	beats per minute
CAA	coronary artery atherosclerosis
CABG	coronary artery bypass graft
CAD	coronary artery disease
CADILLAC	Controlled Abciximab and Device Investigation to Lower Late Angioplasty Complications
CAFE	Conduit Artery Function Evaluation
CAPRIE	Clopidogrel versus Aspirin in Patients at Risk of Ischaemic Events
CASTEL	Cardiovascular Study in the Elderly
CAT	computed axial tomography
CCU	coronary care unit
CETP	cholesteryl ester transfer protein
CHD	coronary heart disease
CHF	congestive heart failure

CI	confidence interval
CK	creatinine kinase
COMET	Carvedilol Or Metoprolol European Trial
CONSORT	Consolidated Standards of Reporting Trials
CRP	C-reactive protein
CT	computed tomography
CV	cardiovascular
CVA	cerebrovascular accident
CVD	cardiovascular disease
CVRF	cardiovascular risk factors
DALY	Disability Adjusted Life Years (a measure of lost years of healthy life)
DASH	Dietary Approaches to Stop Hypertension
DBP	diastolic blood pressure
DECODE	Diabetes Epidemiology: Collaborative analysis of Diagnostic criteria in Europe
DLB	Diffuse Lewy body dementia
DWMH	deep white matter hyperdensity
ECG	electrocardiograph
EF	ejection fraction
EGIR	European Group for Study of Insulin Resistance
ESC	European Society of Cardiology
ESH	European Society of Hypertension
ESRD	end-stage renal disease
EUROASPIRE	European Action on Secondary Prevention through Intervention to Reduce Events
FEV_1	forced expiratory volume in 1 second
FH	familial hypercholesterolaemia
FLAIR	fluid-attenuated inversion recovery
FMD	flow-mediated dilatation
FPF	false-positive fraction
FRISC	Fragmin and fast Revascularization during Instability in Coronary artery disease
GFR	glomerular filtration rate
GREAT	General Rule to Enable Atheroma Treatment
H-FABP	heart-type fatty acid binding protein
HDL	high-density lipoprotein
HDL-c	high-density lipoprotein cholesterol
HOMA-IR	homeostasis model assessment of insulin resistance
HOPE 2	Heart Outcomes Prevention Evaluation-2
HOT	Hypertension Optimal Treatment (study)
HRQL	health-related quality of life
hs-CRP	high-sensitive CRP
ICAM-1	intercellular adhesion molecule 1
ICD	International Classification of Diseases
IFG	impaired fasting glucose
IGT	impaired glucose tolerance
IHD	ischaemic heart disease
IL	interleukin

IMT	intimal–medial thickness
INVEST	INternational VErapamil SR and Trandolapril STudy
JNC7	Seventh Report of the Joint National Committee on Prevention, Detection, Evaluation, and Treatment of High Blood Pressure
LCAT	lecithin-cholesterol-acyl-transferase
LDH	lactate dehydrogenase
LDL	low-density lipoprotein
LLL	lots of little lipoproteins
Lp(a)	lipoprotein (a)
Lp-PLA2	lipoprotein-associated phospholipase
LV	left ventricular
MB	myoglobin
MCP-1	monocyte chemoattractant 1
MDRD	Modification of Diet in Renal Disease
MI	myocardial infarction
MIRACL	Myocardial Ischaemia Reduction with Aggressive Cholesterol Lowering
MMP	matrix metalloproteinase
MONICA	MONitoring trends and determinants in CArdiovascular disease
MPO	myeloperoxidase
MRC	Medical Research Council
MRFIT	Multiple Risk Factor Intervention Trial
MRI	magnetic resonance imaging
NCEP	National Cholesterol Education Program
NHANES	National Health and Nutrition Examination Study
NHLBI	National Heart, Lung, and Blood Institute
NICE	National Institute for Health and Clinical Excellence
NORVIT	Norwegian Vitamin
NYHA	New York Heart Association
OGTT	oral glucose tolerance test
OR	odds ratio
PAI-1	plasminogen activator inhibitor-1
PAPP-A	pregnancy-associated plasma protein A
PCI	percutaneous coronary intervention
PDA	personal digital assistant
PDAY	Pathological Determinants of Atherosclerosis in Youth
PET	positron emission tomography
PlGF	placental growth factor
PRAIS-UK	Prospective Registry of Acute Ischaemic Syndromes in the UK
PRECARD™	computer program used for electronic CVD risk assessment and management
PROCAM	Prospective Cardiovascular Münster (system)
PROGRESS	Perindopril Protection against Recurrent Stroke Study
PROSPER	Prospective Study of Pravastatin in the Elderly at Risk
PTCA	percutaneous transluminal balloon angioplasty
PWA	pulse wave amplitude
PWV	pulse wave velocity
RAAS	renin–angiotensin–aldosterone system
RCT	randomized controlled trial
ROC	receiver operating characteristic

ROR	rollover risk
RR	relative risk
SAA	serum A amyloid
SBP	systolic blood pressure
SCORE	Systemic Coronary Risk Evaluation
SCT	social cognitive theory
SES	socioeconomic status
SHEP	Systolic Hypertension in the Elderly
SHHEC	Scottish Heart Health Extended Cohort
Syst-Eur	European working group on systolic hypertension
TC	total cholesterol
TIA	transient ischaemic attack
TIMP	tissue inhibitor of metalloproteinase
TOD	target organ damage
TPA	tissue plasminogen activator
TPF	true-positive fraction
TVR	target vessel revascularization
UC	ultracentrifugation
UKPDS	United Kingdom Prospective Diabetes Study
VaD	vascular dementia
VLDL	very low-density lipoprotein
WHAS1	Women's Health and Aging Study
WHO	World Health Organization

Index